D0074724

CLINICAL TOXICOLOGY
Principles and Mechanisms

CLINICAL TOXICOLOGY
Principles and Mechanisms

FRANK A. BARILE

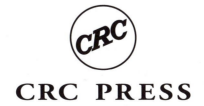

CRC PRESS

Boca Raton   London   New York   Washington, D.C.

Library of Congress Cataloging-in-Publication Data

Barile, Frank A.
  Clinical toxicology: principles and mechanisms/ Frank A. Barile.
      p. cm.
  Includes bibliographical references and index.
  ISBN 0-8493-1582-4
  1. Clinical toxicology.
  [DNLM: 1. Toxicology—standards. 2. Pharmacology, Clinical—standards. 3. Toxicity
Tests—standards. 4. Toxicology—classification. QV 600 B252c 2003] I. Title.
  RA1218.5.B37 2003
  615.9—dc22   2003055716

Visit the CRC Press Web site at www.crcpress.com

© 2004 by CRC Press LLC

No claim to original U.S. Government works
International Standard Book Number 0-8493-1582-4
Library of Congress Card Number 2003055716
Printed in the United States of America 1 2 3 4 5 6 7 8 9 0
Printed on acid-free paper

Dedication

To the memory of Frank Barile, Sr.

Preface

In the last 50 years, the science of clinical toxicology has evolved from an applied science, progressing in the shadows of more highly defined areas of toxicology, to its own recognized discipline. Much like the development of other fields, such as genetic engineering or information technology, the maturity of the subject of clinical toxicology has been sporadic. In particular, its progress has been prompted by public health initiatives and responses. In the 1950s, the discipline established poison control centers primarily as counseling focal points for emergency treatment. With social drug use and rampant drug abuse overwhelming the U.S. in the 1960s, the importance of clinical toxicology became more apparent. Narcotics, psychedelic drugs, stimulants, and other potent illicit compounds flooded the streets at unprecedented rates. Americans of all ages, ethnic backgrounds, and socioeconomic status were inundated with the sudden accessibility of chemicals that could alter mind, mood, behavior, and perception. Large and cumbersome government campaigns to thwart the influx and abuse of illicit drugs interspersed daily routines, from community programs to public service advertisement. Such programs included the interception of illegal importation of heroin and education programs to teach school children about the untoward effects and the addictive power of unwarranted drug use. Poison control centers and emergency departments were occupied with controlling and managing toxic effects and overdoses that quickly followed.

The 1970s witnessed the development of emergency techniques to combat the rising death rates associated with acute overdose. The Scandinavian method for treatment of acute toxicity from depressants (sedative/hypnotics and opioids) was accepted as a reliable emergency procedure. It became apparent that maintenance of respiration and other vital functions, rather than pharmacological antagonism, was paramount in reversing the acute toxicity of these compounds.

The 1980s introduced newer challenges to the resilience of clinical toxicology. "Basement" derivatives of parent illicit drugs released more potent analogs onto the streets. Agents such as PCP and "ecstasy" produced toxic syndromes that were not immediately apparent after ingestion. The cardiovascular toxicity and psychological derangement associated with these newer compounds are, to date, difficult to manage.

The 1990s and the trial of football star O.J. Simpson did more for the sciences of forensic and clinical toxicology than any other event to date. The explanation of the analytical methods of DNA isolation and identification, and the depiction of the ladder-like patterns of DNA profiles appeared on every television news channel for months. For a brief time, reporting on the techniques of forensic and clinical toxicology was so common that it was not necessary to define the terms "DNA" or "genetic material" in the national media reports.

The principles of clinical toxicology do not differ significantly from other toxicology disciplines. Consequently, many of the topics discussed in this text include those commonly broached in general toxicology texts, namely, mechanism of toxicity, medicinal chemistry, and toxicokinetics. Topics such as signs and symptoms and clinical management of acute toxicity are unique to the discipline. However, it is important to note that this book is not an emergency reference text. As such, detailed therapeutic management protocols are not included. Specific antidotes, therapeutic interventions, and general supportive measures are addressed as general guidelines of treatment modalities.

This book examines the complex interactions associated with clinical toxicological events as a result of therapeutic drug administration or deliberate or inadvertent chemical exposure. Special emphasis is placed on signs and symptoms of syndromes and pathology caused by chemical exposure and administration of clinical drugs. Source, pharmacological and toxicological mechanism of action, toxicokinetics, medicinal chemistry, clinical management of toxicity, and detection and identification of the drug or chemical in body fluids, are discussed. Proprietary names are inserted where applicable, and particularly when publicly available. Historically well-known but obsolete drugs are mentioned only as a matter of reference. Contemporary issues in clinical toxicology, including the various means of possible exposure to therapeutic and nontherapeutic agents, an overview of protocols for managing various toxic ingestions, and the antidotes and treatments associated with their pathology, are conveyed. In addition, special chapters are devoted to therapeutic adverse drug reactions (ADRs), chemical and biological threats to public safety, and pharmacology and toxicology of herbal products.

It is hoped that this text instills a greater respect among health profession students as they strive to understand the serious consequences of exposure to therapeutic drugs and environmental and occupational chemicals. As societies become more technologically adept at many levels, the thirst for information about chemicals increases. As a result, the public develops a greater awareness and appreciation for the consequences of ingesting prescription medicines, of exposure to nontherapeutic compounds, of the risk from biological threats, and of the adverse effects of herbal products. As a generation becomes more knowledgeable, its preparedness to respond to the threat of toxins is more formidable.

The Author

Frank A. Barile, Ph.D., is associate professor in the Toxicology Division of the Department of Pharmaceutical Sciences, at St. John's University College of Pharmacy and Allied Health Professions, Jamaica, New York.

Dr. Barile received his B.S. in Pharmacy (1977), M.S. in pharmacology (1980), and Ph.D. in toxicology (1982) at St. John's University. After completing a postdoctoral fellowship in pulmonary pediatrics at the Albert Einstein College of Medicine, Bronx, New York, he moved to the Department of Pathology, Columbia University, St. Luke's Roosevelt Hospital, New York, as a research associate. In these positions he investigated the role of pulmonary toxicants on collagen metabolism in cultured lung cells. In 1984, he was appointed as assistant professor in the Department of Natural Sciences at City University of New York, at York College. Sixteen years later he rejoined St. John's University in the Department of Pharmaceutical Sciences and became an instrumental part of the new six-year pharmacy (Pharm.D.) and toxicology programs in the College of Pharmacy.

Dr. Barile holds memberships in several professional associations, including the U.S. Society of Toxicology, American Association of University Professors, American Association for the Advancement of Science, American Society of Hospital Pharmacists, New York City Pharmacists Society, New York Academy of Sciences, and New York State Council of Health System Pharmacists. He has been appointed as a consultant scientist with several clinical and industrial groups, including the Department of Pediatrics, Pulmonary Division, Schneider's Children's Hospital, Long Island Jewish/Cornell Medical Centers, New Hyde Park, New York.

Dr. Barile has been the recipient of PHS research grants from the National Institutes of Health (NIGMS) for the last 20 years, including awards from the Minority Biomedical Research Support (MBRS) program, the Minority High School Student Research Apprentice (MHSSRAP) program, and Academic Research Enhancement Award (AREA) program.

Dr. Barile has authored and coauthored approximately 75 papers and abstracts in peer-reviewed biomedical and toxicology journals, as well as one book and one contributed chapter. He continues fundamental research on the cytotoxic effects of therapeutic drugs and environmental chemicals on cultured human and mammalian cells.

Contributors

Zhuoxiao Cao, M.D.
Research Fellow
Department of Pharmaceutical Sciences
St. John's University
College of Pharmacy and Allied Health
  Professions
Jamaica, New York

Diane Hardej, Ph.D.
Research Fellow
Department of Pharmaceutical Sciences
St. John's University
College of Pharmacy and Allied Health
  Professions
Jamaica, New York

Yunbo Li, M.D., Ph.D.
Associate Professor
Department of Pharmaceutical Sciences
St. John's University
College of Pharmacy and Allied Health
  Professions
Jamaica, New York

Michael A. Thrush, Ph.D.
Professor
Department of Environmental Health
  Sciences
Bloomberg School of Public Health
The Johns Hopkins University
Baltimore, Maryland

Louis D. Trombetta, Ph.D.
Professor and Chair
Department of Pharmaceutical Sciences
St. John's University
College of Pharmacy and Allied Health
  Professions
Jamaica, New York

Contents

PART II   Toxicity of Therapeutic Agents

PART III   Toxicity of Nontherapeutic Agents

Yunbo Li, Zhuoxiao Cao, and Michael A. Thrush

Part I

*Introduction to Basic
Toxicological Principles*

1 Introduction

1.1 BASIC DEFINITIONS

1.1.1 TOXICOLOGY

The classic definition of toxicology has traditionally been understood as the study of xenobiotics, or simply stated, as the science of poisons — i.e., the interaction of exogenous agents with mammalian physiological compartments. For purposes of organizing the nomenclature, chemicals, compounds, or drugs are often referred to as *agents*. And since such agents induce undesirable effects, they are usually referred to as *toxins*. Consequently, toxicology involves internal and external physiological exposure to toxins and their interactions with the body's components. With time, the term has evolved to include many chemically unrelated classes of agents. What transforms a chemical into a toxin depends more on the length of time of exposure, dose (or concentration) of the chemical, or route of exposure, and less on the chemical structure, product formulation, or intended use of the material. As a result, almost any chemical has the potential for toxicity, and thus, falls under the broad definition of toxicology.

1.1.2 CLINICAL TOXICOLOGY

Traditionally, clinical toxicology was regarded as the specific discipline of the broader field of toxicology concerned with the toxic effects of agents whose intent is to treat, ameliorate, modify, or prevent disease states, or, the effect of drugs which, at one time, were intended to be used as such. These compounds would fall under the classification of therapeutic agents (Part II). A more liberal definition of clinical toxicology involves not only the toxic effects of therapeutic agents but also those chemicals whose intention is not therapeutic. This includes drugs whose exposure has an environmental component (metals), drug use as a result of societal behavior (alcohol and drugs of abuse), chemical by-products of industrial development (gases, hydrocarbons, radiation), or essential components of urban, suburban, or agricultural technologies (pesticides, insecticides, herbicides). These chemicals can be classified as nontherapeutic agents (and constitute Part III of this book), but are in fact associated with a variety of well-known clinical signs and symptoms that warrant discussion as part of a clinical toxicology text.

1.2 TYPES OF TOXICOLOGY

1.2.1 GENERAL TOXICOLOGY

General toxicology involves the broad application of toxins and their interaction with biological systems. Like any scientific or clinical discipline, however, the term general toxicology has lost its popularity and has been replaced by more specialized fields of study. With the development of advanced methodologies in biotechnology, the requirement for increased training in the field, and the involvement of toxicology in legal applications, it became necessary to accommodate the discipline with an expanding body of specialties. Thus evolved a variety of adjectives to further define the specialties.

1.2.2 MECHANISTIC TOXICOLOGY

Mechanistic toxicology refers to the identification of the cause of toxicity of a chemical at the cellular or organismal level. The classification of toxicity of a chemical, therefore, may be expressed in terms of its mechanism of toxicity. A similar expression, mechanism of action, is universally applied in the study of pharmacology. Thus mechanistic toxicology seeks to ascertain the biochemical, physiological, or organic basis of a chemical's effect on mammalian systems.

1.2.3 REGULATORY TOXICOLOGY

Regulatory toxicology refers to the administrative dogma associated with the availability of potential toxins encountered in society. Regulatory toxicology defines, directs, and dictates the rate at which an individual may encounter a synthetic or naturally occurring toxin and establishes guidelines for its maintenance in the environment or within the therapeutic market. The guidelines are generally promulgated by agencies whose jurisdiction and regulations are established by federal, state, and local authorities.

1.2.4 DESCRIPTIVE TOXICOLOGY

Descriptive toxicology is a subjective attempt at explaining the toxic agents and their applications. Descriptive toxicology developed principally as a method for bridging the vacuum between the science and the public's understanding of the field, especially when it became necessary for nonscientific sectors to comprehend the importance of toxicology. For instance, the study of metals in the environment (metals toxicology) has become a popular description for toxicologists interested in examining the role of heavy or trace metals in drinking water. Clinical toxicology may also be considered as a descriptive category. Other descriptive adjectives for the field include: **genetic toxicology** — incorporates molecular biology principles in applications of forensic sciences, such as DNA testing, as legal evidence in court proceedings; **occupational toxicology** — examines hazards associated with toxic exposure in the workplace; *in vitro* **toxicology** — refers to the development of cell culture techniques as alternatives to animal toxicity testing. **Analytical, cellular, molecular,** and **developmental toxicology, immunotoxicology,** and **neurotoxicology** are other descriptive areas. More recently, the field has blossomed into several broad descriptive areas including, but not limited to, the study of apoptosis, receptor-mediated signal transduction, gene expression, proteomics, oxidative stress and toxicogenomics, among others.

TABLE 1.1
Descriptive Areas of Toxicology and
Toxicologists

Types of Toxicology	Types of Toxicologists
General	Forensic
Mechanistic	Clinical
Regulatory	Regulatory
Descriptive	Research

1.3 TYPES OF TOXICOLOGISTS

Table 1.1 summarizes the different specialties of toxicology and the practitioners trained for those specific fields. In general, many toxicologists have roles that overlap within the disciplines. For instance, clinical toxicologists may also be involved in understanding the mechanisms of toxic agents, whether from a clinical application or basic research perspective.

1.3.1 FORENSIC TOXICOLOGIST

From its inception in the medieval era to its maturity as a distinct and separate discipline in the 1950s, toxicology was taught primarily as an applied science. More recently, toxicology has evolved from applications of analytical and clinical chemists whose job definitions were the chemical identification and analysis of body fluids. Thus, the first modern toxicologists were chemists with specialized training in inorganic separation methods, including chromatographic techniques. Later, analytical chemists employed thin-layer and gas chromatography. As the instrumentation evolved, high performance liquid chromatography was incorporated into the analytical methods in order to isolate minute quantities of compounds from complex mixtures of toxicological importance. Forensic toxicologists integrated these techniques to identify compounds from mixtures of sometimes-unrelated poisons as a result of incidental or deliberate exposure. Initially, forensic sciences profited from the application of the principles of chemical separation methods for the identification of controlled substances in body fluids. Later, forensic toxicologists applied biological principles of antigen-antibody interaction for paternity testing. By using the principles of blood grouping and "exclusion" of the possible outcomes of paternal contribution to offspring phenotype, it became possible to eliminate the possibility of a male as the father of a child. Antigen-antibody interactions also became the basis for enzyme-linked immunosorbent assays (ELISA, EMIT), currently used for specific and sensitive identification of drugs in biological fluids. Radioimmunoassays (RIAs) utilize similar antigen-antibody reactions while incorporating radiolabeled ligands as indicators. DNA separation and sequencing techniques have now almost totally replaced traditional paternity exclusion testing. These methods are also the basis for inclusion or exclusion of evidence in criminal and civil cases.

1.3.2 CLINICAL TOXICOLOGIST

Clinical toxicologists have evolved and branched away from their forensic counterparts. The clinical toxicologist is interested in identification, diagnosis, and treatment of a condition, pathology, or disease resulting from environmental, therapeutic, or illicit exposure to chemicals or drugs. Exposure is commonly understood to include individual risk of contact with a toxin but can further be defined to include population risk.*

1.3.3 RESEARCH TOXICOLOGIST

In the academic or industrial arenas, the research toxicologist examines the broad issues in toxicology in the laboratory. Academic concerns include any of the public health areas where progress in understanding toxicological sciences is necessary. These include the elucidation of mechanistic, clinical, or descriptive toxicological theories. In the pharmaceutical industry, research toxicologists are needed to conduct phase I trials — i.e., preclinical testing of pharmaceuticals before clinical evaluation and marketing. Preclinical testing involves toxicity testing of candidate compounds, which are chemically and biochemically screened as potentially useful therapeutic drugs. The toxicity testing procedures include both *in vitro* and animal protocols.

1.3.4 REGULATORY TOXICOLOGIST

Regulatory toxicologists are employed primarily in government administrative agencies. Their role is to sanction, approve, and monitor the use of chemicals by enforcing rules and guidelines. The guiding principles are promulgated through laws enacted by appropriate federal, state, and local jurisdictions that grant the regulatory agency its authority. Thus, through these regulations, the agency determines who is accountable and responsible for manufacturing, procurement, distribution, marketing, and ultimately, release and dispensing of potentially toxic compounds to the public.

REFERENCES

SUGGESTED READINGS

Abraham, J., The science and politics of medicines control, *Drug Saf.*, 26, 135, 2003.
Bois, F.Y., Applications of population approaches in toxicology, *Toxicol. Lett.*, 120, 385, 2001.
Eaton, D.L. and Klassen, C.D., Principles of toxicology, in *Casarett and Doull's Toxicology: The Basic Science of Poisons*, Klaassen, C.D., Ed., 6th ed., McGraw-Hill, New York, 2001, chap 2.
Ettlin, R.A. et al., Careers in toxicology in Europe — options and requirements. Report of a workshop organized on behalf of the individual members of EUROTOX during the EUROTOX Congress 2000 in London (September 17–20, 2000), *Arch. Toxicol.*, 75, 251, 2001.

---

* Risks to groups of persons from exposure to radiation, pollutants, and chemical or biological toxins that would necessitate diagnosis and treatment are classified as population risks.

Gennings, C., On testing for drug/chemical interactions: definitions and inference, *J. Biopharm Stat.*, 10, 457, 2000.

Greenberg, G., Internet resources for occupational and environmental health professionals, *Toxicology,* 178, 263, 2002.

Kaiser, J., Toxicology. Tying genetics to the risk of environmental diseases, *Science,* 300, 563, 2003.

Meyer, O., Testing and assessment strategies, including alternative and new approaches, *Toxicol. Lett.*, 140, 2003.

Tennant, R.W., The National Center for Toxicogenomics: using new technologies to inform mechanistic toxicology, *Environ. Health Perspect.*, 110, A8, 2002.

REVIEW ARTICLES

Aardema, M.J. and MacGregor, J.T., Toxicology and genetic toxicology in the new era of "toxicogenomics": impact of "-omics" technologies, *Mutat. Res.,* 499,13, 2002.

Abraham, J. and Reed, T., Progress, innovation and regulatory science in drug development: the politics of international standard-setting, *Soc. Stud. Sci.,* 32, 337, 2002.

Barnard, R.C., Some regulatory definitions of risk: interaction of scientific and legal principles, *Regul. Toxicol. Pharmacol.,* 11, 201, 1990.

Dayan, A.D., Development immunotoxicology and risk assessment. Conclusions and future directions: a personal view from the session chair, *Hum. Exp. Toxicol.,* 21, 569, 2002.

Eason, C. and O'Halloran, K., Biomarkers in toxicology versus ecological risk assessment, *Toxicology,* 181, 517, 2002.

Harris, S.B. and Fan, A.M., Hot topics in toxicology, *Int. J. Toxicol.*, 21, 383, 2002.

Johnson, D.E. and Wolfgang, G.H., Assessing the potential toxicity of new pharmaceuticals, *Curr. Top. Med. Chem.,* 1, 233, 2001.

Lewis, R.W., et al., Recognition of adverse and nonadverse effects in toxicity studies, *Toxicol. Pathol.*, 30, 66, 2002.

Schrenk, D., Regulatory toxicology: objectives and tasks defined by the working group of the German society of experimental and clinical pharmacology and toxicology, *Toxicol. Lett.*, 126, 167, 2002.

Waddell, W.J., The science of toxicology and its relevance to MCS, *Regul. Toxicol. Pharmacol.*, 18, 13, 1993.

Wolfgang, G.H. and Johnson, D.E., Web resources for drug toxicity, *Toxicology,* 173, 67, 2002.

2 Risk Assessment and Regulatory Toxicology

2.1 RISK ASSESSMENT

Risk assessment is a complex process aimed at determining, evaluating, and predicting the potential for harm to a defined community from exposure to chemicals and their by-products. The tolerance of chemicals in the public domain is initially determined by the need for such chemicals, by the availability of alternative methods for obtaining the desired qualities of the chemicals, and by the economic impact of the presence or absence of chemical agents on the economic status of the region. For example, over the last few decades, the amounts and frequency of use of pesticides and herbicides have increased exponentially, especially in the agricultural industry. The benefits of these chemicals have been proven, with time, to generate greater yields of agricultural products, as a result of reduced encroachment by insects and wild-type plant growth. Indeed, greater availability of food products and more sustainable produce has been realized. The balance between safe and effective use of such chemicals and the risk to the population constantly undergoes reevaluation, to determine whether pesticides or herbicides are associated with developmental, carcinogenic, or endocrine abnormalities.

2.2 REGULATORY TOXICOLOGY

The following administrative government agencies are responsible for the application, enforcement, and establishment of rules and regulations associated with safe and effective chemical and drug use in the U.S. A summary of the regulatory agencies and acts under their jurisdiction is organized in Table 2.1.

2.2.1 NUCLEAR REGULATORY COMMISSION (NRC)

Headed by a five-member commission, the NRC is an independent agency established by the Energy Reorganization Act of 1974 to regulate civilian use of nuclear materials.* The NRC's primary mission is to protect the public health and safety, and the environment, from the effects of radiation from nuclear reactors, materials, and waste facilities. In addition, it monitors national defense and promotes security

---

*The Atomic Energy Act of 1954 established the single agency known as the Atomic Energy Commission. It was responsible for the development and production of nuclear weapons and for both the development and safety regulation of civilian uses of nuclear materials. The Act of 1974 split these functions, assigning to the Department of Energy the responsibility for the development and production of nuclear weapons and other energy-related work, and delegating to the NRC the regulatory work noted above.

TABLE 2.1
Summary of Regulatory Agencies and Acts under Their Jurisdiction

Agency	Act	Regulatory Responsibility
NRC	Energy Reorganization Act of 1974	Established the NRC; development and production of nuclear weapons, promotion of nuclear power, and other energy-related work; provides protections for employees who raise nuclear safety concerns (later amendment)
EPA	Clean Air Act	Air quality, air pollution
	Clean Water Act	Water pollution, waste treatment management, toxic pollutants
	CERCLA	"Superfund"; clean up of hazardous substances released in air, land, water
	FIFRA	Safety and regulation of pesticides
	RCRA	Generation, transportation, and disposal of hazardous waste
	Safe Drinking Water Act	Standards for drinking water; establishes MCLs
	Toxic Substances Control Act	Production, processing, importation, testing, and use of potentially hazardous chemicals; testing for HVHE and HPV chemicals
FDA	Federal Food, Drug, and Cosmetic Act	Safety and/or efficacy of food and color additives, medical devices, premarketing drug approval, cosmetics
DEA	Controlled Substances Act	Manufacture, distribution, dispensing, registration, handling of narcotics, stimulants, depressants, hallucinogens, and anabolic steroids; monitors chemicals used in the illicit production of controlled substances
CPSC	Consumer Product Safety Act	Safety standards for consumer products
	FHSA	Toxic, corrosive, radioactive, combustible, or pressurized labeling requirements for hazardous substances
	PPPA	Packaging of hazardous household products
OSHA	OSHA	Sets occupational safety and health standards, and toxic chemical exposure limits, for working conditions

Note: CERCLA = Comprehensive Environmental Response, Compensation and Liability Act; FIFRA = Federal Insecticide, Fungicide and Rodenticide Act; FHSA = Federal Hazardous Substances Act; HPV and HVHE = high production volume and high volume–high exposure chemicals, respectively; MCLs = maximum contaminant levels for drinking water; OSHA = Occupational Safety and Health Act; PPPA = Poison Prevention Packaging Act; RCRA = Resource Conservation and Recovery Act.

from radiological threat. NRC carries out its mission through the enactment of policy, protection of workers from radiation hazards, development of standards, inspection of facilities, investigation of cases, research and development, licensing in the procurement, storage and use of radiation materials, and adjudication.

2.2.2 ENVIRONMENTAL PROTECTION AGENCY (EPA)

Headed by a presidentially appointed administrator, EPA's mission is to protect human health and safeguard the natural environment. The EPA employs over 18,000 engineers, scientists, environmental protection specialists, and staff members in program offices, regional offices, and laboratories.

EPA's mandate is guided by federal laws protecting human health and the environment. It oversees natural resources, human health, economic growth, energy, transportation, agriculture, industry, and international trade in establishing environmental policy. EPA provides leadership in environmental science, research, education, and assessment efforts and works closely with other federal agencies, state and local governments, and Native American tribes to develop and enforce regulations. EPA sets national standards and delegates responsibility to states and tribes for issuing permits, enforcing compliance, and issuing sanctions. It monitors and enforces a variety of voluntary pollution prevention programs and energy conservation efforts, particularly with industrial concerns.

2.2.3 THE FOOD AND DRUG ADMINISTRATION (FDA)

At the beginning of the twentieth century, revelations about filth in the Chicago stockyards shocked the nation into awareness that, in an industrial economy, protection against unsafe products is beyond any individual's means. The U.S. Congress responded to Upton Sinclair's best-selling book *The Jungle* by passing the Food and Drug Act of 1906, which prohibited interstate commerce of misbranded and adulterated food and drugs. Enforcement of the law was entrusted to the U.S. Department of Agriculture's Bureau of Chemistry, which later became the FDA. The Act was the first of more than 200 laws, some of which are discussed below, that constitute a comprehensive and effective network of public health and consumer protections. FDA's mission, therefore, is to promote and protect public health by ensuring the safety and efficacy of products in the market and monitoring them for continued safety. Overall, the FDA regulates $1 trillion worth of products a year.

FDA is under the jurisdiction of the Department of Health and Human Services (HHS) and consists of seven centers: Center for Biologics Evaluation and Research (CBER), Center for Devices and Radiological Health (CDRH), Center for Drug Evaluation and Research (CDER), Center for Food Safety and Applied Nutrition (CFSAN), Center for Veterinary Medicine (CVM), National Center for Toxicological Research (NCTR), and the Office of Regulatory Affairs (ORA).

The *Code of Federal Regulations* (CFR) is a codification of the rules published in the *Federal Register* by executive departments and agencies of the federal government. The CFR is divided into 50 titles, which represent broad areas subject to federal regulation, with environmental regulations contained mainly in Title 40.

Products regulated by the FDA through the CFR include: food and food additives (except for meat, poultry, and some egg products), medical and surgical devices, therapeutic drugs, biological products (including blood, vaccines and tissues for transplantation), animal drugs and feed, and radiation-emitting consumer and medical products. Furthermore, the CFR acts to prevent the willful contamination of all regulated products and improve the availability of medications to prevent or treat injuries caused by biological, chemical, or nuclear agents.

The Federal Food, Drug, and Cosmetic Act (FD&C) of 1938 (Table 2.1) was passed after a legally marketed toxic elixir killed 107 children and adults. The FD&C Act authorized the FDA to demand evidence of safety for new drugs, issue standards for food, and conduct factory inspections.

The Kefauver-Harris Amendments of 1962 were inspired by the thalidomide tragedy in Europe. The Amendments strengthened the rules for drug safety and required manufacturers to prove drug effectiveness.*

The Medical Device Amendments of 1976 followed a U.S. Senate finding that faulty medical devices had caused 10,000 injuries, including 731 deaths. The law established guidelines for safety and effectiveness of new medical devices.

2.2.4 DRUG ENFORCEMENT ADMINISTRATION (DEA)

The DEA is under the policy guidance of the Secretary of State and the HHS and is headed by an administrator. Its mission is to enforce U.S. controlled substance laws and regulations and prosecute individuals and organizations involved in the growing, manufacture, or distribution of controlled substances appearing in or destined for illicit traffic. It also recommends and supports nonenforcement programs aimed at reducing the availability of illicit controlled substances on the domestic and international markets. The DEA's primary responsibilities include: investigation and preparation for the prosecution of major violators of controlled substance laws operating at interstate and international levels; prosecution of criminals and drug gangs; management of a national drug intelligence program in cooperation with federal, state, local, and foreign officials to collect, analyze, and disseminate strategic and operational drug intelligence information; seizure and forfeiture of assets derived from, traceable to, or intended to be used for illicit drug trafficking; enforcement of the provisions of the Controlled Substances Act (see below) as they pertain to the manufacture, distribution, and dispensing of legally produced controlled substances; and coordination and cooperation with federal, state, and local law enforcement officials on mutual drug enforcement efforts, including the reduction of the availability of illicit abuse-type drugs, crop eradication, and training of foreign officials.

The Controlled Substances Act (CSA), Title II of the Comprehensive Drug Abuse Prevention and Control Act of 1970, is a consolidation of numerous laws. It regulates the manufacture and distribution of narcotics, stimulants, depressants, hallucinogens, anabolic steroids, and chemicals used in the illicit sale or production

---

* Prompted by the FDA's vigilance and monitoring of clinical cases, thalidomide was prevented from entering the U.S. market.

TABLE 2.2
Controlled Substances Schedules and Description

Schedules	Description of Regulated Substances	Some Examples of Listed Substances
I	Drug or substance has a high potential for abuse, has no currently accepted medical use in treatment in the U.S., and there is a lack of accepted safety for its use under medical supervision.	Benzylmorphine, etorphine, heroin, dimethyltryptamine (DMT), marijuana, lysergic acid diethylamide (LSD), mescaline, peyote, psilocybin, cocaine, tetrahydrocannabinols (THC)
II	The drug or substance has a high potential for abuse, has a currently accepted medical use in treatment in the U.S. with or without severe restrictions, and may lead to severe psychological or physical dependence.	Fentanyl, levorphanol. methadone, opium and derivatives
III	The drug or substance has a potential for abuse less than the substances in schedules I and II, has a currently accepted medical use in treatment in the U.S., and may lead to moderate or low physical dependence or high psychological dependence.	Amphetamines, phenmetrazine methylphenidate, phencyclidine, nalorphine, anabolic steroids
IV	The drug or substance has a low potential for abuse relative to those drugs or substances in schedule III, has a currently accepted medical use in treatment in the U.S., and may lead to limited physical dependence or psychological dependence.	Barbital, chloral hydrate, meprobamate, phenobarbital
V	The drug or substance has a low potential for abuse, has a currently accepted medical use in treatment in the U.S., and may lead to limited physical dependence or psychological dependence.	Not >200 mg of codeine/100 ml; not >2.5 mg of diphenoxylate and not <25 mcg of atropine sulfate per dosage unit (Lomotil®)

of controlled substances. The CSA places all regulated substances into one of five schedules, based upon the substance's therapeutic importance, toxicity, and potential for abuse or addiction. Table 2.2 describes the federal schedules and some examples of drugs within these classifications. Proceedings to add, delete, or change the schedule of a drug or other substance may be initiated by the DEA or HHS. Any other interested party may also petition the DEA, including the manufacturer of a drug, a medical society or association, a pharmacy association, a public interest group concerned with drug abuse, a state or local government agency, or individuals.

The CSA also creates a closed system of distribution for those authorized to handle controlled substances. The cornerstone of this system is the registration of all those authorized by the DEA to handle controlled substances. All individuals and firms that are registered are required to maintain complete and accurate inventories and records of all transactions involving controlled substances, as well as security for the storage of controlled substances.

2.2.5 Consumer Product Safety Commission (CPSC)

The CPSC is an independent federal regulatory agency created to protect the public from unreasonable risks of injuries and deaths associated with some 15,000 types of consumer products. Its mission is to inform the public about product hazards through local and national media coverage, publication of booklets and product alerts, through a Web site, a telephone hotline, the National Injury Information Clearinghouse, the CPSC's Public Information Center, and through responses to Freedom of Information Act (FOIA) requests. CPSC was created by Congress in 1972 under the Consumer Product Safety Act.[*]

The CPSC fulfills its mission through the development of voluntary standards with industry and by issuing and enforcing mandatory standards or banning consumer products if no feasible standard adequately protects the public. The CPSC obtains recalls of products or arranges for their repair. In addition, it conducts research on potential product hazards, informs and educates consumers, and responds to consumer inquiries. Some of the product guidelines under CPSC jurisdiction are listed in Table 2.3.

TABLE 2.3
Examples of Some Consumer Products with Established Safety and Monitoring Guidelines under CPSC Jurisdiction

All-terrain vehicles safety	Home heating equipment
Art and crafts safety	Household products safety
Bicycle safety	Indoor air quality
Child safety	Older consumers' safety
Children's furniture	Outdoor power equipment safety
Clothing safety	Playground safety
Consumer product safety review	Poison prevention
Crib safety and SIDS[a] reduction	Pool and spa safety
Electrical safety	Public use products
Fire safety	Recreational and sports safety
General information	Reports
Holiday safety	Toy safety

[a] SIDS = sudden infant death syndrome.

[*] The CPSC is headed by three presidentially nominated commissioners (one of whom is Chairman) who are confirmed by the Senate for staggered seven-year terms. The three commissioners set policy for CPSC. The CPSC is not part of any other department or agency in the federal government. The Congressional Affairs, Equal Employment and Minority Enterprise, General Counsel, Inspector General, Secretary, and Executive Director report directly to the Chairman.

TABLE 2.4
Substances Covered by the PPPA of 1970

Therapeutic Category	Examples of Drugs and Substances
Analgesics	Aspirin, acetaminophen, methyl salicylate
Controlled substances	Opioids, S/H, stimulants
Vitamins and dietary supplements	Iron-containing drugs and other dietary supplements
Local anesthetics	Lidocaine, dibucaine, and minoxidil
Nonprescription NSAIDs	Ibuprofen, naproxen, and ketoprofen
Nonprescription antihistamines	Diphenhydramine (Benadryl®)
Nonprescription antidiarrheal products	Loperamide (Imodium®)
General	Human oral prescription drugs (with some exceptions and exemptions)

Note: S/H = sedative/hypnotics.

The Poison Prevention Packaging Act (PPPA) of 1970 is administered by the CPSC. The PPPA requires child-resistant packaging of hazardous household products and dispensed prescription medicine. There have been significant declines in reported deaths from ingestions of toxic household substances by children since the inception of this act. However, it is estimated that more than one million calls to poison control centers are still registered following unintentional exposure to medicines and household chemicals by children under 5 years of age. Of these, more than 85,000 children are examined in emergency departments (EDs), resulting in almost 50 deaths of children each year.*

Some of the reasons accounting for continuing ingestions are: availability of non-child-resistant packaging, on request, for prescription medication; availability of one non-child-resistant size of over-the-counter medications; inadequate quality control by manufacturers, leading to defective child-resistant closures; misuse of child-resistant packaging in the home (leaving the cap off or unsecured, transferring the contents to a non-child-resistant package); and violations by health professionals. Consequently, the CPSC has designed a textbook to educate health professionals, particularly pharmacists and physicians, about the child-resistant packaging program. It is intended to be incorporated into medical and pharmacy school curricula to bring greater awareness of legal responsibilities. Some of the substances covered by the PPPA regulations are listed in Table 2.4.

2.2.6 Occupational Safety and Health Administration (OSHA)

Created by the Occupational Safety and Health Act of 1970, OSHA assures safe and healthful working conditions for the working public. It accomplishes this task through inspectors and staff personnel. OSHA authorizes the enforcement of the

---

* According to the National Electronic Injury Surveillance System (a CPSC database of emergency room visits) and the American Association of Poison Control Centers (2003).

standards developed under the act in cooperation with 26 states. In addition, it provides for research, information, education, and training in the field of occupational safety and health. As a testament to the impact of the agency and the act, workplace fatalities, occupational injury, and illness rates have been reduced by 40 to 50%, while U.S. employment has doubled from 56 to 111 million workers at 7 million sites since 1971.

The agency fulfills its mandate by setting standards established by regulations. For example, the **OSHA Lead Standards for General Industry and Construction** require employers to provide biological monitoring for workers exposed to airborne lead above the action level. Monitoring must be provided for lead and zinc protoporphyrin (or free erythrocyte protoporphyrin) in blood (see Chapter 24, "Metals," for description). The employer is required to have these analyses performed by a laboratory that meets accuracy requirements specified by OSHA. The **OSHA List of Laboratories Approved for Blood Lead Analysis** is designed to provide a source to locate laboratories that OSHA has determined meet the requirements of the accuracy provisions of the lead standards. Laboratories voluntarily provide proficiency test data to OSHA for evaluation.

REFERENCES

Suggested Readings

Clarkson, T.W., Principles of risk assessment, *Adv. Dent. Res.,* 6, 22, 1992.
Cross, J., et al., Postmarketing drug dosage changes of 499 FDA-approved new molecular entities, *Pharmacoepidemiol. Drug Saf.,* 11, 439, 2002.
Dietz, F.K., Ramsey, J.C., and Watanabe, P.G., Relevance of experimental studies to human risk, *Environ. Health Perspect,* 52, 9, 1983.
Luft, J. and Bode, G., Integration of safety pharmacology endpoints into toxicology studies, *Fundam. Clin. Pharmacol.,* 16, 91, 2002.
Nicoll, A. and Murray, V., Health protection — a strategy and a national agency, *Public Health,* 116, 129, 2002.
Patterson, J., Hakkinen, P.J., and Wullenweber, A.E., Human health risk assessment: selected Internet and World Wide Web resources, *Toxicology,* 173, 123, 2002.

Review Articles

Acquavella, J., et al., Epidemiologic studies of occupational pesticide exposure and cancer: regulatory risk assessments and biologic plausibility, *Ann. Epidemiol.,* 13, 1, 2003.
Baht, R.V. and Moy, G.G., Monitoring and assessment of dietary exposure to chemical contaminants, *World Health Stat. Q.,* 50, 132, 1997.
Barlow, S.M., et al., Hazard identification by methods of animal-based toxicology, *Food Chem. Toxicol.,* 40, 145, 2002.
Boyes, W.K., et al., EPA's neurotoxicity risk assessment guidelines, *Fundam. Appl. Toxicol.,* 40, 175, 1997.
Buchanan, J.R., Burka, L.T., and Melnick, R.L., Purpose and guidelines for toxicokinetic studies within the National Toxicology Program, *Environ. Health Perspect,* 105, 468, 1997.

Carere, A. and Benigni, R., Strategies and governmental regulations, *Teratog. Carcinog. Mutagen,* 10, 199, 1990.

Casciano, D.A., FDA: a science-based agency, *FDA Consum.,* 36, 40, 2002.

Clewell, H.J., III, Andersen, M.E., and Barton, H.A., A consistent approach for the application of pharmacokinetic modeling in cancer and noncancer risk assessment, *Environ. Health Perspect.,* 110, 85, 2002.

Conolly, R.B., The use of biologically based modeling in risk assessment, *Toxicology,* 181, 275, 2002.

Eason, C. and O'Halloran, K., Biomarkers in toxicology versus ecological risk assessment, *Toxicology,* 181, 517, 2002.

Hertz-Picciotto, I., Epidemiology and quantitative risk assessment: a bridge from science to policy, *Am. J. Public Health,* 85, 484, 1995.

Indans, I., The use and interpretation of *in vitro* data in regulatory toxicology: cosmetics, toiletries and household products, *Toxicol. Lett.,* 127, 177, 2002.

Kowalski, L., et al., Overview of EPA Superfund human health research program, *Int. J. Hyg. Environ. Health,* 205, 143, 2002.

Lathers, C.M., Risk assessment in regulatory policy making for human and veterinary public health, *J. Clin. Pharmacol.,* 42, 846, 2002.

Liebsch, M. and Spielmann, H., Currently available *in vitro* methods used in the regulatory toxicology, *Toxicol. Lett.,* 127, 127, 2002.

Lorber, M., Indirect exposure assessment at the United States Environmental Protection Agency, *Toxicol. Ind. Health,* 17, 145, 2001.

Lu, F.C. and Sielken, R.L. Jr., Assessment of safety/risk of chemicals: inception and evolution of the ADI and dose-response modeling procedures, *Toxicol. Lett.,* 59, 5, 1991.

Pirkle, J.L., et al., Using biological monitoring to assess human exposure to priority toxicants, *Environ. Health Perspect,* 103, 45, 1995.

Temple, R., Policy developments in regulatory approval, *Stat. Med.,* 21, 2939, 2002.

3 Therapeutic Monitoring of Adverse Drug Reactions (ADRs)

3.1 ADVERSE DRUG REACTIONS IN CLINICAL PRACTICE

The Institute of Medicine of the National Academy of Sciences estimated in 1999 that medical errors killed as many as 98,000 people per year in the U.S., more than car crashes. About 7,000 of those deaths were attributed to drug errors, including wrong drugs, wrong doses, or fatal combinations. A 2002 study of 368 hospitals cited overworked nursing staff, doctors' handwriting, and computer-entry errors for drug mistakes as the most common reasons for the errors.

Today, as the potency, effectiveness, and specificity of clinical drugs improves, the toxicity associated with them also increases. As a result, prevention and treatment of clinical toxicity is not limited to fortuitous encounters with random chemicals but may take on a more subtle form of exposure. This exposure, commonly referred to as pharmacotoxicology, is related to continuous and chronic use of prescription as well as nonprescription, *over-the-counter* (OTC) medications, for the treatment or prevention of pathologic conditions. The toxicity resulting from therapeutic agents, therefore, generally occurs as a result of a number of factors, which are summarized in Table 3.1 and further described below.

3.1.1 INADEQUATE MONITORING OF PRESCRIBED DRUGS

Inadequate monitoring of prescribed drugs results from the failure of coordination between laboratory therapeutic monitoring of medication blood concentrations and the intended therapeutic goals. It also involves lack of attention to appearance of adverse reactions that may occur during the course of treatment. This practice of monitoring is instituted by the prescriber, and its progress is necessarily continued by other health care professionals who are responsible for the patient. Patients must also be vigilant, as far as they can be relied on, to be aware of and report any subjective untoward reactions. However, this requires that sufficient medical information is explained and discussed with the patient concerning the medication and its influence on the condition. Thus, the health care team approach to monitoring the progress of the patient's treatment is regarded as the cornerstone of effective therapy. The practice of monitoring and coordinating health care, however, sometimes requires more resources than what is practical. When resources are scarce or their implementation is not feasible, serious drug toxicity can result.

TABLE 3.1
Factors That Influence Pharmacotoxicology of Therapeutic Drugs

Inadequate monitoring of prescribed drugs
Improper adherence to directions
Inadequate patient compliance
Overprescribing of medications
Drug-drug interactions
Drug-disease interactions
Drug-nutrition interactions
Allergic reactions
Inadequate attention to medication warnings

3.1.2 IMPROPER ADHERENCE TO PRESCRIBED DIRECTIONS

Improper adherence to prescribed directions is a common cause of drug toxicity. Elderly patients often have trouble reading the small print on medication bottles, often leading to improper dosage administration. Patients also may not adequately follow up on treatment protocols. Frequently they either miss scheduled appointments to discuss the development of any untoward effects or fail to report warning signs. Often, patients take the liberty of adjusting dosage regimens without proper consultation.

3.1.3 OVERPRESCRIBING OF MEDICATIONS

In 2000, over 2.8 billion outpatient prescriptions were written, amounting to ten prescriptions per person in the U.S. It is not unreasonable to conclude, therefore, that health care practitioners in the U.S. and around the world have a tendency to overprescribe medications. Today the public relies heavily on scientific breakthroughs and developments, especially in the field of drug development. This is a justifiable assumption, since biotechnology and its drug development products have increased life expectancy. Consequently, compromising social behaviors, such as poor nutritional habits and lack of daily routine exercise programs, are often substituted by increased drug use.

3.1.4 DRUG–DRUG AND DRUG–DISEASE INTERACTIONS

Further complicating the preponderance and availability of drugs, drug interactions from both prescription and OTC medications can compromise therapy. Accordingly, drug-drug and drug-disease interactions are often difficult to identify, monitor, and adjust. The question then arises if the untoward or unanticipated effect is due to the combination of medications or to exacerbation of the condition. Corrective measures such as adjustment of dosage, removal of one or more medications, substitution of one of the components in the treatment schedule, or further tests may be necessary.

3.1.5 ALLERGIC REACTIONS

Any drug preparation has the potential to elicit an allergic reaction. Even a careful patient medication history may not reveal an allergic tendency. Immediate hypersensitivity reactions occurring within minutes or hours of consumption are often easiest to detect. This is because the patient is more alert to the possibility of a cause-effect response soon after one or two doses are ingested. A patient, however, may not associate the effects of an administered dose with an allergic reaction occurring 72 h later, typical of a *delayed hypersensitivity reaction*. Thus, the patient may not arrive at the critical connection between these events. Careful monitoring of drug toxicity, therefore, is essential to differentiate a true hypersensitivity reaction, immediate or delayed, from any incidental or pathologic complication.*

3.1.6 INADEQUATE ATTENTION TO MEDICATION WARNINGS

Whether buried in the small print of package inserts or on the backs of labels of OTC products, inadequate attention to medication warnings results in significant toxicity. Weight-loss products containing sympathetic stimulants are notorious for causing cardiovascular complications in patients with or without heart disease. As described in subsequent chapters, excessive use of other OTC products can cause cumulative toxicities or further complicate normal physiological function. Such products include aspirin, acetaminophen, and antihistamines, and products used for wakefulness, sleep, cough, colds, and energy.

3.1.7 MEDICATION ERRORS

Medication errors by health professionals account for a large proportion of unanticipated, untoward toxicity. As noted above, with the increased availability of and reliance on drug treatment, the possibility of medication errors is amplified. Table 3.2 lists some common sources of errors by health care professionals. Recently, in an effort to reduce the high rate of medical errors, the U.S. Food and Drug Administration (FDA) announced that it would require bar codes on all medications so that hospitals could use scanners to make sure patients get the correct dose of the right drug. The new requirement is one of several steps the agency has taken to reduce medical errors.

3.1.8 ADVERSE DRUG REACTIONS (ADRs)

ADR is a ubiquitous term, which describes any undesirable effect of medication administration in the course of therapeutic intervention, treatment, or prevention of disease. The FDA defines ADR as "a reaction that is noxious, unintended, and occurs at doses normally used in man for the prophylaxis, diagnosis, or therapy of disease." The term ADR has come to replace the common usage of "side effect" often associated with a drug, although the latter is still popular with the public. An ADR

---

*It is interesting to note that, during the course of obtaining medication histories, health care professionals often do not assess how the patient has concluded that they may have an allergic tendency. Subjective negative reactions to a drug in the past, which may not be associated with an allergy toward the medication, may preclude the inclusion of the drug as part of future treatment.

TABLE 3.2
Common Sources of Errors by Health Care Professionals

Prescriber	Pharmacist	Nurse
Confusion with similar sounding drug names	Illegible prescription order	Illegible prescription order
Prescribing wrong dosage	Lack of follow-up on questionable medication or dosage	Lack of follow-up on questionable medication
Transcribing drug for an unintended patient	Confusion with similar sounding drug names	Confusion with similar sounding drug names
Inadequate familiarity with the product	Dispensing wrong medication or wrong dosage	Administering wrong medication or wrong dosage
Inadequate attention to age, sex, weight of patient	Dispensing medication to the wrong patient	Administering medication to the wrong patient
Misdiagnosis	Lack of attention to follow-up signs and symptoms	Lack of attention to follow-up signs and symptoms
Failure to set a therapeutic endpoint	Lack of attention to drug interactions	Inadequate attention to time of administration
Inadequate counseling	Inadequate counseling	Inadequate counseling

may or may not be anticipated, depending on the patient and the condition in question. It is estimated that 15 to 30% of all hospitalized patients have a drug reaction. In addition, one out of five injuries or deaths to hospitalized patients and 5% of all admissions to hospitals are ascribed to ADRs. Adverse reactions double the length of a hospital stay. Overall, over 2 million ADRs occur annually, of which 350,000 occur in nursing homes. It is the fourth leading cause of death in the U.S. (100,000 deaths), at a cost of $136 billion yearly.

Each medication possesses several descriptive terms which detail any and all toxicities that have been encountered in preclinical and clinical use. Table 3.3 lists the categories of untoward effects and their definitions, collectively known as ADRs, including a separate category referred to as Adverse Reactions, which are understood for all FDA-approved drugs.

3.2 TREATMENT OF ADRs AND POISONING IN PATIENTS

3.2.1 History

Among the first treatment modalities used in the presence of unknown, unsuspected toxicity were the induction of emesis and the use of activated charcoal. Early Greek and Roman civilizations recognized the importance of administering charcoal to victims of poisoning, as well as for treating anthrax and epilepsy. Early American folk medicine called for the use of common refined chalk, obtained from the bark of black cherry trees or peach stones and ground to a powder, mixed with common

TABLE 3.3
Categories of Untoward Effects

Warnings and Precautions	Specify conditions in which use of the drug may be hazardous and establish parameters to monitor during therapy
Drug Interactions	Outline a brief summary of documented, clinically significant drug-drug, drug-lab test and drug-food interactions
Contraindications	Specify those conditions in which the drug should not be used
Adverse reactions	Describe the undesirable results of drug administration in addition to or extension of the desired therapeutic effect (side effect)
Overdosage	Describes the administration of a quantity of drug which is greater than that required for a therapeutic effect

chalk, and administered for the treatment of stomach distress due to unknown ingestion. Bread burned to charcoal, dissolved in cold water, was used as a remedy for dysentery. Induction of emesis was also suggested in early civilizations for reversing the effects of ingested poisons. The use of ipecac was described by South American Indians and first mentioned by Jesuit friars in 1601. Brazilian, Colombian, and Panamanian ipecacs were introduced into Europe in 1672 and well established in medicine by the turn of the century. Today, syrup of ipecac is readily available and should be a part of all household medicine chests.

3.2.2 POISON CONTROL CENTER (PCC)

The first specialized medical units devoted to treating poisoned patients were started in Denmark and Hungary, while poison information services began in the Netherlands in the 1940s. PCCs started in the 1950s in Chicago and were well established by the 1970s. The role of the PCC has evolved significantly in the last 50 years to provide public and professional toxicological services associated with emergency management and prevention. Table 3.4 lists some of the aims of the PCC.

PCCs are staffed by a board-certified medical toxicologist and supportive personnel. Board certification is obtained by passing the certification examination after approval of the required minimum experience. The American Board of Applied Toxicology (ABAT), the American Association of Poison Control Centers (AAPCC),

TABLE 3.4
Role of the Poison Control Center

Provide product ingredient information
Provide information on treatment of poisoned patients
Supply direct information to patients
Provide diagnostic and treatment information to health care professionals
Institute education programs for health care professionals
Sponsor poison prevention activities

the American Academy of Clinical Toxicology (AACT), and the American Board of Medical Subspecialties (for physicians) are positioned to administer and maintain standards and board certification in medical toxicology.

3.2.3 CLINICAL MANAGEMENT OF ADRs

Clinical management of ADRs presents situations that require careful examination by health care professionals or trained emergency department (ED) personnel. In addition, ADRs can be detected through insightful questioning of patients by pharmacists, since very often, they are the first health professionals readily available. Thus, a team-oriented approach, whether in an outpatient or inpatient setting, is critical to ascertaining the nature of potential toxic reactions to therapeutic drugs.

In general, acute, sudden reactions to drugs are usually the result of allergic tendencies, contraindications, or overdosage. Even one therapeutic dose of a medication can result in a serious ADR. These reactions, such as the appearance of a sudden rash, obviously may be of considerable concern to the patient and should be treated without delay. These reactions, however, do not always require an emergency room visit.

Alternatively, ADRs associated with chronic administration of medications are more subtle and insidious. Chronic toxicity occurs as a result of prolonged accumulation, the effects of which will develop into organ-specific toxicity. The adverse reactions in this case may be difficult to differentiate from a coexisting pathologic condition. For example, chronic low-grade digoxin toxicity often mimics symptoms of congestive heart failure, the precise condition it is designed to treat (see Chapter 18).

Overall, the hallmark of effective management of ADRs includes an approach that is not at all different from the "medical ABCs" — i.e., obtaining a detailed patient history, performing a physical examination, arriving at a differential diagnosis, requesting supplementary laboratory tests, reaching a final diagnosis, prescribing of therapy, follow-up, and evaluation of condition.

Included in a general medical history are questions pertaining to the use of drugs (prescription, OTC, or illicit), alcohol, tobacco, and any dietary supplements (vitamins, herbal products). In addition, the time and method of administration should be ascertained.

3.2.4 CLINICAL MANAGEMENT OF TOXICOLOGIC EMERGENCIES

Clinical management of a patient presenting with apparent poisoning involves a stepwise approach to securing effective treatment of the suspected toxicologic emergency. Whether the perceived emergency is in the hospital emergency room or in the field, such as at home or on the street, it is important to begin management of the situation in a systematic manner. This includes: (1) stabilization of the patient; (2) clinical evaluation (including, if possible, history of the events leading to the emergency), physical examination, and laboratory and/or radiological tests; (3) prevention of further absorption, exposure, or distribution; (4) enhancement of elimination of the suspected toxin; (5) administration of an antidote; and (6) supportive care and follow-up.

1. *Stabilization of the patient* involves a general assessment of the situation and the environment, overall appearance of the patient, and maintenance of vital signs. Removal of the victim from the obvious source of contamination, such as from fumes, gas, or spilled liquid, is of primary concern. This is followed by maintenance of the **ABCs** of clinical management; that is, maintain **a**irway, **b**reathing, and **c**irculation, which are crucial to survival. This includes monitoring of blood pressure and heart rate, ensuring that respirations are adequate, checking the status of the pupils, determination of skin temperature, color, and turgor. There may be wide variability in the initial signs and symptoms, especially in the first few minutes post exposure. Stabilization includes not only the return of vital signs to normal but also normal rhythm.

2. *Clinical evaluation* includes documentation of the history of the events leading to the emergency. This is accomplished more easily in the emergency room, or on phone intake, by a witness or the patient who is conscious and able to respond. Determination of the substance ingested can also be obtained by inspection of the area adjacent to the victim and questioning of any potential witnesses. Time of exposure is critical and can influence the course of treatment and prognosis. If time permits, calls to a local pharmacy or physician's office may contribute some valuable information as to the etiologic agent. Location of the victim, neighborhood, and activity in the vicinity, may also divulge some hints as to the nature of the ingested agent.

   Physical examination involves identification of a constellation of clinical signs and symptoms that, together, are likely associated with exposure from certain classes of toxic agents. Also known as the identification of the toxic syndrome or "toxidrome," this compilation of observations allows for the initiation of treatment and progress toward follow-up care and support. Table 3.5 describes five of the most common toxidromes and their clinical signs and symptoms that suggest a particular toxic agent, or category of agents, is responsible. Commonly observed features are listed first, followed by peripheral or more severe signs and symptoms. The agents and the mechanisms responsible for the toxidromes are discussed in subsequent chapters. It is important to note that the clinical picture becomes complicated when multiple drugs or chemicals are involved. The manifestations of one drug may mask or prevent the identification of other chemicals.

   Although stat* tests are available for most clinical drugs, laboratory tests and radiological exams have limited turnaround times for identification of the cause of toxicity. Consequently, substance analysis of biolog-

---

* Quick, immediate, or on emergency order.

TABLE 3.5
Common Toxidromes and Their Clinical Features

Anticholinergic	Dry mucous membranes, flushed skin, urinary retention, decreased bowel sounds, altered mental status, dilated pupils, cycloplegia
Sympathomimetic	Psychomotor and physical agitation, hypertension, tachycardia, hyperpyrexia, diaphoresis, dilated pupils, tremors; seizures (if severe)
Cholinergic	SLUDGE (sialorrhea, lacrimation, urination, diaphoresis, gastric emptying), BBB (bradycardia, bronchorrhea, brochospasms); muscle weakness, intractable seizures
Opioid	CNS depression, miosis, respiratory depression, bradycardia, hypotension, coma
Benzodiazepine	Mild sedation, unresponsive or comatose with stable vital signs; transient hypotension, respiratory depression

ical specimens is generally performed for confirmation of differential diagnosis and follow-up treatment. Initializing emergency measures should not depend on obtaining laboratory results. Qualitative and quantitative analysis of biological specimens, however, may be necessary for optimal patient management for specific drugs, including: acetaminophen, aspirin, digoxin, iron, lead, lithium, and theophylline. Drug screens aid in diagnosis, and sodium (Na^+), chloride (Cl^-), and bicarbonate ions (HCO_3^-), as well as glucose, contribute to determination of the serum osmolarity. High serum concentrations of drugs, enough to cause unstable clinical conditions, alter the osmolarity and create a gap between the osmoles measured by laboratory analysis and the calculated osmoles. This **anion gap** is a nonspecific, yet instrumental, diagnostic manipulation and can be of assistance in monitoring the progression of treatment. Anion gap is calculated according to the following formula:

$$[Na^+ - (Cl^- + HCO_3^-)]$$

where the concentrations of ions are in meq/l. A normal value is less than 12. An elevated anion gap suggests metabolic acidosis. Most common chemical agents that contribute to an elevated anion gap include: alcohol, toluene, methanol, paraldehyde, iron, lactic acid, ethylene glycol, and salicylates. Other conditions suggested by an elevated anion gap include diabetic acidosis and uremia. Paraldehyde, a hypnotic drug, was also frequently encountered but is no longer available (the acronym AT MUD PILES, which includes paraldehyde, may still be of some pneumonic use).

Another nonspecific diagnostic aid used to monitoring the progression of toxicity is the osmolar gap. The following formula is used to calculate the osmolar gap:

$$(2 \times Na^+) + ([glucose]/18) + (BUN/2.8)$$

where glucose and BUN (blood urea nitrogen) concentrations are in mg/dl. The osmolar gap is determined by subtracting the calculated value from the measured osmolarity. The normal osmolar gap is less than 10 mOsm. An increase in the gap above 10 suggests poisoning with ethanol, ethylene glycol, isopropanol, or methanol. It is important to note that, depending on the method used to determine the osmolar gap, a normal value does not rule out poisoning with ethylene glycol or methanol.

3. *Prevention of any further absorption or exposure* to a toxic agent initially involves removing the patient from the environment, especially in the presence of gaseous fumes or corrosive liquids. In the event of dermal exposure to a liquid, removal of the contaminated clothes and thorough rinsing with water are important steps. Rinsing the exposed area with soap and water are of great benefit for acid and phenol burns.

   Limiting exposure of oral intoxication of an agent should be pursued immediately after a known ingestion. In the home or ED, several methods can be employed to limit intestinal absorption, enhance bowel evacuation, or promote emesis. Activated charcoal is the best method to diminish intestinal absorption. A 1- to 2-g/kg dose, as a slurry, is given orally or through a large bore (36 to 40 French) nasogastric tube. The 1000- to 2000-m^2 surface area per gram of activated charcoal can effectively absorb 50% of an orally ingested chemical 1 hour later. The material binds high-molecular-weight organics, by noncovalent forces, more effectively than low-molecular-weight inorganic molecules. Activated charcoal, however, is not effective for metals such as lead or iron, hydrocarbons, acids, and alkalis.

   All households should have syrup of ipecac readily available. Vomiting is induced within 20 to 30 min of a 20-ml dose. Effectiveness of ipecac is limited by its delay of onset and the risk of aspiration of stomach contents. Additionally, treatment is contraindicated in children under six years of age, in the presence of caustic acids or alkalis, and coma.

   Gastric lavage, or "pumping the stomach," has limited value, since it has not been demonstrated to be of much clinical benefit. It is most effective when administered within 1 h of ingestion through an orogastric tube. In addition, the procedure is uncomfortable and, like syrup of ipecac, exposes the patient to the possibility of tracheal aspiration of stomach contents.

4. *Enhancement of elimination* of suspected chemical agents or drugs is accomplished using whole bowel irrigation. In adults, oral administration of polyethylene glycol (Golytely®, Colyte®), at a rate of 2 l/hr, can flush ingested toxic agents through the bowel. Administration of the preparation is continued for 4 to 5 h, or until the bowel effluents are clear. The method is useful for enhanced elimination of sustained-released preparation of capsules or tablets, cellophane packets of street heroin or cocaine, and agents not effectively absorbed with charcoal.

   Hemodialysis has historical and sometimes empirical value in enhancing elimination. The hemodialysis machine pumps the patient's blood through a dialysis membrane, the purpose of which is to decrease the drug's volume of distribution (V_d). Ideally, the compound should be of low molecular weight, higher water solubility, and low protein-binding capacity. The procedure appears to be useful when other measures have failed, especially in the treatment of amphetamine, antibiotic, boric acid, chloral hydrate, lead, potassium, salicylate, and strychnine poisoning.

Alkalinization or acidification of urine, although based on valid chemical pharmacokinetic principles of ion trapping and acid-base reactions, is not clinically recommended. Practically, the concept is not effective and may aggravate or complicate the removal of agents that interfere with acid-base balance.

5. *Administration of an antidote.* As noted above, adherence to the ABC principles and good supportive care are the hallmarks of treatment of the poisoned patient. Once the agent responsible is suspected or identified, administration of an antidote may be necessary. Table 3.6 organizes a variety of toxins according to their classification and available antidotes. Although a small number of antidotes are available, many of these agents can completely reverse the toxicologic consequences of poisoning. Also, specific antidotes are discussed further under the individual chapter headings (chelating agents for metal poisoning are reviewed separately in Chapter 24, "Metals"). However, it should be noted that antidotes are associated with their own adverse reactions and toxicity. In addition, effectiveness of antidotes is compromised in the presence of overdose from multiple agents.

6. *Supportive care and maintenance.* After the primary goal of stabilization of vital signs is achieved, supportive care and maintenance are essential. This may require several more hours in the ED before release or transfer to an intensive care unit. Only a few drugs and chemicals have a tendency for delayed toxicity, including: iron tablets or elixir, salicylates, acetaminophen, opioids, sedative-hypnotics (barbiturates and benzodiazepines), and paraquat. In addition, salicylate and iron toxicity, as well as lead poisoning, may exhibit multiple phases of acute toxicity, interspersed with stages of remission of signs and symptoms. Monitoring in an ICU is essential to ensure complete recovery. In the event of suspected deliberate intoxication, ingestion, or administration, psychiatric assessment, forensic analysis, and police investigation are warranted.

3.3 DRUG IDENTIFICATION AND METHODS OF DETECTION

The analysis of drugs in biological fluids, tissues, or in mixtures with other compounds, is a complex science. Several areas of toxicology rely on identification of drugs and chemicals for monitoring of toxic effects.

TABLE 3.6
Classification of Toxins and Their Specific Antidotes

Classification of Toxins	Examples of Specific Toxic Agents	Antidote
Alcohols	Ethylene glycol	Ethanol, fomepizol, pyridoxine
	Methanol	Ethanol, fomepizol, folic acid, leucovorin
Analgesics	Acetaminophen	N-acetylcysteine
	Aspirin	Sodium bicarbonate, ipecac
Anticholinergics	Cholinergic blockers	Physostigmine
	Tricyclic antidepressants	Sodium bicarbonate
Anticoagulants	Heparin	Protamine
	Warfarin	Vitamin K_1 (phytonadione)
Arthropod bites and stings	Black widow spider bite	*Latrodectus* antivenom
	Brown recluse spider bite	*Loxosceles* antivenom
	Rattlesnake bite	*Crotalidae* antivenom
	Scorpion sting	Antivenin
Benzodiazepines	Diazepam, alprazolam	Flumazenil
Cardiovascular drugs	Digitalis glycosides	Digoxin immune FAB
	β-blockers	Glucagon
	Calcium channel blockers	Calcium, glucagon
Gases	Chlorine gas	Sodium bicarbonate[a]
	Hydrogen sulfide gas	Sodium nitrite
	Carbon monoxide	100% oxygen
	Cyanide	Amyl nitrite, sodium nitrite, sodium thiosulfate
Infectious agents	*Clostridium botulinuum* (botulism)	*Botulinuum* antitoxin
Metals	Arsenic	BAL
	Copper	D-penicillamine
	Mercury	BAL, DMSA
	Iron	Deferoxamine
	Lead	Calium-Na_2-EDTA, dimercaprol, DMSA, BAL, D-penicillamine
Methemoglobinemia-inducing agents	Nitrites, nitrates	Methylene blue
Opiates	Narcotic analgesics and heroin	Naloxone, natrexone, nalmefene
Pesticides	Organophosphate insecticides	Atropine followed by pralidoxime
	Carbamate insecticides	Atropine

Note: BAL = British antilewisite; DMSA = 2,3-dimercaptosuccinic acid; EDTA = ethylenediamine tetraacetate; FAB = fragment antigen-binding.

[a] For treatment of accompanying metabolic acidosis.

TABLE 3.7

Forensic Toxicology Laboratory Initial Testing (Screening) Methods Based on Specimen Availability

Specimen Available	Compounds	Method
Blood or urine	Volatiles (alcohols, acetone); gases (CO)	HS/GC
	Opiates, benzylecgonine	RIA
Urine only	Amphetamines, canabinoids, PCP, methadone, barbiturates	EI
	Salicylates, APAP	CT
	Other basic drugs[a]	GC/MS or GC/NP
Blood only or Tissue only	Volatiles	HS/GC
	Opiates, barbiturates benzylecgonine	RIA
	Salicylates (blood only)	CT
	Other basic drugs[a]	GC/MS or GC/NP

Note: APAP = acetaminophen, CO = carbon monoxide, CT = color test, EI = enzyme immunoassay, GC = gas chromatography, HS = head space, HPLC = high performance liquid chromatography, MS = mass spectrometry, PCP = phencyclidine, SP = spectrophotometry, RIA = radio immunoassay, NP = nitrogen phosphorus detector.

[a] See Table 3.8.

Forensic toxicology laboratories have the responsibility of identifying drug ingredients, predominantly of unknown origin, and separating them from additives and contaminants. The assortment of drug specimens that confront the criminalist presents a formidable task for identifying illicit drugs. The first step in detecting and identifying a suspected chemical agent is the application of a screening test. The results of this procedure determine the next test, or series of tests, to confirm the presence of the specific compound. Initial analytical methods range from simple color tests and chromatography screens to more sophisticated gas chromatographic–mass spectrometry (GC-MS) detection. In addition, extraction techniques are sometimes necessary in order to separate the suspected active constituent from the complex nature of the specimen.

Table 3.7 outlines the approaches, compounds, and methods employed in the forensic toxicology laboratory for screening and identifying common drugs of abuse. Details of the procedures and analytical methods for specific drugs and chemicals are discussed in the references (Suggested Readings). Available methods for identification of classes of compounds in biological specimens are also included in each of the respective chapters.

Clinical toxicology laboratories are involved in detection of drugs in suspected cases of drug abuse, overdosage, or for monitoring of drugs in sports. Drug abuse tests are generally noninvasive and employ mostly screening tests for the more common illicit compounds. Urine is used for large-scale testing because of its ease of acquisition and its noninvasive nature. Analysis for unauthorized use of drugs is performed in a variety of settings. Testing of drug abusers in drug rehabilitation clinics and hospitals is done to monitor the effectiveness of the rehabilitation program for the patient. Monitoring of drug use in the workplace, schools, and in individuals involved in critical jobs (such as police and pilots) is a relatively recent phenomenon. Testing is required or is mandatory in order to protect employees, employers, students, and the public from the harmful consequences of illicit drug use by individuals responsible for public safety. Identification of drugs in drug abuse cases and monitoring of suspected drug use in sports is generally accomplished with rapid screening of urine samples.

Monitoring of drugs in cases of overdosage falls within the realm of the clinical (and sometimes forensic) toxicology lab. The major reason for analysis of fluids in overdose cases is to establish the source and extent of chemical toxicity and to apply an appropriate treatment program. Samples obtained in overdose cases (intentional or accidental) are usually more amenable to preparation and analysis than samples supplied to the forensic toxicology laboratory. Based on the signs and symptoms of the overdose (coma, respiratory depression, hallucinations, cardiac arrest), the range of possible chemical suspects is also narrower. Screening methods and confirmation tests are available for proper management of poisoning cases.

As mentioned above, **therapeutic drug monitoring** is necessary for clinical scrutiny of ADRs. It is also important for managing appropriate therapeutic response to potent medications and for preventing inadequate or toxic responses. Therapeutic drug plasma levels are requested in order to adjust the dose for optimal effect. A variety of more sophisticated analytical techniques have been developed for monitoring therapeutic drugs, including high performance liquid chromatography (HPLC), gas chromatography (GC), and bioassays such as enzyme immunoassays (EI) and radio immunoassays (RIA).

Table 3.8 outlines some of the drugs and the methods used in routine toxicology and therapeutic screens. Basic drugs encompass the majority of compounds detected in toxicology laboratories. Extraction of active constituents from biological specimens is a necessary prerequisite for analysis of drugs by GC/NP (GC coupled with nitrogen phosphorus detector). Acidic or basic drugs are extracted from biological fluids or tissue homogenates by adjusting the medium pH to acidic or basic, respectively. The compounds are then extracted and back-extracted into appropriate inorganic and organic solvents after further adjustment of pH. Calibration curves, negative and positive controls, and internal and external standards are part of the routine procedures. Some examples of drugs that are not routinely tested in toxicology screens include: highly polar drugs (antibiotics, diuretics, lithium), highly volatile compounds (nitrous oxide, hydrocarbons), and highly nonpolar compounds (steroids, digoxin, plant derivatives). Other toxic anions and alkaloids that are difficult to detect, or not routinely screened, are GHB, cyanide, LSD, and the ergotamines. Specific details of the techniques are discussed in referenced Suggested Readings. Analytical methods for specific drugs and chemicals are also located under the headings for the classes of compounds in subsequent chapters.

TABLE 3.8
Drugs Tested in Routine Toxicology and Therapeutic Screens Based on Their Chemical Class

Chemical Class	Compounds	Method
Volatiles and Gases	Ethanol, acetone	HS/GC
	CO	SP, CT
Acidic and Neutral Drugs	APAP, salicylates	CT, HPLC
	Barbiturates	EI, RIA, HPLC
	Anticonvulsants (phenytoin, carbamazepine); digoxin	HPLC, RIA
Basic Drugs	Amitriptyline, amoxapine, chlorpheniramine, diphenhydramine, doxepin, doxylamine, ethylbenzylecgonine, flurazepam, fluoxetine, haloperidol, imipramine, ketamine, lidocaine, meperidine, methorphan, propoxyphene, verapamil	GC, GC/MS
	Benzylecgonine, cocaine, codeine, morphine	EI, RIA, GC/MS
	Chlordiazepoxide, diazepam, methadone, PCP	EI, GC, GC/MS
	Chlorpromazine, thioridazine	CT, GC, GC/MS
	Caffeine, theophylline	GC, GC/MS, HPLC
Hormones and Miscellaneous	Anterior pituitary hormones, thyroid hormones, specific binding proteins, antibiotics, antineoplastics	RIA

Note: APAP = acetaminophen, CO = carbon monoxide, CT = color test, EI = enzyme immunoassay, GC = gas chromatography, MS = mass spectrometry, HS = head space, HPLC = high performance liquid chromatography, PCP = phencyclidine, SP = spectrophotometry, RIA = radio immunoassay.

REFERENCES

SUGGESTED READINGS

Chamberlain, J., *The Analysis of Drugs in Biological Fluids*, 2nd ed., CRC Press, Inc., Boca Raton, FL, 1995.

Meyer, C., *American Folk Medicine*, Plume Books, New American Library, 1973.

Harsman, J.G. and Limbird, L.E., *Goodman & Gilman's The Pharmacological Basis of Therapeutics,* 10th ed., McGraw-Hill Co., New York, 2001, chaps. 32, 33, 34, and 35.

REVIEW ARTICLES

Abbruzzi, G. and Stork, C.M., Pediatric toxicologic concerns, *Emerg. Med. Clin. North Am.,* 20, 223, 2002.

Bond, C.A. and Raehl, C.L., Pharmacists' assessment of dispensing errors: risk factors, practice sites, professional functions, and satisfaction, *Pharmacotherapy,* 21, 614, 2001.

Bowden, C.A. and Krenzelok, E.P., Clinical applications of commonly used contemporary antidotes. A U.S. perspective, *Drug Saf.,* 16, 9, 1997.

Dawson, A.H. and Whyte, I.M., Evidence in clinical toxicology: the role of therapeutic drug monitoring, *Ther. Drug Monit.,* 24, 159, 2002.

Epstein, F.B. and Hassan, M., Therapeutic drug levels and toxicology screen, *Emerg. Med. Clin. North Am.,* 4, 367, 1986.

Fountain, J.S. and Beasley, D.M., Activated charcoal supercedes ipecac as gastric decontaminant, *N. Z. Med. J.,* 111, 402, 1998.

Guernsey, B.G., et al. Pharmacists' dispensing accuracy in a high-volume outpatient pharmacy service: focus on risk management, *Drug Intell. Clin. Pharm.,* 17, 742, 1983.

Henry, J.A. and Hoffman, J.R., Continuing controversy on gut decontamination, *Lancet,* 352, 420, 1998.

Jackson, W.A., Antidotes, *Trends Pharmacol. Sci.,* 23, 96, 2002.

Jacobsen, D. and Haines, J.A., The relative efficacy of antidotes: the IPCS evaluation series. International Programme on Chemical Safety, *Arch. Toxicol. Suppl.,* 19, 305, 1997.

Jones, A., Recent advances in the management of poisoning, *Ther. Drug Monit.,* 24, 150, 2002.

Krenzelok, E.P., New developments in the therapy of intoxications, *Toxicol Lett.,* 127, 299, 2002.

Larsen, L.C. and Cummings, D.M., Oral poisonings: guidelines for initial evaluation and treatment, *Am. Fam. Physician,* 57, 85, 1998.

Lheureux, P., Askenasi, R., and Paciorkowski, F., Gastrointestinal decontamination in acute toxic ingestions, *Acta. Gastroenterol. Belg.,* 61, 461, 1998.

Meredith, T., Caisley, J., and Volans, G., ABC of poisoning. Emergency drugs: agents used in the treatment of poisoning, *Br. Med. J.* 289, 742, 1984.

Neville, R.G., et al. A classification of prescription errors, *J. R. Coll. Gen. Pract.,* 39, 110, 1989.

Rubenstein, H. and Bresnitz, E.A., The utility of Poison Control Center data for assessing toxic occupational exposures among young workers, *J. Occup. Environ. Med.,* 43, 463, 2001.

Schneider, M.P., Cotting, J., and Pannatier, A., Evaluation of nurses' errors associated in the preparation and administration of medication in a pediatric intensive care unit, *Pharm. World Sci.,* 20, 178, 1998.

Seifert, S.A. and Jacobitz, K., Pharmacy prescription dispensing errors reported to a regional poison control center, *J. Toxicol. Clin. Toxicol.* 40, 919, 2002.

Shannon, M., Therapeutics and toxicology, *Curr. Opin. Pediatr.* 11, 253, 1999.

Vernon, D.D. and Gleich, M.C., Poisoning and drug overdose, *Crit. Care Clin.* 13, 647, 1997.

Warner, A., Setting standards of practice in therapeutic drug monitoring and clinical toxicology: a North American view, *Ther. Drug Monit.,* 22, 93, 2000.

4 Classification of Toxins in Humans

4.1 INTRODUCTION

Classification of chemical agents is a daunting task, considering the vast number and complexity of chemical compounds in the public domain. With the variety of chemicals and drugs available, and their varied pharmacological and toxicological effects, an agent may find itself listed in several different categories. Even compounds with similar structures or pharmacological actions may be alternatively grouped according to their toxicological activity or physical state. The following outline of the classification systems is generally accepted for understanding the complex nature of toxins. The mechanisms of toxicity will be discussed in subsequent chapters.

4.2 TARGET ORGAN CLASSIFICATION

4.2.1 AGENTS AFFECTING THE HEMATOLOGIC SYSTEM

Hematotoxicology is the effect of therapeutic and nontherapeutic chemicals on circulating blood components, coagulation processes, and blood-forming tissues (Bloom, 1997). Understanding the toxicity borne by these physiologic systems requires a working knowledge of the hematopoietic process and its cellular constituents. Figure 4.1 illustrates the process of hematopoiesis, including the development and ontogeny of erythrocytes (red blood cells) and leukocytes (white blood cells). Chemicals which affect hematopoiesis, therefore, may interfere with the normal physiologic function of any of its cells and proteins including: erythrocytes and their oxygen carrying capacity residing in hemoglobin; thrombocytes (platelets) and their role in fibrin clot formation; basophils, neutrophils, and eosinophils, and their antimicrobial activities. Chemicals which interfere with white blood cell components and their formation are generally classified as leukemogenic agents and are discussed individually in later chapters.

Figure 4.2 illustrates the intrinsic and extrinsic pathways of coagulation, incorporating the tissue factors and phospholipids associated with the coagulation cascade. Anticoagulants, such as the clinical drug and pesticide warfarin, interfere with the synthesis of coagulation proteins and factors. A detailed explanation of the mechanism of warfarin and other anticoagulants is outlined in Chapter 28, "Rodenticides."

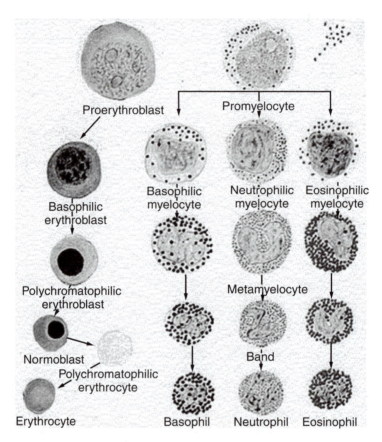

FIGURE 4.1 Hematopoiesis. (From A.W. Ham and D.H. Cormack, *Histology*, Lippincott, New York, 1979, Plate 12.1. With permission.)

4.2.2 IMMUNOTOXIC AGENTS

The immune system and the mechanisms by which the body maintains homeostasis and protection against microorganisms are often the targets of chemical agents and therapeutic drugs. Table 4.1 and Table 4.2 organize the immune system according to the concepts of **innate immunity** (i.e., the immunological protection afforded without the production of antibodies) and **acquired immunity** (the adaptive response induced as a result of exposure to antigen). Familiarity with the role of the immune system allows for an understanding of the mechanisms by which compounds, especially a number of therapeutic immunosuppressive drugs, produce toxicity.

4.2.3 HEPATOTOXIC AGENTS

The liver is a target organ for many chemicals and therapeutic drugs, predominantly because of its high metabolic capacity, its extensive circulation, and sizeable surface area. For instance, the hepatotoxic effects of vinyl chloride and carbon tetrachloride

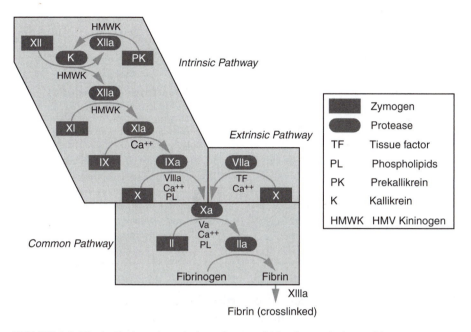

FIGURE 4.2 The intrinsic and extrinsic pathways of blood coagulation and its components. (From Dr. Douglas M. Tollefsen, Washington University Medical School. With permission.)

TABLE 4.1
Characteristics and Properties of Innate Immunity

Innate Immunity	Characteristics and Properties
Susceptibility	Result of genetic influences
Epithelial barriers	Desquamation, dessication, fatty acid secretion, mucosal enzymes
Lymphoid tissue	Bone marrow, thymus, spleen, lymphatics; BALT, GALT, MALT[a]
Inflammatory response	PMN,[a] APP,[a] cytokines and vasoactive mediators; calor, rubor, tumor, dolor.[b]
Complement	Complement proteins and cell lysis
Phagocytosis	Pinocytosis, endocytosis, opsonization, degranulation; cells include granulocytes and the monocyte/macrophage system
Nonspecific extracellular killing	NK[a] cells

[a] BALT = bronchial-associated lymphoid tissue, GALT = gut-associated lymphoid tissue, MALT = mucosa-associated lymphoid tissue, PMN = polymorphonuclear cells, APP = acute phase proteins, NK = natural killer.

[b] Fever, redness, swelling, pain (respectively).

TABLE 4.2
Characteristics and Properties of Acquired Immunity

Acquired Immunity	Subdivision	Characteristics and Properties
Active immunity	Cell-mediated immunity	T-lymphocytes: allogeneic response, cytokine production, tumor cell cytotoxicity, immunologic memory
	Humoral immunity	B-lymphocytes: antigen-antibody response, cytokine production, complement activation, LPS, immunologic memory, vaccination
Passive immunity	Passive immunization: oral, parenteral administration of antiserum	Administration of antitoxin, antivenom; colostrums; placental transfer of antibodies; bone marrow transplant

have been known for decades to be a consequence of industrial exposure. The seriousness of hepatotoxicity of the type-2 antidiabetic drug Rezulin® (troglitazone) was identified only after the drug was prescribed to over 800,000 patients for about six years, which prompted withdrawal from the prescription drug market. Table 4.3 lists the physiological functions and biochemical pathways in the liver, the representative chemicals that interfere with these functions, and resulting injury associated with these pathways.

4.2.4 NEPHROTOXIC AGENTS

It is not unusual that the kidneys bear a significant burden from the assault of xenobiotic exposure, since they are ultimately involved with maintenance of homeostasis. The functions of the kidney in maintaining this role include: monitoring of blood electrolyte composition and concentration, elimination of metabolic waste, regulation of extracellular fluid volume, maintenance of blood pressure, and adjustment of acid-base balance. Metabolically, the kidneys synthesize and secrete important hormones, such as renin and erythropoietin, necessary for regulation of blood pressure and hematopoiesis, respectively. Metabolically, they convert vitamin D_3 to the active 1,25-dihydroxy metabolite. Figure 4.3 illustrates the anatomical arrangement of the nephron, the functional kidney cell unit. Direct or indirect exposure to nephrotoxic agents may result in ultrastructural damage to any of the principal components of the nephron. Consequently, the pathologic response to a toxic insult is not necessarily different for various chemicals affecting alternate parts of the nephron. For example, acute renal failure (ARF) is the most common manifestation of toxic renal exposure, resulting in an abrupt decline in glomerular filtration rate (GFR). The anatomical sites of chemically-induced ARF, and some of the drugs and chemicals associated with injury include:

TABLE 4.3
Functions of the Liver and Characteristics of Chemical Agents Associated with Hepatotoxicity

Physiologic Liver Function	Associated Pathways	Representative Drug or Toxins	Resulting Damage
Biochemical homeostasis	Glucose storage and synthesis	CCL_4, ethanol, insulin	Hypoglycemia
	Cholesterol synthesis and uptake		Hypercholesterolemia, fatty liver
Protein synthesis	Clotting factors, albumin, lipoproteins (LDL, VLDL)[a]	Iron, metals, aspirin	Hemorrhage
			Hypoalbuminemia
			Fatty liver
Bioactivation and detoxification	P450 isozymes	CCL_4, acetaminophen	Increased sensitivity to drug interactions, drug overdose
	Glutathione/GSH levels	Acetaminophen	
	Oxygen-dependent bioactivation	Allyl alcohol, ethanol, iron	
Bile formation and secretion	Bilirubin and cholesterol synthesis; uptake of lipids and vitamins	Amoxicillin	Bile duct damage, malnutrition, gallstones, steatorrhea
Hepatic sinusoids	Exchange of lmw[a] substances between hepatocytes and sinusoid	Metals, anabolic steroids, cyclophosphamide	Jaundice, gallstones, neurotoxicity, interference with secondary male sex characteristics
Direct hepatocyte toxicity	Inflammation, wound healing and repair	Acetaminophen, arsenic, ethanol, vinyl chloride	Cell death, fibrosis, cirrhosis
	Tumors	Aflatoxin, androgens	Hepatocellular carcinoma

[a] LDL = low density lipoproteins; VLDL = very low density lipoproteins; lmw = low molecular weight.

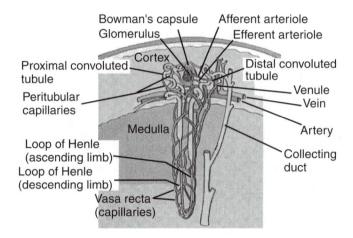

FIGURE 4.3 Schematic diagram of the nephron, the functional cell unit of the kidney. (From Purves, W.K. et al., *Life: The Science of Biology*, 4th ed., Sinauer Associates, Sunderland, MA, 1994, Fig. 44.13C. With permission.)

- **Prerenal** (i.e., prior to entering the glomerulus): diuretics, vasodilator antihypertensive agents, angiotensin-converting enzyme inhibitors
- **Vasoconstriction of afferent/efferent arterioles**: cyclosporin, nonsteroidal anti-inflammatory agents (NSAIDs)
- **Crystalluria**: sulfonamides, acyclovir, ethylene glycol
- **Proximal and distal tubular toxicity**: aminoglycosides, vancomycin
- **Glomerular capillary endothelial injury**: cocaine, quinine, conjugated estrogens
- **Glomerular injury**: gold compounds, NSAIDs, penicillamine

4.2.5 Pulmonary Toxic Agents

There are numerous lung diseases caused by direct exposure to inhalation of toxic airborne products, traditionally referred to as inhalation toxicology. These agents have historically been classified according to occupational diseases because of their association with inhalation and the workplace. Agents that produce pathological changes to the pulmonary system, however, whether airborne or bloodborne, may also be classified according to their pulmonary target-organ toxicity. Today, the differences in organizing chemicals according to their target organ or route of exposure are more subtle, given the ubiquitous nature of environmental pollution. Table 4.4 and Table 4.5 outline some acute or chronic diseases, respectively, associated with direct inhalation or blood exposure to select toxic compounds. Hallmark features that characterize the syndromes are also presented. Some agents lack systematic classification because of the unusual nature of the pulmonary pathology. Such compounds, like monocrotaline, a naturally occurring plant alkaloid found in herbal teas, grains, and honey, produce endothelial hyperplasia with pulmonary arterial hypertension. Naphthalene, a principal component

TABLE 4.4
Acute Pulmonary Responses and Associated Select Toxic Agents

Common Pathology	Characteristic Syndrome	Toxic Agents
Bronchitis	Bronchial inflammatory response	Arsenic, chlorine, chromium (VI)
Hard metal disease	Hyperplasia and metaplasia of bronchial epithelium	Titanium and tungsten carbides
Silicosis	Acute silicosis	Silica
Pulmonary edema	Exudative lung injury with thickening of alveolar-capillary wall	Histamine, paraquat, phosgene, beryllium (berylliosis), nitrogen oxide, nickel
Bronchoconstriction	Decrease in airway diameter and increased airflow resistance	Histamine, cholinergic drugs, prostaglandins, leukotrenes, β-adrenergic inhibitors
Acute pulmonary fibrosis	Increased deposition of collagen in alveolar interstitium	Paraquat, bleomycin

TABLE 4.5
Chronic Pulmonary Responses and Associated Select Toxic Agents

Common Pathology	Characteristic Syndrome	Toxic Agents
Chronic pulmonary fibrosis	Increased deposition of collagen in alveolar interstitium (resembles ARDS[a])	Paraquat, bleomycin, aluminum dust, beryllium, BCNU[a], cyclophosphamide, kaolin (kaolinosis), ozone, talc
Emphysema	Abnormal enlargement of airspaces distal to terminal bronchioles, destruction of alveolar walls, without fibrosis	Cadmium oxide, tobacco smoking, air pollution
Asthma	Narrowing of bronchi due to direct or indirect inhalation of toxicants, increased airway reactivity	Isocyanates, tobacco smoking, air pollution, ozone
Carcinoma	Bronchogenic adenocarcinoma, squamous cell carcinoma	Asbestos fibers (asbestosis), tobacco smoking, metallic dusts, mustard and radon gases, formaldehyde, chromium, arsenic, perchlorethylene
Pulmonary lipidosis	Intracellular macrophages containing abnormal phospholipid complexes	Amiodarone, chlorphentermine

[a] ARDS = adult respiratory distress syndrome; BCNU = 1,3-bis-(2-chloroethyl)-1-nitrosourea.

of tar and petroleum distillates, produces extensive bronchial epithelium necrosis. Oxygen toxicity results in bronchial metaplasia and alveolar destruction (see Chapter 23, "Gases"). Many more industrial chemicals have been associated with pulmonary toxicity, as evidenced from epidemiological data and from studies conducted with experimental animals.

4.2.6 AGENTS AFFECTING THE NERVOUS SYSTEM

Elucidating the mechanisms by which neurotoxicants exert their clinical effects has been instrumental in understanding many concepts of neurophysiology. These mechanisms have prompted breakthroughs, in part, through the development of psychoactive drugs aimed at the same target receptors in common with neurotoxic compounds. Figure 4.4 illustrates a representative diagram of the neuron and some of its components. Examination of the components of the neuron makes it possible to envision the types of damage a neurotoxic agent is capable of eliciting. Some pathologic effects include: neuronopathies, axonopathies, myelinopathies, and interference with neurotransmission. Table 4.6 classifies clinically important neurotoxicants according to these major categories and their sites of action. It is important to note that, although these compounds appear to have an anatomical site specificity, their action may uniformly affect any aspect of the central, autonomic, and peripheral nervous systems, thus leading to a variety of complications and effects.

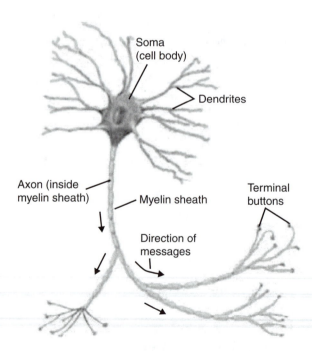

FIGURE 4.4 Schematic diagram of the neuron, the functional cell unit of the nervous system. (www.macalester.edu/~psych/whathap/UBNRP/dreaming/py1

TABLE 4.6
Mechanisms of Neurotoxicity and Associated Select Toxic Agents

Mechanism of Neurotoxicity	Representative Toxic Agents	Anatomical Sites of Toxic Action
Neuronopathy	Doxorubicin, methyl mercury, catecholamines, MPTP[a]	Dorsal root ganglion, autonomic ganglia, visual cortex, cerebellum; midbrain, thalamic, hypothalamic centers
Axonopathy	Carbon disulfide, acrylamide, chloroquine, lithium, organophosphates	Central and peripheral axons, ascending and descending spinal cord axons
Myelinopathy	Hexachlorophene, lead	Central and peripheral myelinated axons
Interference with neurotransmission	Nicotine, cocaine, amphetamines	Central cognitive and motor centers; associative and integrative pathways; dopaminergic, serotonergic, cholinergic systems

[a] MPTP = 1-methyl-4-phenyl-1,2,3,6-tetrahydropyridine (causes Parkinson-like syndrome).

4.2.7 AGENTS AFFECTING THE CARDIOVASCULAR (CV) SYSTEM

Subsequent to significant breakthroughs in the treatment of cancers in the last 25 years, cardiovascular disease is now the primary cause of mortality among adults in the U.S. Simultaneously, a major effort to develop drugs to treat heart disease has resulted in a rapid turnover of these drugs and the establishment of new categories of CV agents. Therefore, adverse drug reactions of therapeutic CV drugs, as well as those of other unrelated chemicals and xenobiotics, have been documented to provoke significant toxic effects on the heart and circulatory system. Toxicity generally occurs as a result of direct and indirect actions on the myocardium, the mechanisms of which are summarized in Table 4.7 and Table 4.8, for some commonly encountered agents. The toxicity of therapeutic drugs, administered with the intention of treating a heart condition, is not necessarily different from adverse drug reactions of compounds not intended to treat heart conditions. Thus, the mechanisms of toxicity are seemingly related.

4.2.8 DERMATOTOXIC AGENTS

The skin boasts the largest surface area of any organ and has traditionally been understood as the first line of defense against microbial and xenobiotic insult. It is reasonable to anticipate, therefore, that this organ is often a target for environmental toxicants. In addition, since many drugs are administered percutaneously, the skin distributes chemicals in a process known as transdermal drug delivery. Consequently, the most common manifestations of dermatotoxic agents include contact dermatitis and, to a lesser extent, phototoxicity. Table 4.9 summarizes the most common agents responsible for skin toxicity and their mechanisms.

TABLE 4.7
Mechanisms of Cardiovascular Toxicity Associated with Select CV and Non-CV Therapeutic Agents

Drug Classification	Representative Agents	Cardiotoxic Effects	Mechanism of Cardiotoxicity
Agents used in the treatment of CV disease			
Antiarrhythmic: Class I	Disopyramide, phenytoin, procainamide	↓ conduction velocity	Na+ channel inhibition
Antiarrhythmic: Class II	Propranolol, metoprolol, atenolol	Heart block	β-adrenergic receptor inhibition
Antiarrhythmic: Class III	Amiodarone, quinidine	↑ duration of AP	K+ channel inhibition
Antiarrhythmic: Class IV	Diltiazem, verapamil	↓ AV conduction	Ca+ channel inhibition
Cardiac glycosides	Digoxin	↓ AV conduction	Na+, K+-ATPase inhibition
Catecholamines	Epinephrine, isoproterenol, norepinephrine	Tachycardia	β1-adrenergic receptor stimulation
Non-CV therapeutic agents			
Antibacterial: aminoglycosides	Gentamicin, kanamycin, streptomycin, tobramycin	Negative inotropy	↓ Ca+ influx
Antibacterial: fluoroquinolones	Ciprofloxacin, levofloxacin, moxifloxacin	↑ AP duration	K+ channel inhibition
Antibacterial: macrolides	Azithromycin, clarithromycin, erythromycin	↑ AP duration	K+ channel inhibition
Antifungal	Amphotericin B	Negative inotropy	Ca+ channel inhibition
Antihistamines	Astemizole, terfenadine	↑ AP duration	K+ channel inhibition
Antineoplastic: anthracyclines	Daunorubicin, doxorubicin	Cardiomyopathy	Oxidative stress, apoptosis
Antiviral: nucleoside analog RTI	Stavudine, zidovudine	Cardiomyopathy	Mitochondrial injury
Appetite suppressants	Amphetamines, fenfluramine, phentermine	Tachycardia	Nonselective β-adrenergic receptor stimulation
Bronchodilators	Albuterol, metaproterenol, salmeterol, terbutaline	Tachycardia	Nonselective β-adrenergic receptor stimulation
General anesthetics	Halothane, enflurane	Negative inotropic effect	Ca+ channel inhibition
Local anesthetics	Cocaine	Myocardial ischemia/infarction	Sympathomimetic stimulant

Drug Classification	Representative Agents	Cardiotoxic Effects	Mechanism of Cardiotoxicity
Methylxanthines	Theophylline	Tachycardia	PDE inhibition
Nasal decongestants	Ephedrine and ephedra alkaloids, phenylephrine, PPA, pseudoephedrine	Tachycardia	Nonselective β-adrenergic receptor stimulation
Phenothiazines	Chlorpromazine, thioridazine	Tachycardia, arrhythmia, ↓ AV conduction	Anticholinergic effects
SSRIs	Fluoxetine, paroxetine, risperidone	Bradycardia	Ca^+ channel inhibition
Thyroid hormones	Thyroxine, triiodothyronine	Tachycardia	Altered Ca^+ homeostasis
Tricyclic antidepressants	Amitriptyline, desipramine, imipramine	ST segment Elevation, QT interval prolongation	Na^+, K^+, Ca^+ channel inhibition

Note: AP = action potential; CV = cardiovascular; PDE = phosphodiesterase; PPA = phenylpropranolamine; RTIs = reverse transcriptase inhibitors; SSRIs = selective serotonin reuptake inhibitors.

Modified from K.S. Ramos et al. (2001). Used with permission.

TABLE 4.8
Mechanisms of Cardiovascular (CV) Toxicity Associated with Select Nontherapeutic Agents

Drug Classification	Representative Agents	Cardiotoxic Effects	Mechanism of Cardiotoxicity
Nontherapeutic agents with CV toxicity			
Alcohols	Ethanol	↓ conductivity	Oxidative stress
Bacterial endotoxins	Gram-negative bacteria	Bacterial endocarditis	Cardiogenic shock
Halogenated hydrocarbons	Carbon tetrachloride, chloroform, trichloroethane	Altered conduction	↑ adrenergic sensitivity
Heavy metals	Cadmium, lead	Negative inotropy	Altered Ca^+ homeostasis
Ketones	Acetone	Altered conduction	↑ adrenergic sensitivity
Solvents	Toluene, xylene	Altered conduction	↑ adrenergic sensitivity

TABLE 4.9
Responses of the Skin to Dermatotoxic Agents

Reaction	Common Chemicals or Toxic Agents Associated with Dermatotoxicity
Allergic contact dermatitis	Topical antibiotics, antiseptics; preservatives, cosmetics; plant resins, leather products, industrial solvents, cleaning products and paints; jewelry and metals
Carcinogenic changes	UV light, ionizing radiation, PAH,[a] arsenic
Chemical burn	Inorganic and organic acids or bases; ammonia; liquids or concentrated vapors of halides, oxides; phenol, phosphorus; organic solvents
Irritant dermatitis	When applied topically, any chemical or drug at low dose has this potential
Photoallergy	Topical salicylic acid derivatives; hexachlorophene; camphor, menthol, phenol as additives; wood and leather oils
Phototoxicity	Furocoumarins (psoralen derivatives); PAH,[a] tetracyclines; sulfonamides; eosin dyes
Pigmentary disturbances:	
Hyperpigmentation	Anthracene; hydroquinones, metals, psoralens; UV light; amiodarone, chloroquine, tetracyclines
Hypopigmentation	BHT,[a] hydroquinones, phenolic compounds
Urticaria	Antibacterial antibiotics; food preservatives (BHT, benzoic acid) and additives (CMC,[a] pectin); plants, weeds; latex (natural rubber gloves); lectins (grains, nuts, fruit), pectin (fruit), and a variety of meats, poultry, fish, vegetables, grains, and spices

[a] BHT = butylhydroxytoluene; CMC = carboxymethylcellulose; PAH = polycyclic aromatic hydrocarbons (coal tar, anthracene derivatives).

Among the more common dermal reactions, contact dermatitis and photosensitivity predominate. Contact dermatitis reactions include:

1. Irritant dermatitis — a nonimmune reaction of the skin as a result of toxic exposure, characterized by eczematous itching or thickened eruptions.
2. Chemical burn — coagulative necrosis resulting from extreme corrosivity from a reactive chemical, characterized by potent skin corrosivity, exothermic reaction, blistering, scar formation, and systemic absorption.
3. Allergic contact dermatitis — a type IV, delayed hypersensitivity reaction, possessing dose-dependent intensity and requiring initial sensitization, adaptation, and subsequent rechallenge; the reaction ranges from mild irritation, eczematous reactions, eruptions and flaring, to full systemic immune manifestations.

Photosensitivity involves:

1. Phototoxicity — an abnormal sensitivity to ultraviolet and visible light produced as a result of systemic or topical exposure; it is characterized by red, blistering eruptions, as well as hyperpigmentation and thickening.
2. Photoallergy — represents a type IV delayed hypersensitivity reaction.

Other dermatotoxic responses include: *chloracne*, a disfiguring form of acne characterized by comedones,* papules, pustules or cysts, not limited to the facial region; *pigmentary disturbances*, represented as hyper- or hypopigmentation; *urticaria*, commonly known as hives; and, *carcinogenic changes*.

4.2.9 AGENTS AFFECTING THE REPRODUCTIVE SYSTEM

In the last 50 years, the effects of environmental and occupational exposure to industrial chemicals have posed alarming risks to human health and safety. Like other endocrine organs, the male and female gonads act to maintain the reproductive integrity of the species. Thus, chemicals and drugs currently identified as environmental estrogens, whether or not they are structurally similar to the hormone, have the potential for endocrine disruption — i.e., the ability of nonheavy metals to alter steroidogenesis. Although the etiology of their adverse effects is unclear, their mechanisms influence maternal and paternal dynamics. Table 4.10 and Table 4.11 outline several classes of drugs and chemicals (endocrine disruptors) that alter male and female reproductive systems, respectively. Their target mechanisms and possible adverse effects are noted.

4.2.10 AGENTS AFFECTING THE ENDOCRINE SYSTEM

Endocrine glands coordinate activities that maintain homeostasis throughout the body. Through their hormonal secretions, and in cooperation with the nervous system, these specialized organs regulate the action of their target cells, increasing or decreasing their respective activities. Consequently, many toxicants have the potential for disrupting hormonal pathways, either by site-specific toxicity at the endocrine level, or by interference with the feedback mechanisms. A list of the endocrine organs, the potential toxicants, and their effects is summarized in Table 4.12. Some of the toxicants exert their effects by causing proliferative changes, resulting in hyperplastic and neoplastic transformation, while other agents inhibit steroid hormone synthesis and secretion.

4.3 CLASSIFICATION ACCORDING TO USE IN THE PUBLIC DOMAIN

4.3.1 PESTICIDES

The U.S. Environmental Protection Agency (EPA) defines pesticides as substances or mixtures of substances intended for preventing, destroying, repelling, or mitigating any pest. In general, pesticides are classified according to the biological target or organism killed. Four major classes of pesticides include insecticides, herbicides, fungicides, and rodenticides (Table 4.13 and Table 4.14). Because of the physiological and biochemical similarities between target species and mam-

---

* A comedone is a dilated hair follicle infundibulum filled with keratin, squamae, and sebum; it is the primary lesion of acne vulgaris.

TABLE 4.10
Representative Drugs and Chemicals That Affect the Male Reproductive System

Classification	Representative Agents	Target	Adverse Effects
Alkylating agents	Busulfan, chlorambucil, cyclophosphamide, nitrogen mustard	Gonadogenesis	Testicular development
Androgen derivatives	Danocrine	Steroidogenic enzymes	Testicular atrophy
Chlorphenoxy herbicides	TCDD	Spermatogenesis	Testicular development
Diuretics	Spironolactone	Steroidogenic enzymes	Testicular atrophy
Heavy metals	Cadmium	Sertoli cell	Testicular toxicity
	Lead	Spermatocytes	Spermatocidal, infertility
Plasticizers	Phthalate esters	Sertoli cell	Testicular toxicity

Note: TCDD = 2,3,4,8-tetrachlorodibenzo-*p*-dioxin.

TABLE 4.11
Representative Drugs and Chemicals That Affect the Female Reproductive System

Classification	Representative Agents	Target	Adverse Effects
Alkylating agents	Busulfan, chlorambucil, cyclophosphamide, nitrogen mustard	Gonadogenesis	Ovarian development
Androgen derivatives	Danocrine	Steroidogenic enzymes	Disrupts gonadotropin cycles
Steroids and derivatives	Estrogens, progestins	Hypothalamic–pituitary–ovarian axis	Disrupts gonadotropin action

TABLE 4.12
Target Endocrine Organs and Potential Toxicants

Organ	Representative Toxicants[a]	Target Cell Mechanism	Adverse Effects
Adrenal cortex	Acrylonitrile	Necrosis	Adrenal atrophy
	Anilines	Lipidosis	
	Corticosteroids	Proliferative lesions	
Adrenal medulla	Atenolol, excess dietary calcium intake, nicotine, reserpine, vitamin D$_3$	Proliferative lesions	Adrenal hypersecretion and atrophy
Parathyroid gland	Aluminum	Inhibits PTH secretion	Hypocalcemia
	Ozone	Hyperplasia	Parathyroid atrophy
Pituitary	Calcitonin, estrogens	Hyperplasia, neoplasia	Pituitary tumors, hypersecretion
Thyroid gland	Thiouracil, sulfonamides	Proliferative changes	Thyroid tumors
	Thiocynate, thiourea, methimazole, PTU	Inhibits thyroid hormone synthesis	Hypertrophy
	Excess iodide, lithium	Inhibits thyroid hormone secretion	Hypertrophy and goiter

Note: PTH = parathyroid hormone, PTU = propylthiouracil.

[a] Most of the evidence is from studies performed with laboratory animals.

TABLE 4.13
Classification of Insecticides

Classification	Representative Agents	Mechanism of Toxicity in Mammalian Species
Organophosphorus esters	Ethyl parathion, malathion, mevinphos, sarin, soman, tabun, TEPP	Acetylcholinesterase inhibition
Organochlorine compounds	Aldrin, DDT, chlordane, dieldrin, endrin, lindane, methiochlor, methoxychlor	Selective neurotoxicity
Carbamate esters	Aldicarb, carbofuran, carbaryl (Sevin), propoxur (Baygon)	Reversible acetylcholinesterase inhibition
Pyrethroid esters	Cismethrin, pyrethrin I	Topical inflammatory reaction
Avermectins	Avermectin B1a, ivermectin	Interferes with neuronal transmission
Botanical derivatives	Nicotine	Autonomic NS, neuromuscular stimulant
	Rotenoids	Inhibits neuronal transmission

Note: DDT = dichlorodiphenyltrichloroethane, NS = nervous system, TEPP = tetraethyl pyrophosphate.

malian organisms, there is an inherent toxicity associated with pesticides in the latter. In addition, within each classification, compounds are identified according to mechanism of action, chemical structure, or semisynthetic source. For instance, although many fungicide categories exist, fungicidal toxicity in humans is mostly of low order. Similarly, fumigants range from carbon tetrachloride to ethylene oxide and are used to kill insects, roundworms, and fungi in soil, stored grain, fruits, and vegetables. Their toxicity, however, is limited to occasional occupational exposure.

4.3.2 FOOD AND COLOR ADDITIVES

Direct food or color additives are intentionally incorporated in food and food processing for the purpose of changing, enhancing, or masking color. They are also used for a variety of functionalities ranging from anticaking agents to stabilizers, thickeners, and texturizers. This area falls within the field of food toxicology, and the reader is referred to any of the review articles concerning food ingredients and contaminants.

4.3.3 THERAPEUTIC DRUGS

Toxicological classification of therapeutic agents follows their pharmacological mechanisms of action or their principal target organs of toxicity. Part II of this book addresses clinical toxicology of therapeutic drugs as an extension of their adverse reactions, as well as their direct effect resulting from excessive or overdosage.

TABLE 4.14
Classification of Herbicides and Rodenticides

Classification	Representative Agents	Mechanism of Toxicity in Mammalian Species
Herbicides		
Chlorphenoxy compounds	2,4-D; 2,4,5-T; TCDD (dioxin)	Neuromuscular, carcinogenic, teratogenic[a]
Bipyridyl derivatives	Diquat, paraquat	Single electron reduction, free radical generation
Chloroacetanilides	Alachlor, metolachlor	Probable human carcinogens
Phosphonomethyl amino acids	Glufosinate, glyphosate	Metabolic enzyme inhibition
Rodenticides		
Anticoagulants	Warfarin	Inhibits vitamin K-dependent newly synthesized clotting factors
α-Naphthyl thiourea (ANTU)	ANTU	Interferes with microsomal monooxygenases
Miscellaneous	Zinc phosphide	Cellular necrosis
	Fluoroacetic acid	Interferes with tricarboxylic acid cycle
	Red squill	Digitalis-like activity
	Phosphorus	Inhibits carbohydrate, lipid and protein metabolism
	Thallium	Chelates sulfhydril-containing enzymes

Note: 2,4-D = 2,4-dichlorophenoxyacetic acid; 2,4,5-T = 2,4,5-trichlorophenoxyacetic acid; TCDD = 2,3,7,8-tetrachlorodibenzo-p-dioxin.

[a] Mechanism is still debatable.

4.4 CLASSIFICATION ACCORDING TO SOURCE

4.4.1 BOTANICAL

Contact dermatitis caused by poison ivy is a well-characterized syndrome of acute inflammation. Today, many compounds of botanical origin are classified as herbal supplements, implying that their origin is botanical. Their importance in maintaining health has also been related to their natural derivation. The toxicities of these agents, however, are poorly understood. A detailed discussion of herbal supplements and related products is addressed in Chapter 21, "Herbal Remedies."

4.4.2 ENVIRONMENTAL

As a result of industrialization, many chemicals are associated and classified according to their continuous presence in the environment — i.e., water, land, and soil. The phenomenon is not limited to Western developed nations, but is also a rising problem among developing Asian and African countries.

Environmental toxicology is a distinct discipline encompassing the areas of air pollution and ecotoxicology. A discussion of air pollution necessarily includes: outdoor and indoor air pollution, presence of atmospheric sulfuric acid, airborne particulate matter, interaction of photochemicals with the environment, and chemicals found in smog. Ecotoxicology is that branch of environmental toxicology that investigates the effects of environmental chemicals on the ecosystems in question. The reader is referred to the review articles for further discussion.

4.5 CLASSIFICATION ACCORDING TO PHYSICAL STATE

An apparently simple classification scheme involves categorizing chemicals according to their physical state. The importance of such classification for clinical toxicology lies in the knowledge of the physical nature of the substance and the contribution in determining the availability of the compound, the route of exposure and the onset of action.

4.5.1 SOLIDS

Most therapeutic drugs are available as solid powders in the form of tablets or capsules. This deliberate drug design is intended for facility of administration, ease of packaging, and convenience. As a result, most clinical toxicity results from oral ingestion of solid dosage forms. Solids, however, are subject to the peculiarities of gastrointestinal absorption, pH barriers, and solubility — factors that ultimately influence toxicity.

4.5.2 LIQUIDS

For *nontherapeutic* categories, compounds in their liquid state are readily accessible. Their presence in the environment, food, drinking water, or household products allows for immediate oral or dermal exposure. The availability of liquid dosage forms of *therapeutic* agents is intended for pediatric oral use, injectables, and for those special situations where liquid ingestion is more convenient, such as when it is easier for a patient to swallow a liquid dose of medication. As with solid dosage forms, liquids are also subject to bioavailability upon oral ingestion.

4.5.3 GASES

The gaseous state of a chemical represents the fastest route of exposure outside intravenous injection. Inhaled therapeutic or nontherapeutic agents readily permeate upper and lower respiratory tracts and transport across alveolar walls, gaining access to capillary circulation. In addition, immediate absorption also occurs with penetration of the mucous membranes, before diffusion of the gas to the lower respiratory tract. Both routes of exposure bypass most gastrointestinal absorption and first-pass (hepatobiliary) detoxification phenomena. Consequently, exposure to toxic gases should be approached in all instances as a clinical emergency.

4.6 CLASSIFICATION ACCORDING TO BIOCHEMICAL PROPERTIES

4.6.1 CHEMICAL STRUCTURE

Drugs and chemicals are initially identified, synthesized, and screened for activity according to their chemical classification. Because drug and chemical development depends upon the availability of parent compounds, the synthesis of structurally related compounds is an important process for the industry. Thus, understanding the chemical structure of a compound allows for reasonable prediction of many of its anticipated and adverse effects. Some examples of agents that are categorized according to their molecular structures include: benzodiazepines (sedative-hypnotics), imidazolines (tranquilizers), floroquinolones (antibiotics), organophosphorus insecticides, and heavy metals.

4.6.2 MECHANISM OF ACTION OR TOXICITY

Similarly, it is convenient to organize drugs and chemicals according to their physiologic or biochemical target. Such examples include: β-adrenergic agonists, methemoglobin-producing agents, or acetylcholinesterase inhibitors.

REFERENCES

SUGGESTED READINGS

Bloom, J.C., Introduction to hematotoxicology, in *Comprehensive Toxicology*, Sipes, I.G., McQueen, C.A., and Gandolfi, A.J., Eds, Vol. 4, Oxford Pergamon Press, New York, 1997, chap. 1.
Ramos, K.S., et al., Toxic responses of the heart and vascular systems, in *Casarett and Doull's Toxicology: The Basic Science of Poisons*, 6th ed., Klaassen, C.D., Ed., McGraw-Hill, New York, 2001, chap. 18.

REVIEW ARTICLES

Baker, V.A., Endocrine disrupters — testing strategies to assess human hazard, *Toxicol. In Vitro*, 15, 413, 2001.
Basketter, D.A., et al., Factors affecting thresholds in allergic contact dermatitis: safety and regulatory considerations, *Contact Dermatitis*, 47, 1, 2002.
Boudou, A. and Ribeyre, F., Aquatic ecotoxicology: from the ecosystem to the cellular and molecular levels, *Environ. Health Perspect.*, 105, 21, 1997.
Dewhurst, I.C., Toxicological assessment of biological pesticides, *Toxicol. Lett.*, 120, 67, 2001.
Feron, V.J., et al., International issues on human health effects of exposure to chemical mixtures, *Environ. Health Perspect.*, 110, 893, 2002.
Gerner, I. and Schlede, E., Introduction of *in vitro* data into local irritation/corrosion testing strategies by means of SAR considerations: assessment of chemicals, *Toxicol. Lett.*, 127, 169, 2002.
Goldman, L.R., Epidemiology in the regulatory arena. *M. J. Epidemiol.*, 154, 18, 2001.

Hattan, D.G. and Kahl, L.S., Current developments in food additive toxicology in the U.S.A., *Toxicology,* 181, 417, 2002.

Herbarth, O., et al., Effect of sulfur dioxide and particulate pollutants on bronchitis in children — a risk analysis, *Environ. Toxicol.,* 16, 269, 2001.

McCarty, L.S., Issues at the interface between ecology and toxicology, *Toxicology,* 181, 497, 2002.

Pauluhn, J., et al., Acute inhalation toxicity testing: considerations of technical and regulatory aspects, *Arch. Toxicol.,* 71, 1, 1996.

Ren, S. and Schultz, T.W., Identifying the mechanism of aquatic toxicity of selected compounds by hydrophobicity and electrophilicity descriptors, *Toxicol. Lett.,* 129, 151, 2002.

Salem, H. and Olajos, E.J., Review of pesticides: chemistry, uses and toxicology, *Toxicol. Ind. Health,* 4, 291, 1988.

Wexler, P. and Phillips, S., Tools for clinical toxicology on the World Wide Web: review and scenario, *J. Toxicol. Clin. Toxicol.,* 40, 893, 2002.

Winter, C.K., Electronic information resources for food toxicology, *Toxicology,* 173, 89, 2002.

Wolf, H.U. and Frank, C., Toxicity assessment of cyanobacterial toxin mixtures, *Environ. Toxicol.,* 17, 395, 2002.

5 Exposure

5.1 INTRODUCTION

Given the proper circumstances, any chemical has the potential for toxicity — i.e., the same dose of a chemical or drug may be harmless if limited to oral exposure but toxic if inhaled or administered parenterally. Thus, the route and site of exposure have a significant influence in determining the toxicity of a substance. More frequently, a therapeutic dose for an adult may be toxic for an infant or child. Similarly, a substance may not exert adverse effects until a critical threshold is achieved. Thus, in order to induce toxicity, it is necessary for the chemical to accumulate in a physiological compartment at a concentration sufficiently high to reach the threshold value. Finally, repeated administration, over a specific period of time, also determines the potential for toxicity. The following chapter details the circumstances for exposure and dosage of a drug that favor or deter the potential for clinical toxicity.

5.2 ROUTE OF EXPOSURE

5.2.1 ORAL

By far, oral administration of drugs and toxins is the most popular route of exposure. Oral administration involves the presence of several physiological barriers that must be penetrated or circumvented if an adequate blood concentration of the compound is to be achieved. The mucosal layers of the oral cavity, pharynx, and esophagus consist of stratified squamous epithelium, which serves to protect the upper gastrointestinal (GI) lining from the effects of contact with physical and chemical agents. Simple columnar epithelium lines the stomach and intestinal tracts that function in digestion, secretion, and some absorption. Immediately underlying the epithelium is the lamina propria, a mucosal layer rich in blood vessels and nerves. Mucosa-associated lymphoid tissue (MALT) is layered within this level, where prominent lymphatic nodules sustain the presence of phagocytic macrophages and granulocytes. Salivary and intestinal glands contribute to the digestive process by secreting saliva and digestive juices. The submucosa, muscularis, and serosa complete the strata that form the anatomical envelope of the GI tract. Enteroendocrine and exocrine cells in the GI tract secrete hormones and, in the stomach, secrete acid and gastric lipase.

The primary function of the stomach is mechanical and chemical digestion of food. Absorption is secondary. Consequently, several factors influence the transit and stability of a drug in the stomach, thereby influencing gastric emptying time (GET). The presence of food delays absorption and dilutes the contents of the stomach, thus reducing subsequent drug transit. An increase in the relative pH of the stomach causes a negative feedback inhibition of stomach churning and motility, which also results in delay of gastric emptying. Any factor that slows stomach motility will increase the amount of time in the stomach, prolonging the GET. Thus, the longer the GET, the greater the duration of a chemical within the stomach, and the more susceptible to gastric enzyme degradation and acid hydrolysis. In addition, prolonged GET delays passage to, and subsequent absorption in, the intestinal tract.

5.2.2 INTRANASAL

Intranasal insufflation is a popular method for therapeutic administration of corticosteroids and sympathomimetic amines and for the illicit use of drugs of abuse, such as cocaine and opioids. In the former, the dosage form is usually aerosolized in a metered nasal inhaler. In the latter case, the crude illicit drugs are inhaled through the nares ("snorted") as fine or coarse powders. In either case, absorption is rapid, due to the extensive network of capillaries in the lamina propria of the mucosal lining within the nasopharynx. Thus the absorption rate rivals that of pulmonary inhalation.

5.2.3 INHALATION

The vast surface area of the upper and lower respiratory tracts allows for wide and immediate distribution of inhaled powders, particulates, aerosols, and gases. Figure 5.1 illustrates the thin alveolar wall that separates airborne particulates from access to capillary membranes. Once a drug is ventilated to the alveoli, it is transported across the alveolar epithelial lining to the capillaries, resulting in rapid absorption.

5.2.4 PARENTERAL

Parenteral administration includes epidermal, intradermal, transdermal, subcutaneous (s.c.), intramuscular (i.m.), and intravenous (i.v.) injections. Parenteral routes, in general, are subject to minimal initial enzymatic degradation or chemical neutralization, thus bypassing the hindrances associated with passage through epithelial barriers. Figure 5.2 illustrates the layers of the skin: the epidermis, the outermost

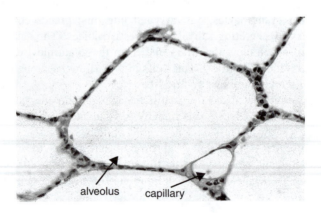

FIGURE 5.1 Diagram of pulmonary alveolus.

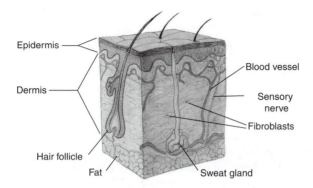

FIGURE 5.2 Epidermis, dermis, and underlying (subcutaneous) layers of the skin. (From Artificial Skin, News Features and Articles, NIH, NIGMS.)

layer, and the underlying dermis and subcutaneous (hypodermis) layers. Epidermal and upper dermal injections have the poorest absorption capabilities of the parenteral routes, primarily because of limited circulation. The deeper dermal and subcutaneous layers provide entrance to a richer supply of venules and arterioles. A subcutaneous injection forms either a depot within the residing adipose tissue with subsequent leakage into the systemic circulation, or the majority of the injection can enter the arterioles and venules. Intramuscular injections ensure access to a more extensive vascular network within skeletal muscle, accounting for more rapid exposure than subcutaneous. Intravenous injection is prompt and the most rapid method of chemical exposure, since access to the circulation is direct and immediate. For instance, when ingested orally, a single 40-mg long-acting tablet of Oxycontin® (oxycodon HCl) produces a blood concentration for sufficient analgesia over a 24-h period. When the same tablet is crushed and injected i.v. by illicit drug users, a naïve victim risks respiratory depression and arrest from the same single tablet. Consequently, the route of exposure contributes as much to toxicity as the dose.

5.3 DURATION AND FREQUENCY

In clinical toxicology, as in pharmacology, duration and frequency depend on the chemical as much as on the route. Thus, for the most part, acute and chronic exposures are relative terms intended for comparative purposes.

5.3.1 Acute Exposure

In general, any exposure less than 24 h may be regarded as *acute*. Exposure to most toxic gases requires less than 24 h for toxicity (carbon monoxide, hydrogen cyanide). In clinical toxicology, however, 72 h may still be an acute exposure, such as in continuous low-dose exposure to acetaminophen in children. In addition, a single i.v. injection of a chemical is certainly classified as an acute exposure. Subacute exposure generally refers to repeated exposure to a chemical longer than 72 h but less than 1 month.

5.3.2 Chronic Exposure

Chronic exposure is any relative time period for which continuous or repeated exposure, beyond the acute phase, is required for the same chemical to induce a toxic response. *Subchronic* is also understood to involve a time period between acute and chronic. The traditional time of subchronic exposure is understood to be a period of 1 to 3 months. In the arena of clinical toxicity, however, a subchronic exposure may include repeated exposure for a period less than 1 month. Thus, the terms are flexible adaptations to define the onset of chemical intoxication. In addition, there is some considerable overlap in judgment when assigning labels to exposure periods.

Frequency of administration involves repeated doses of the drug or toxin during the exposure period. Repeated administration of the same dose of a drug beyond the accepted therapeutic frequency, within the time period defined as acute or chronic, establishes a greater potential for adverse effects. Similarly, continuous repeated exposure to a toxin, especially during an acute time period, has greater toxic potential.

5.4 ACCUMULATION

Dose, duration, frequency, and route of exposure contribute to chemical toxicity in part through accumulation of the compound in physiological compartments. A normal dosage schedule is determined according to a chemical's half-life ($t_{1/2}$) in plasma and its intended response — i.e., the time required for plasma levels to decrease to one-half of the measured or estimated concentration. Thus, if the frequency of administration exceeds the $t_{1/2}$ of the chemical, its concentration in a compartment is likely to increase beyond the desirable level. Accumulation results from overloading of a drug within this compartment.

5.4.1 According to Physiological Compartment

The body as a unit is considered a one-compartment model. Ideally, a drug capable of distributing uniformly throughout the body would maintain steady-state levels for the exposure period. Blood levels* of the compound may also decrease uniformly, assuming a constant rate of elimination. The body, however, is not a homogeneous chamber. A chemical, once absorbed, can distribute and/or bind to one or more of the many physiological sites. The distribution of the chemical depends largely on its physicochemical characteristics (see Chapter 10, "Toxicokinetics," for detailed descriptions of absorption, distribution, metabolism, and elimination). The compartments include: whole blood, serum and serum proteins, plasma and plasma proteins, adipose tissue, interstitial and extracellular fluids, alveolar air space, and bone marrow. In addition, any tissue or organ may preferentially accumulate a chemical, thus acting as a discrete compartment. For instance, many therapeutic drugs, such as warfarin (a vitamin K antagonist anticoagulant), nonspecifically bind to circulating plasma proteins, resulting in

---

* The terms *blood levels* and *plasma levels* are often used interchangeably, although blood and plasma are distinct anatomical compartments.

apparently lower blood concentrations than anticipated. Heavy metals preferentially accumulate in adipose tissue. Consequently their toxicity may be experienced for prolonged periods of time as the compounds are slowly released from this compartment, years after exposure has ceased. Accumulation, therefore, can be predicted based on a chemical's apparent volume of distribution (V_d), which is estimated as the total dose of drug in the body divided by the concentration of drug in the plasma, for a given time period. In general, the greater the V_d, the greater the potential for accumulation in some physiological compartment.[*]

5.4.2 ACCORDING TO CHEMICAL STRUCTURE

Accumulation is also determined by the chemical's structure and its interaction within the physiological compartment. This phenomenon is guided by the chemical's predominant state of existence in a physiological fluid — i.e., its existence in the fluid compartment as an ionic or nonionic species. In general, at physiological pH, lipid-soluble compounds will preferentially remain in their nonionic state, preferring to bind to, and accumulate in, membranes of tissues and organs. Conversely, water-soluble compounds remain as ionic species at the pH of the blood. Thus, because they are less prone to tissue binding, the ions are readily available for renal secretion and elimination (see Chapter 10, "Toxicokinetics," for a complete discussion).

REFERENCES

SUGGESTED READINGS

Acquavella, J., et al., Epidemiologic studies of occupational pesticide exposure and cancer: regulatory risk assessments and biologic plausibility, *Ann. Epidemiol.*, 13, 1, 2003.
Carnevali, O. and Maradonna, F., Exposure to xenobiotic compounds: looking for new biomarkers, *Gen. Comp. Endocrinol.*, 131, 203, 2003.
Eaton, D.L. and Klassen, C.D., Principles of toxicology, in *Casarett and Doull's Toxicology: The Basic Science of Poisons*, 6th ed., Klaassen, C.D., Ed., McGraw-Hill, New York, 2001, chap. 2.

REVIEW ARTICLES

Berry, M.R., Advances in dietary exposure research at the United States Environmental Protection Agency-National Exposure Research Laboratory, *J. Expo. Anal. Environ. Epidemiol.*, 7, 3, 1997.
Efroymson, R.A. and Murphy, D.L., Ecological risk assessment of multimedia hazardous air pollutants: estimating exposure and effects, *Sci. Total Environ.*, 274, 219, 2001.
Furtaw, E.J., Jr., An overview of human exposure modeling activities at the USEPA's National Exposure Research Laboratory, *Toxicol. Ind. Health,* 17, 302, 2001.
McCurdy, T., et al., The national exposure research laboratory's consolidated human activity database, *J. Expo. Anal. Environ. Epidemiol.,* 10, 566, 2000.

---

[*] A standard measure for accumulated internal dose of a chemical is the *body burden,* which refers to the amount of chemical stored in one or several physiological compartments, or in the body as a whole.

Moschandreas, D.J. and Saksena, S., Modeling exposure to particulate matter, *Chemosphere*, 49, 1137, 2002.

Moya, J. and Phillips, L., Overview of the use of the U.S. EPA exposure factors handbook, *Int. J. Hyg. Environ. Health,* 205, 155, 2002.

Schneider, T., et al., Conceptual model for assessment of dermal exposure, *Occup. Environ. Med.,* 56, 765, 1999.

Strickland, J.A. and Foureman, G.L., US EPA's acute reference exposure methodology for acute inhalation exposures, *Sci. Total Environ.,* 288, 51, 2002.

Thron, R.W., Direct and indirect exposure to air pollution, *Otolaryngol. Head Neck Surg.,* 114, 281, 1996.

6 Effects

6.1 GENERAL CLASSIFICATION

As noted in Chapter 4 ("Classification of Toxins in Humans"), chemicals and drugs can be categorized, in part, according to their toxic effects. Prediction of toxicity of a chemical lies in the ability to understand its potential effects based on factors not necessarily related to physicochemical properties. This chapter explores a variety of local and systemic reactions elicited by chemical exposure and the physiological and immunological basis of those effects.

6.1.1 CHEMICAL ALLERGIES

Four types of immunological hypersensitivity (allergic) reactions include: **type I** antibody-mediated reactions, **type II** antibody-mediated cytotoxic reactions, **type III** immune complex reactions, and, **type IV** delayed-type hypersensitivity — cell-mediated immunity.

Type I antibody-mediated reactions occur as three phases. The initial phase, the *sensitization phase,* is triggered by contact with a previously unrecognized antigen. This reaction entails binding of the antigen to immunoglobulin E (IgE) present on the surface of mast cells and basophils. A second phase, the *activation phase*, follows after an additional dermal or mucosal challenge with the same antigen. This phase is characterized by degranulation of mast cells and basophils, with a subsequent release of histamine and other soluble mediators. The third stage, the *effector phase,* is characterized by accumulation of preformed and newly synthesized chemical mediators that precipitate local and systemic effects. Degranulation of neutrophils and eosinophils completes the late-phase cellular response.

Antigens involved in type I reactions are generally airborne pollens, including mold spores and ragweed, as well as food ingredients. Ambient factors, such as heat and cold, drugs (opioids, antibiotics) and metals (silver, gold), precipitate chemical allergies of the type I nature. Because of their small molecular weight, the majority of drugs and chemicals, as single entities, generally circulate undetected by immune surveillance systems. Consequently, in order to initiate the sensitization phase of an antigenic response, chemicals are immunologically handled as haptens.* Some examples of type I hypersensitivity syndromes are described in Table 6.1, and typical effects of chemical allergies are listed in Table 6.2. The effects of chemical allergies are usually acute and appear immediately, compared to other hypersensitivity reactions (described below).

---

* Haptens are small molecular weight chemical entities (<1000 kD) that nonspecifically bind to larger circulating polypeptides or glycoproteins. Binding of the chemical induces a conformational change in the original larger complex. The chemical entity bound to the larger molecule is no longer recognized as "self," rendering it susceptible to immune attack. Under these criteria it has antigenic potential.

TABLE 6.1
Examples of Type I Hypersensitivity Syndromes, Causes, Effects, and Signs and Symptoms

Syndrome	Causes	Effects	Signs and Symptoms
Allergic rhinitis (hay fever)	Pollen, mold spores	↑ capillary permeability in nasal and frontal sinuses and mucosal membranes, ↑ vasodilation	Congestion, sneezing, headache, watery eyes
Food allergies	Lectins and proteins present in nuts, eggs, shellfish, dairy products	↑ capillary permeability, ↑ vasodilation, ↑ smooth muscle contraction	Congestion, sneezing, headache, watery eyes, nausea, vomiting
Atopic dermatitis (allergic dermatitis)	Localized exposure to drugs and chemicals	Initial local mast cell release of cytokines, followed by activation of neutrophils and eosinophils	Local erythematous reaction
Asthma	Chemicals; environmental, behavioral	Chronic obstructive reaction of LRT involving airway hyperactivity and cytokine release	Dyspnea, edema resulting from mucous hypersecretion, bronchoconstriction, airway inflammation

Note: LRT = lower respiratory tract.

TABLE 6.2
Descriptive Inflammatory Effects of Chemical Allergies

Effect	Description
Bullous	Large dermal blisters
Erythema	Redness or inflammation of skin due to dilation and congestion of superficial capillaries (eg. sunburn)
Flare	Reddish, diffuse blushing of the skin
Hyperemia	Increased blood flow to tissue or organ
Induration	Raised, hardened, thickened skin lesion
Macule	Flat red spot on skin due to increased blood flow
Papule	Raised red spot on skin due to increased blood flow and antibody localization
Petechial	Small, pinpoint dermal hemorrhagic spots
Pruritis	Itching
Purulent	Suppuration; production of pus containing necrotic tissue, bacteria, inflammatory cells
Urticaria	Pruritic skin eruption characterized by wheal formation
Vesicular	Small dermal blisters
Wheal	Raised skin lesion due to accumulation of interstitial fluid

Type II antibody-mediated cytotoxic reactions differ from type I in the nature of antigen, the cytotoxic character of the antigen-antibody reaction, and the type of antibody formed (IgM or IgG). In general, antibodies are formed against target antigens that are *altered cell membrane determinants*. Examples of type II reactions include: complement-mediated reactions (CM), antibody-dependent cell-mediated cytotoxicity (ADCC), antibody-mediated cellular dysfunction (AMCD), transfusion reactions, Rh incompatibility reactions, autoimmune reactions, and drug-induced reactions, the last of which is of greater interest in clinical toxicology.

As with type I reactions, drug-induced type II cytotoxicity requires that the agent behaves as a hapten. The chemical binds to the target cell membrane and proceeds to operate as an altered cell membrane determinant. This determinant changes the conformational appearance of a component of the cell membrane, not unlike the effect of a hapten. Thus, it induces a series of responses that terminate in antibody induction. The determinant attracts a variety of immune surveillance reactions including complement-mediated cytotoxic reaction, recruitment of granulocytes, or deposit of immune complexes within the cell membrane. Examples of drugs that traditionally induce type II reactions, and their pathologic effects, are noted in Table 6.3.

Type III immune complex reactions are localized responses mediated by antigen-antibody immune complexes. Type III reactions are stimulated by microorganisms and involve activation of complement. Systemic (serum sickness) and localized (arthus reaction) immune complex disease, infection-associated immune complex disease (rheumatic fever), and occupational diseases (opportunistic pulmonary fungal infections) induce complement-antibody-antigen complexes. These complexes then trigger release of cytokines and recruitment of granulocytes, resulting in increased vascular permeability and tissue necrosis.

TABLE 6.3
Drug-Induced Type II Antibody-Mediated Cytotoxic Reactions

Drug	Classification	Pathologic Effect
Chloramphenicol	Antibiotic (bacterial)	Produces agranulocytosis through binding to WBCs
Chlorpropamide	Antidiabetic	Cholestatic jaundice
Erythromycin estolate	Antibiotic (bacterial)	Cholestatic jaundice
Estrogen/progesterone	Oral contraceptives	Induces SLE syndrome through the production of antinuclear antibodies; cholestatic jaundice
Gentamicin, carbenicillin	Antibiotics (bacterial)	Nephrotoxic immune complex reaction
Hydralazine	Antihypertensive	Induces SLE syndrome through the production of antinuclear antibodies
Isoniazid	Antibiotic (*Mycobacteria* sp.)	Induces cell-to-cell immune complex reactions
Methyldopa	Antihypertensive	Produces a positive DAT in 15 to 20% of patients and AHA in 1%
NSAIDs	Analgesic/anti-inflammatory	Induces cell-cell immune complex reactions
Penicillins, cephalosporins	Antibiotics (bacterial)	Induce hemolysis by binding to RBCs
Phenacetin	Analgesic	Induces hemolytic anemia through binding to RBCs
Phenytoin	Antiepileptic	Induces SLE syndrome through the production of anti-nuclear antibodies
Procainamide	Antiarrhythmic	Induces SLE syndrome through the production of antinuclear antibodies
Quinidine	Antiarrhythmic	Induces cell-cell immune complex reactions
Testosterone	Anabolic steroids	Cholestatic jaundice

Note: WBC = white blood cells; RBCs = red blood cells; DAT = direct antiglobulin test; AHA = autoimmune hemolytic anemia; SLE = systemic lupus erythematosus.

Type IV (delayed-type) hypersensitivity cell-mediated immunity involves antigen-specific T-cell activation. The reaction starts with an intradermal or mucosal challenge (*sensitization stage*). CD4+ T-cells then recognize MHC-II (major histocompatibility class-II) antigens on antigen-presenting cells (such as Langerhans cells) and differentiate to T_H1 cells. This sensitization stage requires prolonged local contact with the agent, usually for at least two weeks. A subsequent repeat challenge stage induces differentiated T_H1 (memory) cells to release cytokines, further stimulating attraction of phagocytic monocytes and granulocytes. The release of lysosomal enzymes from the phagocytes results in local tissue necrosis. Contact hypersensitivity resulting from prolonged exposure to plant resins and jewelry, for example, is caused by the lipophilicity of the chemical in oily skin secretions, thus acting as a hapten.

6.1.2 IDIOSYNCRATIC REACTIONS

Idiosyncratic reactions are abnormal responses to drugs or chemicals generally resulting from uncommon genetic predisposition. An exaggerated response to the skeletal muscle relaxant properties of succinylcholine (SC), a depolarizing neuro-muscular blocker, classifies as a typical idiosyncratic reaction. In some patients, a congenital deficiency in plasma cholinesterase results in a reduction in the rate of SC deactivation. As SC accumulates, respiration fails to return to normal during the postoperative period. Similarly, the cardiotoxic action of cocaine is exaggerated in cases of congenital deficiency of plasma esterases, which are necessary for metabolism of the drug. A paucity of circulating enzymes allows for an uncontrolled, sympathetically mediated tachycardia, vasoconstriction, and subsequent heart failure in naïve or habitual cocaine users.

6.1.3 IMMEDIATE VS. DELAYED EFFECTS

In contrast to immune hypersensitivity reactions, some chemical effects are immediate or delayed, depending on the mechanism of toxicity. The acute effects of sedative-hypnotics are of immediate consequence, where an overdose raises the risk of death from respiratory depression. The effects of carcinogens, however, may not be demonstrated for generations. An important example of this has been demonstrated with the link between diethylstilbesterol (DES) administration to child-bearing women in the 1950s and the subsequent development of clear cell adenocarcinoma vaginal cancers in their offspring.

6.1.4 REVERSIBLE VS. IRREVERSIBLE

In general, the effects of most drugs or chemicals are reversible until a critical point is reached — i.e., when vital function is compromised or a teratogenic or carcinogenic effect develops. In fact, the carcinogenic effect of chemicals, such as those present in tobacco smoke, may be delayed for decades until irreversible cellular transformation occurs. Reversibility of a chemical effect may be enacted through the administration of antagonists, by enhancement of metabolism or elimination, by delaying absorption, by intervening with another toxicological procedure that decreases toxic blood concentrations, or by terminating the exposure.

6.1.5 LOCAL VS. SYSTEMIC

As discussed in Chapter 5 ("Exposure"), local or systemic effects of a compound depend on site of exposure. The integument (skin) or lungs are frequent targets of chemical exposure, since these organs are the first sites of contact with environmental chemicals. Oral exposure requires absorption and distribution of the agent prior to the development of systemic effects. Hypersensitivity reactions types I and IV are precipitated by local activation of immune responses following a sensitization phase, while drug-induced type II reactions are elicited through oral or parenteral administration.

6.2 CHEMICAL INTERACTIONS

6.2.1 POTENTIATION

Potentiation of toxicity occurs when the toxic effect of one chemical is enhanced in the presence of a toxicologically unrelated agent. The situation can be described numerically as "0 + 2 > 2," where a relatively nontoxic chemical alone has little or no effect ("0") on a target organ, but may enhance the toxicity of another coadministered chemical ("2"). The hepatotoxicity of carbon tetrachloride, for instance, is greatly increased in the presence of isopropanol.

6.2.2 ADDITIVE

Two or more chemicals whose combined effects are equal to the sum of the individual effects, are described as additive interactions. Such is the case with the additive effects of the combination of sedative-hypnotics and ethanol (drowsiness, respiratory depression). Numerically, this is summarized as "2 + 2 = 4."

6.2.3 SYNERGISTIC

By definition, synergistic effect is indistinguishable from potentiation except that, in some references, both chemicals must have cytotoxic activity. Numerically, synergism occurs when the sum of the effects of two chemicals is greater than the individual effects, such as that experienced with the combination of ethanol and antihistamines ("1 + 2 > 3"). Often, synergism and potentiation are used synonymously.

6.2.4 ANTAGONISTIC

The opposing actions of two or more chemical agents, not necessarily administered simultaneously, are considered antagonistic interactions. Different types of antagonism include:

- *Functional antagonism* — the opposing physiological effects of chemicals, such as with central nervous system stimulants vs. depressants.
- *Chemical antagonism* — drugs or chemicals that bind to, inactivate, or neutralize target compounds, such as with the action of chelators in metal poisoning.
- *Dispositional antagonism* — interference of one agent with the absorption, distribution, metabolism, or excretion (ADME) of another; examples of agents that interfere with absorption, metabolism, and excretion include activated charcoal, phenobarbital, and diuretics, respectively.
- *Receptor antagonism* — refers to the occupation of pharmacological receptors by competitive or noncompetitive agents, such as the use of tamoxifen in the prevention of estrogen-induced breast cancer.

REFERENCES

SUGGESTED READINGS

Ashby, J., The leading role and responsibility of the international scientific community in test development, *Toxicol. Lett.*, 140, 37, 2003.

Hammes, B. and Laitman, C.J., Diethylstilbestrol (DES) update: recommendations for the identification and management of DES-exposed individuals, *J. Midwifery Womens Health*, 48, 19, 2003.

REVIEW ARTICLES

Bolt, H.M. and Kiesswetter, E., Is multiple chemical sensitivity a clinically defined entity? *Toxicol. Lett.*, 128, 99, 2002.

Bradberry, S.M. and Vale, J.A., Multiple-dose activated charcoal: a review of relevant clinical studies, *J. Toxicol. Clin. Toxicol.*, 33, 407, 1995.

Buckley, N.A., Poisoning and epidemiology: 'toxicoepidemiology,' *Clin. Exp. Pharmacol. Physiol.*, 25, 195, 1998.

Damstra, T., Potential effects of certain persistent organic pollutants and endocrine disrupting chemicals on the health of children, *J. Toxicol. Clin. Toxicol.*, 40, 457, 2002.

Foster, J.R., The functions of cytokines and their uses in toxicology, *Int. J. Exp. Pathol.*, 82, 171, 2001.

Hastings, K.L., Implications of the new FDA/CDER immunotoxicology guidance for drugs, *Int. Immunopharmacol.*, 2, 1613, 2002.

Isbister, G.K., Data collection in clinical toxinology: debunking myths and developing diagnostic algorithms, *J. Toxicol. Clin. Toxicol.*, 40, 231, 2002.

Kimber, I., Gerberick, G.F., and Basketter, D.A., Thresholds in contact sensitization: theoretical and practical considerations, *Food Chem. Toxicol.*, 37, 553, 1999.

Kimber, I., et al., Chemical allergy: molecular mechanisms and practical applications, *Fundam. Appl. Toxicol.*, 19, 479, 1992.

Kimber, I., et al., Toxicology of protein allergenicity: prediction and characterization, *Toxicol. Sci.*, 48, 157, 1999.

Palmer, J.R., et al., Risk of breast cancer in women exposed to diethylstilbestrol in utero: preliminary results (U.S.), *Cancer Causes Control*, 13, 753, 2002.

Tanaka, E., Toxicological interactions between alcohol and benzodiazepines, *J. Toxicol. Clin. Toxicol.*, 40, 69, 2002.

Van Loveren, H., Steerenberg, P.A., and Vos, J.G., Early detection of immunotoxicity: from animal studies to human biomonitoring, *Toxicol. Lett.*, 77, 73, 1995.

7 Dose-Response

7.1. GENERAL ASSUMPTIONS

7.1.1 TYPES OF DOSE-RESPONSE RELATIONSHIPS

The discussion of effects of chemicals as a result of exposure to a particular dose (Chapter 6) necessarily must be followed by a discussion of the path by which that dose elicits that response. This relationship has traditionally been known as the **dose-response** relationship.[*] The result of exposure to the dose can be any measurable, quantifiable, or observable indicator. The response depends on the quantity of chemical exposure or administration within a given time period. Two types of dose-response relationships exist, depending on number of subjects and doses tested. The **graded dose-response** describes the relationship of an individual test subject or system to increasing and/or continuous doses of a chemical. Figure 7.1 illustrates the effect of increasing doses of several chemicals on cell proliferation *in vitro*. The concentration of the chemical is inversely proportional to the number of surviving cells in the cell culture system.

Alternatively, the **quantal dose-response** is determined by the distribution of responses to increasing doses in a population of test subjects or systems. This relationship is generally classified as an "all-or-none effect" where the test system or organisms are quantified as either "responders" or "nonresponders." A typical quantal dose-response curve is illustrated in Figure 7.2 by the LD_{50} (lethal dose 50%) distribution. The LD_{50} is a statistically calculated dose of a chemical that causes death in 50% of the animals tested. The doses administered are also continuous, or at different levels, and the response is generally mortality, gross injury, tumor formation, or some other criteria by which a standard deviation or "cut-off" value can be determined. In fact, other decisive factors, such as therapeutic dose or toxic dose, can be determined using quantal dose-response curves, from which the ED_{50} (effective dose 50%) and the TD_{50} (toxic dose 50%) are derived.

Graded and quantal curves are generated based on several assumptions. The time period at which the response is measured is chosen empirically or selected according to accepted toxicological practices. For instance, empirical time determinations may be established using a suspected toxic or lethal dose of a substance, and the response is determined over several hours or days. This time period is then set for all determinations of the LD_{50} or TD_{50} for that time period.[**] The frequency of administration is assumed to be a single dose administered at the start of the time period when the test subjects are acclimated to the environment.

---

[*] In certain fields of toxicology, particularly mechanistic and *in vitro* systems, the term dose-response is more accurately referred to as concentration-effect. This change in terminology makes note of the specific effect on a measurable parameter that corresponds to a precise plasma concentration.

[**] This time period is commonly set at 24 h for LD_{50} determinations.

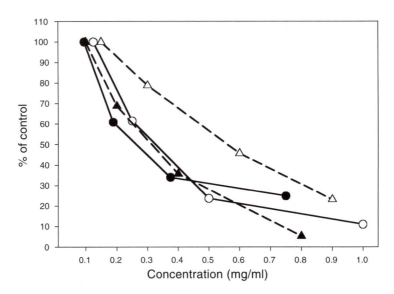

FIGURE 7.1 Graded dose-response curve for caffeine HCl (o), chloramphenicol HCl (•), atropine sulfate (△), and phenol (▲). The graph illustrates the percent of viable human lung cells capable of proliferating in a cell culture system in response to increasing concentrations of the chemicals. (Modified from Yang, A. et al. Subacute cytotoxicity testing with cultured human lung cells, *Toxicol. In Vitro*, 16, 33, 2002.)

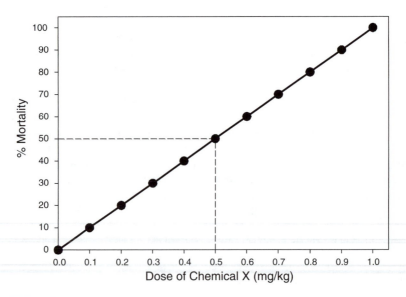

FIGURE 7.2 Quantal dose-response curve showing the experimental derivation and graphic estimation of the LD_{50}.

7.1.2 CONCENTRATION-EFFECT AND PRESENCE AT THE RECEPTOR SITE

It is assumed that, at the conclusion of an experiment, the measured or observed effect is, in fact, due to the presence of the chemical. The establishment of this causal relationship is critical if valid conclusions are drawn from the dose-response curve. It is also presumed that the chemical in question is present at the receptor site or molecular target responsible for the effect. Support for this assumption follows from measurement of concentrations at the cellular or organ level. In fact, as the concentration of a chemical in the affected compartment increases, the degree of response must increase proportionately if this assumption is valid. For this reason, some references have suggested the use of the term "concentration-effect" curve as an alternative label to dose-response. The former is purported to be a more ingenuous description of the causal relationship and more accurately reflects the parameters measured.

7.1.3 CRITERIA FOR MEASUREMENT

Except for lethality, the selection of a measurable or observable endpoint is crucial. A desirable biomarker may be one that accurately reflects the presence of the chemical at the molecular site or suggests that the toxic effect originates from the target organ. Selection of a measurable endpoint thus depends on the suspected mechanism of toxicity, if known, or on empirical determinations based on the chemical formula. Some biomarkers are also subjective, such as reliance on histo-logical grading, calculation of the degree of anesthesia, pain, motor activity, or behavioral change. Thus, the standards for quantifying the endpoint are determined and established prior to the experimental setup.

7.2 LD$_{50}$ (LETHAL DOSE 50%)

7.2.1 DEFINITION

As noted above, the LD$_{50}$ is a statistically calculated dose of a chemical that causes death in 50% of the animals tested, based on the objective observation of lethality. This "all-or-none" effect uses lethality as an absolute, unequivocal measurement. The usefulness of the test provides a screening method for toxic evaluation, partic-ularly useful for new unclassified substances. The determination however is anti-quated, requires large numbers of animals, does not provide information regarding mechanistic effects or target organ, and does not suggest complementary or selective pathways of toxicity. It is also limited by the route and duration of exposure. Consequently, its routine use in drug testing has become the subject of continuous debate and regulatory review in toxicity testing.

7.2.2 EXPERIMENTAL PROTOCOL

A predetermined number of animals, at least ten animals per dose and ten doses per chemical, are selected. Groups of animals are subjected to increasing single doses of the test substance (the dose is calculated as mg of substance per kg of body weight, mg/kg). The number of animals that expire within the group at the end of a predetermined time period (usually 24 to 96 h) are counted and converted to a percentage of the total animals exposed to the chemical. A dose-response relationship is constructed and the 50% extrapolation is computed from the curve (see Figure 7.2 above).

Alternatively, testing of chemicals for biological effects sometimes requires that the response to a chemical is normally distributed — i.e., that the highest number of respondents are gathered in the middle dosage range. Figure 7.3 represents a normal frequency distribution achieved with increasing dosage of a chemical vs. the cumulative percent mortality. The bars represent the percentage of animals that died at each dose minus the percentage that died at the immediately lower dose. As is shown by the normal (gaussian) distribution, the smallest percentage of animals died at the lowest and highest doses, accounted for by biological variation (hypersensitive vs. resistant animals, respectively).

7.2.3 Factors That Influence the LD_{50}

Several factors influence the reliability of the LD_{50} determination including: the selection of species, the route of administration, and the time of day of exposure and observation. In general, reproducibility of an LD_{50} relies on adherence to the same criteria in each trial experiment. The same species must be of the same age, sex, strain, weight, and breeder. The route of administration, as well as the time of administration, is critical. Also, the animal care maintenance should be similar in each run, with

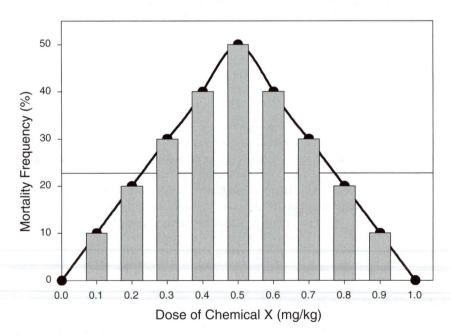

FIGURE 7.3 Normal frequency distribution of mortality frequency (%) vs. dose.

attention to light and dark cycles, feeding, and waste disposal schedules. Variability in LD_{50} is largely due to changes in parameters between experiments.

7.3 ED_{50} (EFFECTIVE DOSE 50%), TD_{50} (TOXIC DOSE 50%), AND TI (THERAPEUTIC INDEX)

7.3.1 RELATIONSHIP TO LD_{50}

The ED_{50} is analogous to the LD_{50} with the important exception that the former uses an endpoint designed to determine a desirable effect of the test substance occurring in 50% of the animals tested. Such desirable effects might include sedation with a sedative-hypnotic drug or analgesia with an opioid derivative. Similarly, the TD_{50} is calculated based on the measurement of a toxic nonlethal endpoint, such as respiratory depression. The relationship between lethal (or toxic dose) and effective dose is calculated and expressed as the therapeutic index (TI):

$$TI = LD_{50} \ (or \ TD_{50})/ED_{50}$$

The formula is generally accepted as an approximation of the relative safety of a chemical and is used as a guide for therapeutic monitoring. The TI is illustrated in Figure 7.4 as a graphic representation of the relationship between the LD_{50} and the ED_{50}.

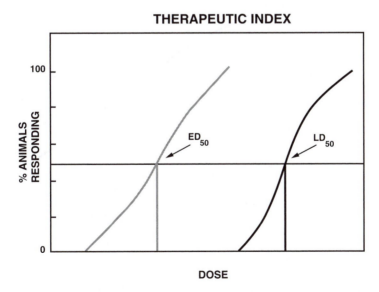

FIGURE 7.4 Graph of therapeutic index (TI). The TI is used to determine the difference between an effective dose and a toxic (or lethal) dose. The TI increases as the difference between the effective (therapeutic) dose and the toxic (or lethal) dose is amplified. The calculation allows for an estimation of the potential usefulness of the agent as a therapeutic tool.

7.3.2 ASSUMPTIONS USING THE TI

The derivation of the TI assumes the measurement of median doses in the experimental protocol.[*] The median dose is calculated according to the desired effect observed in 50% of the animals tested, and represents a quantitative, but relative, estimation of the margin of safety of a chemical. This information may be valuable in establishing guidelines for estimating potential human risk. As with the determination of the LD_{50}, the TI does not provide information on the slopes of the curves (as with Figure 7.2), mechanism of toxicity, or pharmacological action.

7.4 IC_{50} (INHIBITORY CONCENTRATION 50%)

7.4.1 DEFINITION

The concentration necessary to inhibit 50% of a measured response in an *in vitro* system is known as the IC_{50} (similarly as with IC_{75} and IC_{25} that are sometimes computed as "cut-off" values). The number is calculated based on the slope and linearity of a typical concentration-effect curve (Figure 7.5). The symmetry of the curve is mathematically

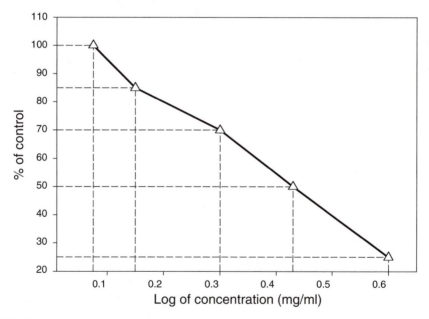

FIGURE 7.5 Graded dose-response (concentration-effect) curve for xylene on cultured human lung cells for 72 h. The measured parameter (% of control) is cell proliferation. The diagram illustrates extrapolation of the IC_{50} (0.43 mg/ml), as well as the IC_{75} (0.6 mg/ml), IC_{30} (0.3mg/ml), and IC_{15} (0.15 mg/ml). The latter represent "cut-off" values corresponding to 25, 70, and 85% of control. (Modified from Yang, A. et al. Subacute cytotoxicity testing with cultured human lung cells, *Toxicol. In Vitro*, 16, 33, 2002.)

---

[*] The median is the middle value in a set of measurements. Like the mean, but not identical to it, it is a measure of central tendency.

estimated from *regression analysis* of the plot, "percentage of control" vs. "log of concentration." The values for "percentage of control" are derived by converting the absolute values of the measured response to a fraction of the control value — i.e., responses measured in the group without chemical treatment. Using the control value as the 100% level, all subsequent groups are transformed into relative percentage values. This manipulation has the advantage of allowing comparison of results between different experiments and different laboratories, even when the absolute values are not identical.

7.4.2 EXPERIMENTAL DETERMINATION

IC_{50} determinations are traditionally performed using cell culture methodology or other *in vitro* methods. Manipulation of cells in culture, whether with continuous or finite cell lines or primary cultures, requires attention to several steps employed in the screening assay. For example, a typical procedure begins with inoculation of cells in multiwell plates at a rate of 10^4 cells per cm^2. Contact-inhibited cultures are grown to stationary phase in appropriate complete media. Monolayers are then incubated with increasing concentrations of sterile, soluble solutions of each chemical for a predetermined period of time. Incubation criteria for mammalian cells generally also dictate 37°C in a gaseous, humidified atmosphere defined by the requirements of the medium. Prior to the end of the incubation period, indicators, dyes, fixatives, or reactive substrates are added as needed and allowed to incubate. The cultures are then processed, and reaction product is quantified according to the protocol.

7.4.3 IN VITRO SYSTEMS

Determination of IC_{50} in *in vitro* systems is analogous to the calculation of the LD_{50} or TD_{50} in animal testing. Unlike LD_{50} or TD_{50}, however, which represents a median lethal or toxic dose, IC_{50} allows for comparisons of **concentrations** of chemicals necessary to inhibit any measurable parameter, such as cell proliferation, protein synthesis, or DNA synthesis. Thus, it becomes a valuable tool for estimating toxic effects. Using IC_{50} for estimating toxicity, international validation programs have now successfully proposed the use of *in vitro* methods to supplement or replace animal toxicity testing programs. In addition, *in vitro* methods are more cost-efficient than animal experimentation. It is conceivable, therefore, that animal toxicity testing in the foreseeable future will be augmented with incorporation of data obtained from *in vitro* systems. Such testing may prove to be more predictive of assessing human clinical toxicity than current animal testing protocols.

REFERENCES

SUGGESTED READINGS

Balls, M., ECVAM and the promotion of international co-operation in the development, validation and acceptance of replacement alternative test methods, *ALTEX*, 16, 280, 1999.

Clemedson, C., et al., MEIC evaluation of acute systemic toxicity. Part VII. Prediction of human toxicity by results from testing of the first 30 reference chemicals with 27 further *in vitro* assays. *Altern. Lab. Anim. (ATLA)*, 28, 161, 2000.

Eaton, D.L. and Klassen, C.D., Principles of Toxicology, in *Casarett and Doull's Toxicology: The Basic Science of Poisons*, 6th ed., Klaassen, C.D., Ed., McGraw-Hill, New York, 2001, chap. 2.

Goldberg, A.M., Development of alternative methods, *J. Toxicol. Sci.*, 20, 443, 1995.

Hoel, D.G., Animal experimentation and its relevance to man, *Environ. Health Perspect*, 32, 25, 1979.

Yang, A., Cardona, D.L., and Barile, F.A., *In vitro* cytotoxicity testing with fluorescence-based assays in cultured human lung and dermal cells, *Cell Biol. Toxicol.*, 18, 97, 2002.

Yang, A., Cardona, D.L., and Barile, F.A., Subacute cytotoxicity testing with cultured human lung cells, *Toxicol. In Vitro,* 16, 33, 2002.

Review Articles

Boyd, E.M., 100-day LD 50 index of chronic toxicity, *Clin. Toxicol.*, 4, 205, 1971.

Crettaz, P., et al., Assessing human health response in life cycle assessment using ED10s and DALYs: part 1 — Cancer effects, *Risk Anal.*, 22, 931, 2002.

Crump, K.S., Dose response problems in carcinogenesis, *Biometrics,* 35, 157, 1979.

Edler, L. and Kopp-Schneider, A., Statistical models for low dose exposure, *Mutat. Res.*, 405, 227, 1998.

Flecknell, P., Replacement, reduction and refinement, *ALTEX*, 19, 73, 2002.

Gaylor, D.W. and Kodell, R.L., Dose-response trend tests for tumorigenesis adjusted for differences in survival and body weight across doses, *Toxicol. Sci.*, 59, 219, 2001.

Green, S., Goldberg, A., and Zurlo, J., TestSmart-high production volume chemicals: an approach to implementing alternatives into regulatory toxicology, *Toxicol. Sci.*, 63, 6, 2001.

Guerrero Munoz, F. and Fearon, Z., Sex related differences in acetaminophen toxicity in the mouse, *J. Toxicol. Clin. Toxicol.*, 22, 149, 1984.

Hakkinen, P.J. and Green, D.K., Alternatives to animal testing: information resources via the Internet and World Wide Web, *Toxicology*, 173, 3, 2002.

Hanson, M.L. and Solomon, K.R., New technique for estimating thresholds of toxicity in ecological risk assessment, *Environ. Sci. Technol.*, 36, 3257, 2002.

Melnick, R.L. and Kohn, M.C., Dose-response analyses of experimental cancer data, *Drug Metab. Rev.*, 32, 193, 2000.

Pennington, D., et al., Assessing human health response in life cycle assessment using ED10s and DALYs: part 2 — noncancer effects, *Risk Anal.*, 22, 947, 2002.

Worth, A.P. and Balls, M., The importance of the prediction model in the validation of alternative tests, *Altern. Lab. Anim. (ATLA)*, 29, 135, 2001.

8 Descriptive Animal Toxicity Tests

8.1 CORRELATION WITH HUMAN EXPOSURE

8.1.1 HUMAN RISK ASSESSMENT

The information derived from descriptive animal toxicity testing is useful in determining the potential toxicity of a compound to humans. The objective of these tests is to identify toxic chemicals at an early stage of chemical development, especially if the substance is already commercially available. Together with *in vitro* tests, animal tests are applied as biological markers of chemically induced risks, whether synthetic or naturally occurring. These validated batteries of tests are used by regulatory agencies to screen for or predict human toxic effects, in an attempt to establish a significant frame of reference for monitoring environmental chemical threats, therapeutic adverse reactions, and commercial toxicity.

8.1.2 PREDICTIVE TOXICOLOGY AND EXTRAPOLATION TO HUMAN TOXICITY

The ability to predict toxicity in humans with a responsible level of safety is probably the most trying conclusion of animal testing. Correlation of results of toxicity testing described in animals with human exposure requires careful consideration of the parameters of the animal tests, including the selection of species with similar physiology. The variety of tests available to reach valid conclusions with a particular chemical must be systematically chosen according to the guidelines of the regulatory agencies.

8.2 SPECIES DIFFERENTIATION

8.2.1 SELECTION OF A SUITABLE ANIMAL SPECIES

Among the mammalian species available to toxicologists for testing of chemicals, the rodent is the most useful and convenient. Notwithstanding the ostensible difference in size and a few minor anatomical distinctions, rodent physiology is almost identical to human. The rodent, therefore, is a suitable animal species that mimics the human. In addition, the species must be able to reflect diverse toxicological challenges, including behavioral, neurological, and cognitive reactions to chemical insult. Thus, rodents are the first species of consideration in general toxicity testing. Other animal species are selected based on the sensitivity of the animal to particular classes of chemicals or for particular organ similarity. For instance, because of their dermal sensitivity, guinea pigs are used for testing of local irritants. Rabbits have traditionally been employed for testing of ocular irritants, as their eyes are anatomically and physiologically similar to humans. Larger species, such as dogs, are useful subjects of specific toxicity testing involving cardiovascular and pulmonary agents. The use of primates for testing behavioral, immunological, microbiological, and neurological response to chemicals is controversial but is often necessary for interpretation of human risk assessment.

8.2.2 Cost-Effectiveness

One of the most important criteria for selecting an appropriate animal species is cost. Animal testing is more costly than *in vitro* methods. The budget for animal testing must account for:

1. Procurement of animals, housing, and maintenance within the animal care facility
2. Daily animal requirements of food, water, bedding
3. Training and employing animal care staff
4. Veterinarian on-call or on-staff
5. Adherence to proper procedures for removal and disposal of specimens and waste

8.2.3 Institutional Animal Care and Use Committee (IACUC)

The Public Health Service (PHS) Policy on Humane Care and Use of Laboratory Animals was promulgated in 1986 to implement the Health Research Extension Act of 1985 (Public Law 99-158), "Animals in Research." The Office of Laboratory Animal Welfare (OLAW) at the National Institutes of Health (NIH), which has responsibility for the general administration and coordination of policy on behalf of the PHS, provides specific guidance, instruction, and materials to institutions on the utilization and care of vertebrate animals used in testing, research, and training. This policy requires institutions to establish and maintain proper measures to ensure the appropriate care and use of all animals involved in research, research training, and biological testing activities conducted or supported by the PHS. In addition, any activity involving animals must provide a written assurance acceptable to the PHS, setting forth compliance with this policy. Assurances are submitted to OLAW at the NIH, and are evaluated by OLAW to determine the adequacy of the institution's proposed program for the care and use of animals in PHS-conducted or supported activities. In summary, the program assurance includes:

1. A list of every branch and major component of the institution.
2. The lines of authority and responsibility for administering the program.
3. The qualifications, authority, and responsibility of the veterinarian(s) who will participate in the program.

4. The membership list of the IACUC committee established in accordance with the requirements.
5. The procedures that the IACUC will follow to fulfill the requirements.
6. The health program for personnel who work in laboratory animal facilities or who have frequent contact with animals.
7. A synopsis of training or instruction in the humane practice of animal care and use. Training or instruction in research or testing methods that minimize the number of animals required to obtain valid results and minimize animal distress must be offered to scientists, animal technicians, and other personnel involved in animal care, treatment, or use.
8. The gross square footage of each animal facility, the species housed and the average daily inventory of animals in each facility; and any other pertinent information requested by OLAW.

Other functions of the IACUC include periodic review of the institution's program, inspection of facilities, preparation of reports, and submittal of suggestions and recommendations on improving the program.

8.3 DESCRIPTIVE TESTS

8.3.1 Required LD_{50} and Two Routes

In accordance with FDA regulations establishing current drug testing protocols using animal experiments, the LD_{50} is required for a substance using at least two routes of exposure, usually oral and parenteral routes. Depending on the nature of the substance, the route can be modified to include testing for inhalation, local, or other selective exposure. In addition, the animals are also monitored for gross appearance, behavior, morbidity, and time of onset of any signs and symptoms. The upper limit dose is 2 g/kg of body weight by any route.

8.3.2 Chronic and Subchronic Exposure

Besides acute 24-h exposures, several exposure periods may be incorporated into the protocols. Subchronic exposure usually involves a 90-day exposure period, with or without repeated doses. Chronic exposure studies are more difficult, cumbersome, and expensive to conduct. These experiments are reserved for carcinogenicity testing or accumulation studies. The rat is the animal of choice in chronic experiments. Hematology, clinical chemistry, and histological analysis also become important parameters to monitor in chronic programs.

8.3.3 Types of Tests

Routine oral or parenteral 24-h studies in a rodent species are performed along with other types of tests, depending on the chemical substance. Local toxicity testing for dermal toxicity or sensitization is conducted with chemicals destined for local use. Cosmetics, nasal or pulmonary inhalation products, toiletries, therapeutic or cosmetic creams, ointments, and lotions, are tested for local hypersensitivity reactions. As

TABLE 8.1
Other Types of Descriptive Animal Techniques and Their Potential for Use in Toxicity Testing Protocols

Methods	Descriptive Protocol	Preferred Species
Dermal testing	Local irritancy	Guinea pig
Draize method	Ocular irritancy	Rabbit
Fertility and reproductive tests	Developmental toxicity	Rabbit and rodent litters
Immunotoxicity studies	Toxicity related to immune function	Rodent
Mammalian mutagenesis	Altered foci induction[a]; skin neoplasm, pulmonary neoplasm, and breast cancer induction	Rodent
Mammalian teratology, whole embryo culture	Teratogenicity	Rabbit, rodent
Perinatal and postnatal studies	Developmental toxicity	Rabbit, rodent
Toxicokinetic studies	Influence on A,D,M,E[a]	Rodent and larger mammals

Note: A,D,M,E = absorption, distribution, metabolism, elimination.

[a] In rodent liver.

noted above, the guinea pig is the species of choice for dermal testing because of skin sensitivity and anatomical resemblance to humans.

Other animal testing techniques are listed in Table 8.1 and include methods for the determination of ocular irritation, local irritation, teratogenicity, developmental toxicity, perinatal and postnatal toxicity, mutagenicity, immunotoxicity, and toxicokinetics. Among these tests, the determination of potential ocular toxicity from chemicals and solvents has been traditionally evaluated in rabbits using the Draize method. This controversial test measures eye irritancy and has been the standard method for six decades. Recently, its replacement by *in vitro* tests has been recommended.

REFERENCES

SUGGESTED READINGS

Bayne, K.A., Environmental enrichment of nonhuman primates, dogs and rabbits used in toxicology studies, *Toxicol. Pathol.*, 31, 132, 2003.

REVIEW ARTICLES

Barrow, P.C., Reproductive toxicology studies and immunotherapeutics, *Toxicology*, 185, 205, 2003.

Bucher, J.R., The National Toxicology Program rodent bioassay: designs, interpretations, and scientific contributions, *Ann. N.Y. Acad. Sci.*, 982, 198, 2002.

James, M.L., IACUC training: from new-member orientation to continuing education, *Lab. Anim. (N.Y.)*, 31, 26, 2002.

Jenkins, E.S., Broadhead, C., and Combes, R.D., The implications of microarray technology for animal use in scientific research, *Altern. Lab. Anim.*, 30, 459, 2002.

Meyer, O., Testing and assessment strategies, including alternative and new approaches, *Toxicol. Lett.*, 140, 21, 2003.

Pauluhn, J., Overview of testing methods used in inhalation toxicity: from facts to artifacts, *Toxicol. Lett.*, 140, 183, 2003.

Pitts, M., A guide to the new ARENA/OLAW IACUC guidebook, *Lab. Anim. (N.Y.)*, 31, 40, 2002.

Rogers, J.V. and McDougal, J.N., Improved method for *in vitro* assessment of dermal toxicity for volatile organic chemicals, *Toxicol. Lett.*, 135, 125, 2002.

Silverman, J., Animal breeding and research protocols — the missing link, *Lab. Anim. (N.Y.)*, 31, 19, 2002.

Smialowicz, R.J., The rat as a model in developmental immunotoxicology, *Hum. Exp. Toxicol.*, 21, 513, 2002.

Spielmann, H., Validation and regulatory acceptance of new carcinogenicity tests, *Toxicol. Pathol.*, 31, 54, 2003.

Steneck, N.H., Role of the institutional animal care and use committee in monitoring research, *Ethics Behav.*, 7, 173, 1997.

Stephenson, W., Institutional animal care and use committees and the moderate position, *Between Species*, 7, 6, 1991.

Whitney, R.A., Animal care and use committees: history and current policies in the United States, *Lab. Anim. Sci.*, 37, 18, 1987.

9 *In Vitro* Alternatives to Animal Toxicity

9.1 *IN VITRO* METHODS

9.1.1 CELL CULTURE METHODS

Techniques used to culture animal and human cells and tissues on plastic surfaces or in suspension have contributed significantly to the development of toxicity testing. Cell culture techniques are fundamental for understanding mechanistic toxicology, as well, and have been used with increasing frequency in all biomedical disciplines. In particular, the mechanisms underlying clinical toxicity have been elucidated with the development of *in vitro* methods. In addition, the necessity to clarify the toxic effects of chemicals and drugs that are developed and marketed at rapid rates has provoked the need for fast, simple, valid, and alternative methods to animal toxicity testing.

9.1.2 ORGAN SYSTEM CYTOTOXICITY

Homogeneous cell populations isolated from the framework of an organ present unique opportunities to study the toxic effects on a single cell type. Among the organs which have proven to be of particular interest as target organs of toxicity are lung, liver, skin, kidney, hematopoietic, nervous, and immune systems. Primary cultures, representing freshly isolated cells from target organs, and established cell lines are valuable in assessing target organ toxicity. Often, classes of chemicals are tested so that their toxicity can be compared within the same system. This permits for the establishment of toxicity data to be used as a reference for previously unknown toxicity of similar classes of chemicals. Essential to this testing principle are hepatocyte cultures, because of the important role that the liver enjoys in xenobiotic metabolism — i.e., metabolism of exogenous substances. Other cell types that are employed for assessing target organ toxicity include lung macrophages and epithelial cells, cardiac, renal, neuronal, and muscle cells.

9.1.3 APPLICATIONS TO CLINICAL TOXICOLOGY

Although primary cultures offer sensitive and specific avenues for detecting target organ toxicity, the system has several disadvantages:

1. Primary cultures require sacrificing animals to establish the cells.
2. Primary cultures are limited to understanding the mechanisms of only one of the many possible organ pathologies that could be determined using animals.
3. Primary systems established from human donors are not standardized, unless efforts are made to match the age and sex of the donors.
4. Response of primary cultures to chemical insult may not reflect the complex nature of chemical-target interaction as inherent in animal species.

Nevertheless, regulatory agencies in Europe and the U.S. have promulgated the use of select *in vitro* tests to be incorporated into routine industrial toxicity testing programs. Among the systems that are currently under evaluation is the EpiOcular™ (MatTek Corporation, Ashland, MA) protocol for ocular irritation. This procedure is a useful *in vitro* alternative for the Draize test.

Established continuous and finite cell lines are also employed to analyze a wide spectrum of mechanisms and effects and are generally used to detect general toxicity. In contrast to animal studies, these systems measure the concentration of a substance that damages components, alters structures, or influences biochemical pathways within specific cells. The range of injury is further specified by the length of exposure (incubation time) and the parameter used to detect an insult (indicator). Careful validation of test methods and repetitive interlaboratory confirmation allows the tests to be predictive for risks associated with toxic effects *in vivo*, for those concentrations of the effective substances tested. All established cell lines, however, are prone to dedifferentiate in culture with time, thus limiting their usefulness for assessing effects other than general toxicity.

9.1.4 RELATIONSHIP TO ANIMAL EXPERIMENTS

Clinical toxicity of chemicals is known to involve various physiological targets interacting with a variety of complex toxicokinetic factors. Chemicals induce injury through an assortment of toxic mechanisms. As a result, *in vitro* testing requires several relevant systems, such as human hepatocytes, heart, kidney, lung and nerve cells, as well as other cell lines of vital importance, to obtain information necessary for human risk assessment. These cell systems are also used to measure basal cytotoxicity — i.e., the toxicity of a chemical that affects basic cellular functions and structures common to all human specialized cells. Basal cytotoxicity of a chemical may reflect the measurement of cell membrane integrity, mitochondrial activity, or protein synthesis, since these are examples of basic metabolic functions common to all cells. The level of activity varies from one organ to another, depending on its metabolic rate and contribution to homeostasis, but the processes do not differ qualitatively among organs. Recent multicenter studies have now shown that human cell lines predict basal cytotoxicity to a greater extent than animal cell lines. These *in vitro* tests are as accurate in screening for chemicals with toxic potential as LD_{50} methods performed in rodents. In addition, validation studies have proposed that these tests be used to supplement animal testing protocols when screening for toxic substances.

9.2 CORRELATION WITH HUMAN EXPOSURE

9.2.1 RISK ASSESSMENT

Together with animal testing, with genotoxicity tests, with toxicokinetic modeling studies, and with microarray technology, *in vitro* cellular test batteries could be applied as biological markers of chemically induced risks. Such tests include biomonitoring for environmental toxicants and biohazards and for the development of specific antagonists. The batteries of tests can be validated for their ability to screen for or predict human toxic effects, as the measurements can establish a database for monitoring of environmental and clinical biohazards and general toxicity.

9.2.2 EXTRAPOLATION TO HUMAN TOXICITY

Standardized batteries of *in vitro* tests have been proposed for assessing acute local and systemic toxicity. This battery of selected protocols may serve as a primary screening tool before the implementation of routine animal testing. The correlation of *in vitro* with *in vivo* data functions as a basis for predicting human toxicity. As it becomes apparent that several batteries of tests reflect the acute toxicity of defined classifications of substances, significant numbers of animals in toxicity testing will be reduced.

9.2.3 PREDICTIVE TOXICOLOGY

Many relatively common and widely available chemicals have never been tested in any system. *In vitro* systems offer the possibility for use as screening methods for carcinogenic, mutagenic, or cumulative toxicity. It is possible to reduce or replace toxicity testing of **existing** chemicals with risk assessment based on the results from these batteries. In combination with clinical studies of dermal and ocular irritancy, and cumulative regressive and progressive longitudinal studies, *in vitro* test databases can contribute to reliable, clinically relevant human toxicity information.

REFERENCES

SUGGESTED READINGS

Acosta, D., *Cellular and Molecular Toxicology and In Vitro Toxicology*, CRC Press, Boca Raton, FL, 1990.

Barile, F.A., *Introduction to In Vitro Cytotoxicology: Mechanisms and Methods*, CRC Press, Boca Raton, FL, 1994.

Ecobichon, D.J., *The Basis of Toxicity Testing*, 2nd ed., CRC Press, Boca Raton, FL, 1997.

Gad, S. and Chengelis, C.P., *Acute Toxicology Testing: Perspectives and Horizons*, CRC Press, Boca Raton, FL, 1988.

Salem, H. and Katz, S.A., *Alternative Toxicological Methods*, CRC Press, Boca Raton, FL, 2003.

REVIEW ARTICLES

Blaauboer, B.J., The integration of data on physico-chemical properties, *in vitro*-derived toxicity data and physiologically based kinetic and dynamic as modelling a tool in hazard and risk assessment. A commentary, *Toxicol. Lett.*, 138, 161, 2003.

Carere, A., Stammati, A., and Zucco, F., *In vitro* toxicology methods: impact on regulation from technical and scientific advancements, *Toxicol. Lett.*, 127, 153, 2002.

Combes, R.D., The ECVAM workshops: a critical assessment of their impact on the development, validation and acceptance of alternative methods, *Altern. Lab. Anim. (ATLA)*, 30, 151, 2002.

Forsby, A., *In vitro* toxicity: mechanisms, alternatives and validation — a report from the 19th annual scientific meeting of the Scandinavian Society for Cell Toxicology, *Altern. Lab. Anim. (ATLA)*, 30, 307, 2002.

Fry, J., George, E., *In vitro* toxicology in the light of new technologies, *Altern. Lab. Anim. (ATLA)* 29, 745, 2001.

Hakkinen, P.J. and Green, D.K., Alternatives to animal testing: information resources via the Internet and World Wide Web, *Toxicology*, 173, 3, 2002.

Indans, I., The use and interpretation of *in vitro* data in regulatory toxicology: cosmetics, toiletries and household products, *Toxicol. Lett.*, 127, 177, 2002.

Jacobs, J.J., et al., An *in vitro* model for detecting skin irritants: methyl green-pyronine staining of human skin explant cultures, *Toxicol. In Vitro,* 16, 581, 2002.

Jones, P.A., et al., Comparative evaluation of five *in vitro* tests for assessing the eye irritation potential of hair-care products, *Altern. Lab. Anim. (ATLA)*, 29, 669, 2001.

Liebsch, M. and Spielmann, H., Currently available *in vitro* methods used in the regulatory toxicology, *Toxicol. Lett.*, 127, 127, 2002.

Pazos, P., Fortaner, S., and Prieto, P., Long-term *in vitro* toxicity models: comparisons between a flow-cell bioreactor, a static-cell bioreactor and static cell cultures, *Altern. Lab. Anim. (ATLA)*, 30, 515, 2002.

Putnam, K.P., Bombick, D.W., and Doolittle, D.J., Evaluation of eight *in vitro* assays for assessing the cytotoxicity of cigarette smoke condensate, *Toxicol. In Vitro,* 16, 599, 2002.

Snodin, D.J., An EU perspective on the use of *in vitro* methods in regulatory pharmaceutical toxicology, *Toxicol. Lett.*, 127, 161, 2002.

Stacey, G. and MacDonald, C., Immortalisation of primary cells, *Cell Biol. Toxicol.*, 17, 231, 2001.

Worth, A.P. and Cronin, M.T., Prediction models for eye irritation potential based on endpoints of the HETCAM and neutral red uptake tests, *In Vitro Mol. Toxicol.*, 14, 143, 2001.

10 Toxicokinetics

10.1 TOXICOKINETICS

10.1.1 RELATIONSHIP TO PHARMACOKINETICS

The study of drug disposition in physiological compartments is traditionally referred to as pharmacokinetics. Toxicokinetics includes the more appropriate study of exogenous compounds (xenobiotics), the adverse effects associated with their concentrations, passage through the physiological compartments, and the chemicals' ultimate fate. Compartmental toxicokinetics involves administration or exposure to a chemical, rapid equilibration to the central compartment (plasma and tissues), followed by distribution to peripheral compartments. Consequently, the principles of pharmacokinetics and toxicokinetics historically have been used interchangeably.

10.1.2 ONE-COMPARTMENT MODEL

A one-compartment model is the simplest representation of a system that describes the *first-order* extravascular absorption of a xenobiotic. The absorption rate is constant (k_a) and allows for entry into a central compartment (plasma and tissues). A constant *first-order elimination* (k_{el}) follows. The reaction is illustrated below (Reaction 1). Few compounds follow one-compartment modeling; agents such as creatinine equilibrate rapidly, distribute uniformly between blood, plasma, and tissues, and are eliminated as quickly.

$$\text{Reaction 1: Chemical} \xrightarrow{k_a} \text{One-Compartment} \xrightarrow{k_{el}} \text{Excreted}$$

Drug or toxin elimination processes, in general, follow zero-order or first-order kinetics. **First-order elimination**, or first-order kinetics, describes the rate of elimination of a drug in proportion to the drug concentration — i.e., an increase in the concentration of the chemical results in an increase in the rate of elimination. This rate usually occurs at **low** drug concentrations. Alternatively, **zero-order elimination** refers to the removal of a fixed amount of drug independent of the concentration — i.e., increasing plasma concentration of the chemical does not proceed with a corresponding increase in elimination. Zero-order kinetics usually occurs when biotransforming enzymes are saturated. Clinically, this situation is the most common cause of drug accumulation and toxicity. **Michaelis-Menton kinetics** occurs when a compound is metabolized according to both processes. For instance, at low concentrations, ethanol is metabolized by first-order kinetics (dose-dependent). As the blood alcohol concentration (BAC) increases, it switches to zero-order (dose-independent) elimination.

10.1.3 Two-Compartment Model

In a two-compartment model, the xenobiotic chemical requires a longer time for the concentration to equilibrate with tissues and plasma. Essentially, molecules enter the central compartment at a constant rate (k_a) and may also be eliminated through a constant *first-order elimination* (k_{el}) process. However, a parallel reaction (Reaction 2) occurs where the chemical enters and exits peripheral compartments through first-order rate constants for distribution (k_{d1} and k_{d2}, respectively). The distribution phases are variable but rapid, relative to elimination. Most drugs and xenobiotics undergo two- or multicompartment modeling behavior.

$$\text{Reaction 2: Chemical} \xrightarrow{k_a} \text{First-Compartment} \xrightarrow{k_{el}} \text{Excreted}$$

$$k_{d1} \downarrow \uparrow k_{d2}$$

$$\text{Second Compartment}$$

10.1.4 Application to Clinical Toxicology

Clinical applications of kinetics and the phenomena of absorption, distribution, metabolism, and elimination (ADME), are useful in the monitoring of pharmacological and toxicological activity of drugs and chemicals. Assigning a compound to compartmental systems, particularly a two-compartment, or the more complex multicompartment model, allows for prediction of adverse effects of the agents based on distribution and equilibration within the body. The ADME factors that influence the fate of a chemical are discussed below.

10.2 ABSORPTION

10.2.1 Ionic and Nonionic Principles

How do ionic or nonionic species of a chemical relate to absorption? Figure 10.1 illustrates the fluid mosaic model of the cell membrane. The membrane is characterized as a flexible, semipermeable barrier that maintains a homeostatic environment for normal cellular functions by preventing chemicals, ions, and water from traversing through easily.

The membrane consists of phospholipid polar heads, glycolipids, and integral proteins organized toward the periphery of the membrane, with the nonpolar tails and cholesterol directed inward. The rest of the membrane is interspersed with transmembrane channel proteins and other intrinsic proteins. The fluidity of the membrane is due to the presence of cholesterol and integral proteins. The phospholipid polar groups and nonpolar tails are derived from triglycerides. Figure 10.2 illustrates the structure of a triglyceride, detailing the positions of the polar environment contributed by the carboxyl moieties, relative to the nonpolar saturated carbon chains.

Because of the selectively permeable arrangement of the cell membrane, the ability of a chemical to bind to or penetrate intact membranes is determined by its

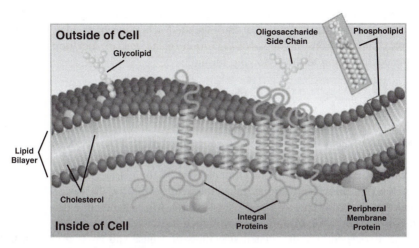

FIGURE 10.1 Fluid mosaic model of the cell membrane. (From Purves, W.K. et al., *Life, the Science of Biology*, 6th ed., Sinauer Associates, Sunderland, MA, 2001. With permission).

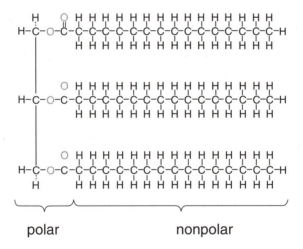

FIGURE 10.2 Structure of triglyceride showing the positions of polar and nonpolar contributions.

polar or nonpolar existence in solution. In turn, the relative contribution of a chemical to its polarity is influenced by the acidic or basic nature of the chemical in solution, which is determined by the proportion of the chemical's ability to dissociate or associate. According to the Bronsted-Lowry theory of acids and bases, an acidic compound dissociates — i.e., donates a proton — and a basic molecule associates — i.e., accepts a proton. The dissociation constant for an acid can be summarized according to the following formula:

$$K_a = \frac{([H^+][A^-])}{[HA]}$$

where K_a is the dissociation constant for an acid; $[H^+]$, $[A^-]$, and $[HA]$ represent the hydrogen ion, conjugate acid, and undissociated acid concentrations, respectively. The pK_a, derived from the negative logarithm of the acid dissociation constant, is calculated according to the following formula:

$$pK_a = -\log K_a$$

The pK_a of a drug, therefore, is defined as the pH at which 50% of the compound is ionized. Similarly, pK_b is the negative logarithm of the base dissociation constant (K_b). In general, acids and bases are classified according to their ability to dissociate, relative to the pH of the solution. Independent of the pH (for now), however, the lower the pK_a of an acid, the stronger the acid. Similarly, the lower the pK_a (or higher the pK_b) of a base, the stronger the base. Most therapeutic drugs are weak acids or bases, neutral, or amphoteric compounds.

The associated and dissociated structures of a base and an acid are illustrated in Figure 10.3, with aniline and benzoic acid, possessing strong basic and acidic characteristics, respectively. The structure of benzoic acid shows the carboxyl anion after dissociation. Since its $pK_a = 4$, the $K_a = 1 \times 10^{-4}$, resulting in a higher dissociation constant and possessing strong acidic properties. Similarly, aniline is a highly protonated species, with a pK_b of 10 and corresponding K_b of 1×10^{-10} (pK_a + pK_b = 14; thus, although it is a base, the pK_a of aniline can also be expressed as 4). The low dissociation constant of the base indicates that the H^+ ions are closely held to the nitrogen and contribute to its strong basic nature.

10.2.2 HENDERSON–HASSELBACH EQUATION

The relationship between the ionization of a weakly acidic drug, its pK_a, and the pH of the solution is given by the Henderson-Hasselbach equation. The equation allows for the prediction of the nonionic and ionic state of a compound at a given pH. For acids and bases, the formulas are:

$$\text{acid: } pH = pK_a + \log ([A^-]/[HA])$$

$$\text{base: } pH = pK_a + \log ([HA]/[A^-])$$

The equations are derived from the logarithmic expression of the dissociation constant formula above. Small changes in pH near the pK_a of a weakly acidic or basic

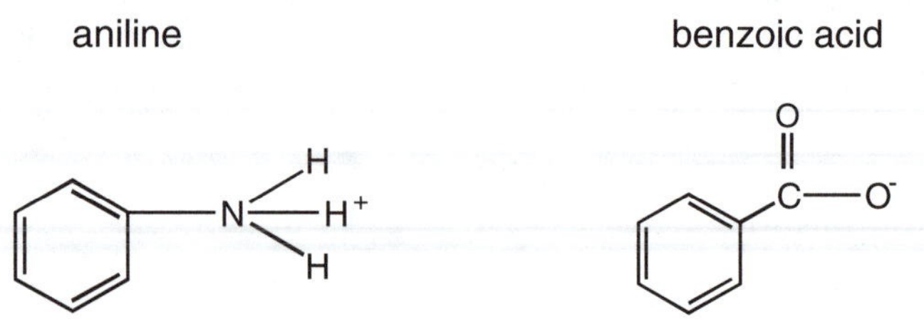

aniline   benzoic acid

FIGURE 10.3 Structures of aniline and benzoic acid.

drug markedly affect its degree of ionization. This is more clearly shown with rearrangement of the Henderson-Hasselbach equations, such that:

$$\text{for an acid: } pK_a - pH = \log ([HA]/[A^-])$$

$$\text{for a base: } pK_a - pH = \log ([A^-]/[HA])$$

For an acidic compound present in the stomach (e.g., $pK_a = 4$, in an average pH = 2), inserting the numbers into the Henderson-Hasselbach equation results in a relative ratio of *nonionized to ionized* species of 100:1. This transforms the compound predominantly to the nonionic form within the acidic environment of the stomach, rendering it more lipophilic. Lipophilic compounds have a greater tendency for absorption within that compartment.[*]

In the proximal small intestine areas of the duodenum and jejunum, where the pH is approximately 8, the same compound will be predominantly in the ionized state. The relative ratio of nonionized to ionized species is reversed ($1:10^4$). Thus, within the weakly basic environment of the proximal intestine, a strongly acidic drug is less lipophilic, more ionized, and slower to be absorbed.

Conversely, for a strong basic compound with a $pK_a = 4$ ($pK_b = 10$) in the stomach, the Henderson-Hasselbach equation predicts that the ratio of *ionized to nonionized* species equals 100:1. Thus, a basic compound is more ionized, less lipophilic, and slower to be absorbed in the stomach. In the basic environment of the proximal intestine (pH = 8), however, the ionized to nonionized species is $1:10^4$, rendering it more lipophilic and imparting a greater propensity for absorption.

The knowledge of the pK_a of a therapeutic drug is useful in predicting its absorption in these compartments. In addition, as explained below, this information is helpful in determining distribution and elimination functions. Table 10.1 and Table 10.2 summarize the chemical properties and behavior of strong acidic and basic drugs, such as aspirin and amphetamine hydrochloride, respectively. Based on the extremely acidic environment of an empty stomach, such compounds are either completely nonionized and highly lipophilic or ionized and hydrophilic. In the basic environment of the small intestine, although some ionization is present, amphetamine absorption is favored over that of aspirin. Conversely, the behavior of weakly basic or acidic drugs, such as morphine sulfate and sodium phenobarbital, respectively, can be predicted depending on the pH of the environment (Table 10.3 and Table 10.4).

It should be noted that some of the pharmacokinetic principles that govern drug absorption are not always significant factors in the determination of toxic effects. This is primarily due to the circumstances surrounding toxic chemical exposure. Consequently, some of the circumstances that influence drug absorption in a therapeutic setting will not be considered here. These factors include: formulation and physical characteristics of the drug product; drug interactions; presence of food in the intestinal tract; gastric emptying time; and concurrent presence of gastrointestinal diseases. Individual categories of toxic substances and special circumstances that alter their effects will be considered in their respective chapters.

---

[*] It should be noted that the absorption rate of the stomach is limited and is secondary to its digestion and churning functions.

TABLE 10.1
Structure, Chemical Properties and Behavior in the Stomach Environment (pH = 2) of Aspirin and Amphetamine Hydrochloride

Compound Properties	ASA	Amphetamine HCl
Structure		

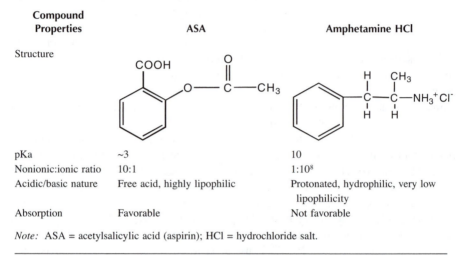

pKa	~3	10
Nonionic:ionic ratio	10:1	$1:10^8$
Acidic/basic nature	Free acid, highly lipophilic	Protonated, hydrophilic, very low lipophilicity
Absorption	Favorable	Not favorable

Note: ASA = acetylsalicylic acid (aspirin); HCl = hydrochloride salt.

TABLE 10.2
Structure, Chemical Properties and Behavior in Proximal Small Intestine (pH = 8–10) of Aspirin and Amphetamine Hydrochloride

Compound Properties	ASA	Amphetamine HCl
Structure		
pKa	~3	10
Nonionic:ionic ratio	$10^{-5}:1$ to $10^{-7}:1$	$10^{-2}:1$ to 1:1
Acidic/basic nature	Proton donor, very low lipophilicity	Some ionization, lipophilic
Absorption	Not favorable	Favorable

Note: ASA = acetylsalicylic acid (aspirin); HCl = hydrochloride salt.

TABLE 10.3
Structure, Chemical Properties and Behavior in Stomach Environment (pH = 2) of Morphine Sulfate and Sodium Phenobarbital

Compound Properties	Morphine SO₄	Na Phenobarbital
Structure		
pKa	8.2–9.9	7.3
Nonionic:ionic ratio	$1:10^7$	$10^5:1$
Acidic/basic nature	Amphoteric nature (weak base), some ionization, low lipophilicity	Weak acid, nonionic, lipophilic
Absorption	Not favorable	Favorable

Note: Na = sodium salt; SO₄ = sulfate salt.

10.2.3 Absorption in Nasal and Respiratory Mucosa

The vestibule of the nasal cavity and nasopharynx is covered by olfactory epithelium. This mucous membrane lining consists of an extensive network of capillaries and pseudostratified columnar epithelium interspersed with goblet cells. Inspired air enters the nasal conchae and is warmed by circulating blood in the capillaries, while mucous secreted by the goblet cells moistens the air and traps airborne particles. Thus, several factors facilitate rapid dissolution and absorption of drugs administered through the nasal route: (1) the vast surface area provided by the capillary circulation and epithelial cells in the mucous membranes; (2) the ability to trap dissolved and particulate substances; and (3) the phospholipid secretions of the nasal mucosa (resulting in a relatively neutral pH). Nonionized drugs are more rapidly absorbed in this compartment relative to their ionized counterparts.

The upper and lower respiratory tracts extend from the nasal cavity to the lungs. The **conducting portion**, responsible for ventilation, consists of the pharynx, larynx, trachea, bronchi, bronchioles, and terminal bronchioles. The **respiratory portion,** the main sites for gas exchange, consists of the respiratory bronchioles, alveolar ducts, alveolar sacs, and alveoli. Most of the upper and lower tracts are covered by ciliated secretory epithelial cells. Aside from the nasal epithelium, however, significant absorption of airborne substances does not occur above the level of the respiratory bronchioles. As respiratory bronchioles penetrate deeply into the lungs, the epithelial lining changes from simple cuboidal to simple

TABLE 10.4
Structure, Chemical Properties and Behavior in Proximal Small Intestine
(pH = 8–10) of Morphine Sulfate and Sodium Phenobarbital

Compound Properties	Morphine SO$_4$	Na Phenobarbital
Structure		
pKa	8.2–9.9 (mean = 9.0)	7.3
Nonionic:ionic ratio	10:1 to 10^{-1}:1	10^{-1}:1 to 10^{-3}:1
Acidic/basic nature	Amphoteric nature (acts as very weak acid), mostly protonated, lipophilic	Weak acid, some ionization, low lipophilicity
Absorption	Favorable	Some absorption over length of intestinal tract

Note: Na = sodium salt; SO$_4$ = sulfate salt.

squamous, enhancing the surface absorptive capability of the mucosa. In addition, the thin 0.5 µm respiratory membrane is composed of 300 million alveoli, and further supported by an extensive network of capillary endothelium. This anatomy allows rapid diffusion of chemicals delivered as gases, within aerosols, or carried by humidified air.

10.2.4 TRANSPORT OF MOLECULES

Absorption of chemicals requires basic mechanisms of transporting the molecules across fluid barriers and cell membranes. These transport vehicles include: *diffusion, active transport, facilitated diffusion, and filtration.*

The simplest mechanism for transportation of molecules involves *diffusion,* defined as the transport of molecules across a semipermeable membrane. The most common pathway of diffusion is *passive transport.* In passive transport, molecules are transported from an area of high to low solute concentration — i.e., down the concentration gradient. It is not an energy-dependent process, and no electrical gradient is generated. Lipophilic molecules, small ions, and electrolytes generally gain access through membrane compartments by passive diffusion, since they are not repelled by the phospholipid bilayer of the cell membrane. Most passive diffusion processes, however, are not molecularly selective.

In contrast to passive transport, polar substances, such as amino acids, nucleic acids, and carbohydrates are moved by an *active transport* process. The mechanism shuttles ionic substances from areas of low solute concentration to high solute concentration — i.e., against a concentration gradient. Active transport is an energy-dependent process and requires macromolecular carriers. The latter two requirements render this process susceptible to metabolic inhibition and, consequently, a site for pharmacological or toxicological influence. In addition, active transport processes are saturable systems, implying that they have a limited number of carriers, making them competitive and selective.

Facilitated diffusion resembles active transport, with the exception that substrate movement is not compulsory against a concentration gradient and it is not energy dependent. For example, macromolecular carriers augment the transfer of glucose across gastrointestinal epithelium through to the capillary circulation.

Filtration allows for the movement of solutes across epithelial membrane barriers, along with water movement. The motive force here is hydrostatic pressure. In general, the molecular weight cutoff for solutes transported along with water is about 100 to 200 mw units. Under normal circumstances, several membranes throughout the body with pores or fenestrations averaging 4 Å in diameter, are designed to allow entry for larger molecules. These special membranes permit coarse filtration of lipophilic or hydrophilic substances. Such filtration processes are described for the nephron and illustrated in Figure 10.4. The filtration slits, formed by the interdigitating podocytes in the glomerular apparatus and Bowman's capsule, prevent the passage of cells and solutes above 45 kD. Under normal circumstances, most smaller molecules pass through the filter, only to be reabsorbed in the proximal and distal convoluted tubules and collecting tubules.

Many organs exhibit passive filtration as fundamental processes for the passage of water. Intestinal absorption of water involves a transport method where water and dissolved nutrients are coarsely filtered and absorbed through the intestinal lumen. At the tissue level, the inotropic action of the cardiac system is the driving force for capillary perfusion. For instance, the thin endothelial/epithelial membranes forming the walls of the pulmonary alveoli represent the only barrier for the diffusion of gases from the alveolar spaces into the alveolar capillaries.

10.3 DISTRIBUTION

10.3.1 FLUID COMPARTMENTS

Anatomically, the body is not a homogeneous entity. Since approximately 70% of total body weight is composed of water, the physiological water compartments play significant roles in drug distribution and its ultimate fate. Table 10.5 illustrates the composition and contribution of water-based compartments relative to body weight. As such, the ability of a compound to gain access to these compartments is determined by a number of factors that influence the compounds' subsequent fate. The distribution of the substance to the target organ (receptor site), as well as to the sites of metabolism and excretion, can be reasonably predicted by such factors. These include: (1) the **physicochemical properties** of the substance, such as lipid solubility

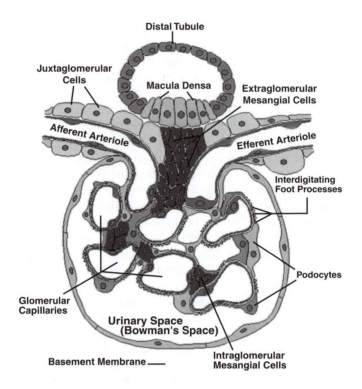

FIGURE 10.4 Diagram of glomerular apparatus of the nephron illustrating the podocytes and interdigitating foot processes that comprise the filtering unit (courtesy of UVA Medical Education).

TABLE 10.5
Components and Relative Percentages of Water-Based Compartments of Total Body Weight

Compartment	Description	Relative % of Body Weight
Plasma water (PL)	Noncellular water component of blood	10%
Interstitial water (IS)	Fluids relating to the interstices (spaces) of tissue	15%
Extracellular water (EC)	PL + IS	25%
Intracellular water (IC)	Confined to cytosol (within cells)	45%
Total body water (TBW)	EC + IC	70%
Solids	Tissue binding capacity	30%
Total body weight	Solids + TBW	100%

and ionic/nonionic principles; (2) **binding to macromolecules**; and (3) the **physiological forces** of blood flow and capillary perfusion. The cooperation of these forces determines the relative bioavailability of a compound. These concepts are further discussed below.

10.3.2 IONIC AND NONIONIC PRINCIPLES

The same mechanisms that govern absorption of molecules across semipermeable membranes also determine the bioavailability of a compound. Thus, a compound with a propensity for a nonionic existence is more likely to be lipophilic. Consequently, it has greater ability to penetrate phospholipid membranes and more access for distribution to liver, kidney, muscle, adipose, and other tissues. Conversely, molecules that are highly ionic in plasma have diminished access to organs and tissues. As with absorption, pH and pK_a have similar influence over the ionization, or lack of, at the tissue level. As an indicator of distribution to organs, the apparent volume of distribution (V_d) is used as a measure of the amount of chemical in the entire body (mg/kg) relative to that in the plasma (mg/L) over a specified period of time. Thus, V_d (l/kg) is useful in estimating the extent of distribution of a substance in the body. Table 10.6 shows the V_d for 50 chemicals whose toxicity is well established. Examination of these numbers indicates that a compound with a large V_d (e.g., chloroquine phosphate, 200 l/kg) is highly lipophilic and sequesters throughout tissue compartments. It necessarily demonstrates a low plasma concentration relative to dose. Alternatively, a compound with a low V_d (warfarin, 0.15 l/kg) is highly bound to circulating plasma proteins and, thus, has a plasma concentration seven times that of the mean total body concentration.

Another criterion for estimating bioavailability is the calculation of the area under the plasma concentration vs. time curve (shaded area, AUC, Figure 10.5). Dividing AUC after an oral dose by AUC after an intravenous dose and multiplying by 100 yields percent bioavailability. This value is used as an indicator for the fraction of chemical absorbed from the intestinal tract that reaches the systemic circulation after a specified period of time. As is explained below, other factors, such as first pass metabolism, rapid protein uptake, or rapid clearance, may alter the calculation. The ability to distribute to target tissues is then determined by the V_d.

10.3.3 PLASMA PROTEIN BINDING

Polar amino acids projecting from the surface of circulating proteins induce nonspecific, reversible binding of many structurally diverse small molecules. Circulating proteins transport chemicals through the circulation to target receptor sites. Such proteins include: serum albumin; hemoglobin (binds iron); $\alpha 1$ globulins (such as transcortin — binds steroid hormones and thyroxin); $\alpha 2$ globulins (ceruloplasmin — binds various ions); $\beta 1$ globulins (transferrin — binds iron); lipoproteins; and red blood cells. The factors that decide the extent of protein binding are dictated by nonionic and ionic forces of the radicals. Most binding is reversible and displaceable, primarily because it involves noncovalent, hydrogen, ionic, or van der Waals forces. The binding renders the molecule nonabsorable and unable to attach to the target receptor site.

TABLE 10.6
Human V_d of 50 Chemicals Tested in the Multicenter Evaluation
for *in Vitro* Cytotoxicity (MEIC) Program

MEIC Chemicals	V_d	MEIC Chemicals	V_d
Paracetamol	1.0	Acetylsalicylate	0.18
Ferrous sulfate	1.0	Diazepam	1.65
Amitriptyline	8.0	Digoxin	6.25
Ethylene glycol	0.65	Methanol	0.6
Ethanol	0.53	Isopropanol	0.6
1,1,1-TCE	1.0	Phenol	1.0
NaCl	1.0	Na fluoride	0.6
Malathion	1.0	2,4-DCP	0.1
Xylene	1.0	Nicotine	1.0
K Cyanide	1.0	Lithium SO_4	0.9
Theophylline	0.5	*d*-propoxyphene HCl	19.0
Propranolol HCl	4.0	Phenobarbital	0.55
Paraquat	1.0	Arsenic O_3	0.2
Copper SO_4	1.0	Mercuric Cl_2	1.0
Thioridazine HCl	18.0	Thallium SO_4	1.0
Warfarin	0.15	Lindane	1.0
Chloroform	2.6	Carbon tetrachloride	1.0
Isoniazid	0.6	Dichloromethane	1.0
Barium nitrate	1.0	Hexachlorophene	1.0
Pentachlorophenol	0.35	Verapamil HCl	4.5
Chloroquine PO_4	200	Orphenadrine HCl	6.1
Quinidine SO_4	2.4	Fenytoin	0.65
Chloramphenicol	0.57	Na oxalate	1.0
Amphetamine SO_4	4.4	Caffeine	0.4
Atropine SO_4	2.3	K chloride	1.0

Modified from Barile et al., 1994.

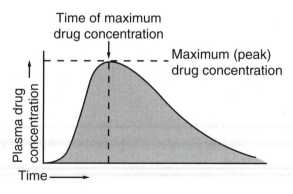

FIGURE 10.5 Plasma concentration vs. time curve for drug X. The shaded region represents the area under the curve (AUC).

Clinically, serum albumin poses significant alteration of drug toxicokinetics and pharmacokinetics by virtue of its high affinity for acidic drugs, such as warfarin and penicillin. The binding of a substance to a circulating transport protein forms a drug-protein complex, such that its activity, metabolism, and rate of elimination is determined by the strength of this bond and diffusion into various compartments. The rate at which a drug-protein complex dissociates, therefore, determines its toxicological, pharmacological, and metabolic fate.

The plasma concentration of a chemical is driven to equilibrium by the rate of cardiac output, and, assuming steady-state conditions, reaches a plateau concentration. In addition, consider that only unbound drug can diffuse into tissues for access to receptor sites or for biotransformation, since a drug-protein complex cannot pass through semipermeable cell membranes. Then, as the unbound transformed molecule is excreted, the dissociation of drug-protein complex increases, shifting the equilibrium toward unbound chemical. This shift continues until the free drug concentration is equal to that in plasma and tissues (i.e., steady state). Thus, this complex acts as a depot, releasing enough active ingredient, as determined by its chemical properties.

Chemicals that are extensively bound to circulating or tissue proteins pose a significant toxicological risk. Toxic effects of such chemicals extend well beyond acute exposures. Chronic, subclinical exposure to lead, for instance, has significant long-term neurological consequences by virtue of its affinity for depositing in bone. Therapeutically, steady state concentrations of warfarin are easily disrupted when another acidic drug, such as acetylsalicylic acid (aspirin), displaces it from circulating albumin binding sites. Since warfarin is extensively protein bound (97%), a displacement of as little as 3% can double the amount of warfarin available for interaction with target organs, resulting in significant adverse hemodynamic events. Consequently, displacement of protein-bound chemicals results in increased unbound drug concentration in plasma, increased pharmacological and toxicological effects, followed by enhanced metabolism.[*]

10.3.4 LIPIDS

Distribution of chemicals is also determined, in part, by their lipid/water partition coefficient. Two chemicals with similar pK_a values, such as amphetamine (9.8) and chlorpromazine (9.3), have different lipid affinities in their nonionized forms. At basic pH (8 to 9), both chemicals are completely nonionized. However, at pH 10 or above, the partition coefficient of chlorpromazine in lipid medium (K_d =$10^{6.3}$) is $10^{4.5}$ times greater than that of amphetamine ($K_d = 10^{1.8}$), allowing for greater absorption of the former in the contents of the intestinal tract. Similarly, the polychlorinated biphenyls (PCBs) and the contact insecticide DDT have high lipid solubilities, dissolve in neutral fats, and thus can readily accumulate in adipose tissue.

---

[*] It is important to note that availability of chemical at the receptor site is influenced more by rate of diffusion (V_d) than by rate of dissociation. This is especially true when the displacement of an acidic drug, with a small apparent V_d, displays clinically important consequences.

10.3.5 LIVER AND KIDNEY

The high capacity of the liver and kidney for binding and concentrating toxicants, coupled with their extensive circulation and metabolic activity, render these organs susceptible to chemical attack. Further details of the metabolic roles that the liver and kidney play in chemical detoxification are addressed below.

10.3.6 BLOOD–BRAIN BARRIER

Formed by the tight junctions of capillary endothelial cells and surrounded by basement membrane and an additional layer of neuroglial cells, the blood-brain barrier (BBB) imposes a formidable hindrance to the passage of molecules. Although often misconstrued as an anatomical structure, it is primarily a physiologically functional entity, selectively allowing passage of few water-soluble molecules, ions, and glucose (by active transport). It is sufficiently impermeable to most compounds, including cells, proteins, and chemicals. Lipid-soluble chemicals, such as oxygen, carbon dioxide, alcohol, anesthetics, and the opioid analgesics, enjoy relatively easy access to the central nervous system via the intact BBB. When the BBB loses its barrier function, as in bacterial or viral encephalitis, the compromised membrane is then susceptible to unregulated entry.

10.3.7 PLACENTA

The placenta is fully developed by the third month of pregnancy and is formed by the embryonic chorion (synctial trophoblast) and the maternal endometrium (decidua basalis). Although gases, vitamins, amino acids, small sugars, ions, as well as waste products, diffuse across or are stored in the placental membrane, viruses and lipid-soluble chemicals can access the fetus. Thus, the same principles of ionization that govern absorption of chemicals influence distribution and passage through the placenta. Nonionized, lipid-soluble substances gain access more easily than ionized, water-soluble materials. In addition, passage through to the fetal membranes does not depend on the number of placental layers formed as the fetus matures. Biotransformation properties of the placenta are addressed below.

10.4 METABOLISM (BIOTRANSFORMATION)

10.4.1 PRINCIPLES OF DETOXIFICATION

Biotransformation refers to the alteration of a chemical (xenobiotic) in biological systems.* Xenobiotic transformation plays a crucial role in maintaining homeostasis during chemical exposure. This is accomplished by converting lipid-soluble (nonpolar), nonexcretable xenobiotics to polar, water-soluble compounds accessible for elimination in the bile and urine. Thus, the outcomes of biotransformation include: facilitation of excretion, conversion of toxic parent compounds to nontoxic metab-

---

* Exogenous chemicals are often referred to as xenobiotics, when foreign substances access biological systems.

olites (known as detoxification), conversion of nontoxic parent compounds to toxic metabolites (known as bioactivation), and conversion of nonreactive compounds to reactive metabolites (pharmacological bioactivation).

10.4.2 BIOCHEMICAL PATHWAYS

Catalysts for xenobiotic transformation are incorporated into *phase I* and *phase II* reactions. Although occurring primarily in the liver, other organs such as the kidney, lung, and dermal tissue have large capacities for these reactions.

Phase I reactions involve hydrolysis, reduction, and oxidation of chemicals to more hydrophilic, usually smaller, entities. *Phase II* reactions follow with glucuronidation, sulfation, acetylation, methylation, and conjugation with amino acids of the phase I metabolites. Phase II enzymes act on hydroxyl, sulfhydril, amino, and carboxyl functional groups present on either the parent compound or the phase I metabolite. Therefore, if a functional group is present on the parent compound, phase I reactions are circumvented.*

10.4.3 ENZYMES

Enzymes used in hydrolysis phase I reactions include carboxylesterase, azo and nitro reductases, and quinone reductases. Carboxylesterases cleave carboxylic acid esters, amide, or thioesters. Azo and nitro reduction reactions incorporate two enzymes: azo (–N=N–) reductases, from intestinal flora, and liver cytochrome P450 reductases. Quinone reduction reactions involve quinone reductases and NADPH cytochrome P450 reductases. The former are involved in *two-electron* reduction reactions (detoxification), and the latter in *one-electron* reduction reactions (bioactivation).

Oxidative enzymes include alcohol dehydrogenases and cytochrome P450 oxidases. For example, alcohol dehydrogenase (ADH) and aldehyde dehydrogenases convert alcohols to corresponding aldehydes and acids, respectively.

Among *phase I* biotransformation enzymes, the cytochrome P450 system is the most versatile and ubiquitous. The enzymes are predominantly monooxygenase, heme-containing proteins, found mostly in liver microsomes and mitochondria. The enzymes are classified into families, subfamilies, or subtypes of subfamilies, according to their amino acid sequences. The enzymes catalyze the incorporation of one atom of oxygen, or facilitate the removal of one atom of hydrogen, in the substrate. Other types of enzymes involved in the P450 system are hydroxylases, dehydrogenases, esterases, N-dealkylation and oxygen transferases.

Phase II biotransformation enzymes include UDP-glucuronosyl transferase, sulfotransferases, acetyltransferases, methyltransferases, and glutathione S-transferases. Except for acetylation and methylation reactions, phase II reactions, along with enzyme cofactors, interact with different functional groups to increase hydrophilicity. Glucuronidation is the main pathway for phase II reactions. It converts nonpolar, lipid-soluble compounds to polar, water-soluble metabolites. Sulfation

---

*For instance, because of the presence of hydroxyl groups, morphine undergoes direct phase II conversion to morphine-3-glucuronide, whereas codeine must endure transformation with both phase I and II reactions.

reactions involve the transfer of sulfate groups from PAPS* to the xenobiotic, yielding sulfuric acid esters that are eliminated into the urine.

Glutathione (GSH) conjugation is responsible for detoxification (or bioactivation) of xenobiotics. GSH conjugates are excreted intact in bile, or converted to mercapturic acid in kidneys and excreted in the urine.

10.5 EXCRETION

10.5.1 URINARY

Urinary excretion represents the most important route of drug, chemical, and waste elimination in the body. Normal glomerular filtration rate (GFR, ~110 to 125 ml/min) is determined by the endothelial fenestrations (pores) formed by the visceral layer of the specialized endothelial cells of the glomerulus. The pores are coupled with the overlying glomerular basement membrane and the filtration slits of the pedicels. This "three-layer" membrane permits the passage of noncellular material, with a molecular weight cutoff of ~45 to 60 K. The filtrate is then collected in Bowman's capsule. Reabsorption follows in the proximal convoluted tubules (PCT), loop of Henle, and distal convoluted tubules (DCT). The collecting ducts have limited reabsorption and secretion capabilities. Control of the transfer of molecules back to the capillary circulation or elimination in the final filtrate depends predominantly on reabsorption and secretion processes.

As with absorption through biological membranes and distribution in physiological compartments, urinary elimination of toxicants is guided by ionic and nonionic principles. While Na^+ and glucose are actively transported or facilitated by symporters across the proximal tubules, other larger polar compounds are prevented from reabsorption back to the capillary circulation. They are eventually eliminated in the urine. Nonionic, nonpolar compounds are transported by virtue of their ability to move across phospholipid membranes. Clinically, these principles are somewhat susceptible to manipulation for reducing chemical toxicity. For instance, it has long been proposed that treatment of overdose of barbiturates (pK_a between 7.2 and 7.5) could be effectively treated with sodium bicarbonate. The mechanism of this therapeutic intervention relies, in theory, on the alkalinization of the urine, rendering the acidic drug ionic, water soluble, and more amenable to elimination. In practice, however, the buffering capacity of the plasma, coupled with a large dose of the depressant, makes this a treatment modality of last resort. Practically, abusers of cocaine or narcotic analgesics, both of which are weak bases, have taken advantage of the principles of elimination. In order to prolong intoxication with the drugs, the addictive behavior dictates ingesting large amounts of antacid preparations, thus alkalinizing the urine and increasing their reabsorption potential.

Other organic ions undergo active tubular secretion. Organic anion transporter proteins (*oat*, organic acid transporters) and organic cation transporter proteins (*oct*) both actively secrete polar molecules from capillaries to the PCT lumen. Some classic examples include the active tubular secretion of para-aminohippuric acid

---

* 3'-phosphoadenosine-5'-phosphosulfate.

(PAH) by *oat* proteins, as well as sulfonamide antibiotics and methotrexate, which compete for the same secretory pathways. Probenecid, a uricosuric agent used in the treatment of gout, competes for *oat* proteins as part of its therapeutic mechanism. While small doses of the drug actually depress the excretion of uric acid by interfering with tubular secretion but not reabsorption, larger doses depress the reabsorption of uric acid and lead to increased excretion and fall in serum levels. Similarly, small doses of probenecid decrease the renal excretion of penicillins, which compete with the same *oat* proteins, necessitating an adjustment of the antibiotic dosage regimen.

10.5.2 FECAL

With the exception of cholestyramine, a cholesterol-binding drug, and the herbicide paraquat, the presence of nonabsorbable, nontransformed xenobiotics in the feces is rare. This is because many metabolites of compounds formed in the liver are excreted into the intestinal tract via the bile. Furthermore, organic anions and cations are biotransformed and actively transported into bile by carrier mechanisms similar to those in the renal tubules.

Orally administered drugs and compounds enter the hepatic portal system and liver sinusoids, only to be extensively cleared by the liver. This pharmacokinetic phenomenon is known as *hepatic first pass elimination*. According to the principles of elimination, compounds may be classified based on their bile-to-plasma (B/P) ratio. Table 10.7 outlines the classification of representative chemicals based on this ratio. Substances with high B/P ratios are readily eliminated in bile. Drugs such as propranolol and phenobarbital are extensively removed by the liver, which explains why the oral bioavailability of these drugs is low despite complete absorption. Other drugs such as lidocaine, a local anesthetic, are extensively eliminated by first pass elimination, such that oral administration is precluded. Compounds with low B/P values are not subject to this phenomenon and maintain relatively high plasma and other compartmental concentrations.

10.5.3 PULMONARY

Gases, aerosolized molecules, and liquids with low vapor pressure are eliminated by simple diffusion via exhalation. The rate of pulmonary elimination is inversely proportional to the blood solubility of the compound. Thus, compounds with low

---

TABLE 10.7
Bile-to-Plasma Ratio of Representative Xenobiotics

Classification	Bile-to-Plasma Ratio (B/P)	Representative Compounds
Class A	1–10	Na^+, K^+, glucose
Class B	10–1000	Arsenic, bile acids, lidocaine, phenobarbital, propranolol
Class C	less than 1	Albumin, zinc, iron, gold, chromium

blood solubility, such as ethylene dioxide, have high vapor pressure, and are readily volatilized and eliminated as pulmonary effluents. Conversely, compounds with high blood solubility, such as ethanol, carbon tetrachloride, and chloroform, have low vapor pressures. Their elimination through the lungs is more a function of concentration than of solubility. Similarly, lipid-soluble general anesthetic agents have long half-lives in plasma because of their low vapor pressure and high plasma solubility.

10.5.4 MAMMARY GLANDS

The mammary glands are modified sudoriferous glands that produce lipid-laden secretion (breast milk) that is excreted during lactation. The lobules of the glands consist of alveoli surrounded by one or two layers of epithelial and myoepithelial cells anchored to a well-developed basement membrane. Unlike the BBB or the placenta, the cells do not interpose a significant barrier to transport of molecules. In addition, breast milk is a watery secretion with a significant lipid component. Consequently, both water-soluble and lipid-soluble substances are transferred through the breast milk. In particular, basic chemicals readily accumulate in the weakly acidic/alkaline environment of breast milk (pH 6.5 to 7.5). Accordingly, nursing infants are exposed to almost any substance present in the maternal circulation.

10.5.5 SECRETIONS

Elimination of chemicals through saliva, tears, hair follicles, or sudoriferous/sebaceous (sweat) glands is a function of the plasma concentration. Elimination is also influenced by liver metabolism, passage through the intestinal tract and pulmonary system, and by limited access to local glandular secretions. Thus, secretion of compounds through mucous, ophthalmic, and dermal glands is not significant. In forensic toxicology, however, some chemicals may be detected in minute concentrations in hair follicles and nails when plasma levels seem to be nonexistent. Chronic arsenic and lead poisoning have been detected by measurement of the metals bound to hair follicles and hair shafts.

REFERENCES

SUGGESTED READINGS

Medinsky, M.A. and Valentine, J.L., Principles of toxicology, in *Casarett and Doull's Toxicology: The Basic Science of Poisons*, 6th ed., Klaassen, C.D., Ed, McGraw-Hill, New York, 2001, chap. 7.

Urso, R., Blardi, P., and Giorgi, G., A short introduction to pharmacokinetics, *Eur. Rev. Med. Pharmacol. Sci.*, 6, 33, 2002.

Wijnand, H.P., Pharmacokinetic model equations for the one- and two-compartment models with first-order processes in which the absorption and exponential elimination or distribution rate constants are equal, *J. Pharmacokinet. Biopharm.*, 16, 109, 1988.

Review Articles

Barile, F.A., Dierickx, P.J., and Kristen, U., *In vitro* cytotoxicity testing for prediction of acute human toxicity, *Cell Biol. Toxicol.*, 10, 155, 1994.

Bodo, A., et al., The role of multidrug transporters in drug availability, metabolism and toxicity, *Toxicol. Lett.*, 140, 133, 2003.

Buchanan, J.R., Burka, L.T., and Melnick, R.L., Purpose and guidelines for toxicokinetic studies within the National Toxicology Program, *Environ. Health Perspect.*, 105, 468, 1997.

Cheng, H.Y. and Jusko, W.J., Relationships between steady-state and single-dose plasma drug concentrations for pharmacokinetic systems with nonlinear elimination, *Biopharm. Drug Dispos.*, 10, 513, 1989.

El-Tahtawy, A.A., et al., Evaluation of bioequivalence of highly variable drugs using clinical trial simulations. II: Comparison of single and multiple-dose trials using AUC and Cmax, *Pharm. Res.*, 15, 98, 1998.

Ikeda, M., Application of biological monitoring to the diagnosis of poisoning, *J. Toxicol. Clin. Toxicol.*, 33, 617, 1995.

Ishii, K., et al., A new pharmacokinetic model including *in vivo* dissolution and gastrointestinal transit parameters, *Biol. Pharm. Bull.*, 18, 882, 1995.

Krzyzanski, W. and Jusko, W.J., Mathematical formalism for the properties of four basic models of indirect pharmacodynamic responses, *J. Pharmacokinet. Biopharm.*, 25, 107, 1997.

Lacey, L.F., et al., Evaluation of different indirect measures of rate of drug absorption in comparative pharmacokinetic studies, *J. Pharm. Sci.*, 83, 212, 1994.

Lin, J.H., Dose-dependent pharmacokinetics: experimental observations and theoretical considerations, *Biopharm. Drug Dispos.*, 15, 1, 1994.

Lin, J.H., Species similarities and differences in pharmacokinetics, *Drug Metab. Dispos.*, 23, 1008, 1995.

Lock, E.A. and Smith, L.L., The role of mode of action studies in extrapolating to human risks in toxicology, *Toxicol. Lett.*, 140, 317, 2003.

Mahmood, I. and Miller, R., Comparison of the Bayesian approach and a limited sampling model for the estimation of AUC and Cmax: a computer simulation analysis, *Int. J. Clin. Pharmacol. Ther.*, 37, 439, 1999.

Meineke, I. and Gleiter, C.H., Assessment of drug accumulation in the evaluation of pharmacokinetic data, *J. Clin. Pharmacol.*, 38, 680, 1998.

Perri, D., et al., The kidney — the body's playground for drugs: an overview of renal drug handling with selected clinical correlates, *Can. J. Clin. Pharmacol.*, 10, 17, 2003.

Plusquellec, Y., Courbon, F., and Nogarede, S., Consequence of equal absorption, distribution and/or elimination rate constants, *Eur. J. Drug Metab. Pharmacokinet.*, 24, 197, 1999.

Poulin, P. and Theil, F.P., Prediction of pharmacokinetics prior to *in vivo* studies. II. Generic physiologically based pharmacokinetic models of drug disposition, *J. Pharm. Sci.*, 91, 1358, 2002.

Ramanathan, M., Pharmacokinetic variability and therapeutic drug monitoring actions at steady state, *Pharm. Res.*, 17, 589, 2000.

Repetto, M.R. and Repetto, M., Concentrations in human fluids: 101 drugs affecting the digestive system and metabolism, *J. Toxicol. Clin. Toxicol.*, 37, 1, 1999.

Rogers, J.F., Nafziger, A.N., and Bertino, J.S. Jr., Pharmacogenetics affects dosing, efficacy, and toxicity of cytochrome P450-metabolized drugs, *Am. J. Med.*, 113, 746, 2002.

Schall, R. and Luus, H.G., Comparison of absorption rates in bioequivalence studies of immediate release drug formulations, *Int. J. Clin. Pharmacol. Ther. Toxicol.,* 30, 153, 1992.

Scharman, E.J., Methods used to decrease lithium absorption or enhance elimination, *J. Toxicol. Clin. Toxicol.,* 35, 601, 1997.

Part II

Toxicity of Therapeutic Agents

11 Sedative/Hypnotics

11.1 BARBITURATES

11.1.1 History and Classification

From the beginning of the twentieth century, bromides enjoyed a significant role in the U.S. as sedatives. With the advent of barbiturates in the 1940s, the use of bromides waned. Since then, barbiturates have been used traditionally for the alleviation of pain, anxiety, hypertension, epilepsy, and psychiatric disorders. Eventually, use of barbiturates would be replaced by other sedative-hypnotics (S/H) of comparable strength, namely chloral hydrate and meprobamate. Benzodiazepines would replace the traditional S/H as more effective, less toxic, and less addictive anxiolytics (sedatives). Today, the most popular therapeutic agents for anxiety (used for sedation), hypnosis (used for sleep), or anesthesia (for deep sleep) include buspirone (Buspar®) and zolpidem (Ambien®). Benzodiazepines are still frequently employed. With the strict enforcement of federal and state controlled substances regulations, barbiturates have lost significant influence in both the therapeutic and illicit drug markets. Nevertheless, they are still the cause of 50,000 accidental and intentional poisonings per year, and their synergistic effects with ethanol are one of the leading causes of hospital admissions.

11.1.2 Medicinal Chemistry

Barbiturates are malonylurea derivatives (diureides), synthesized from malonic acid and urea (Figure 11.1). The electron negative carbonyl carbons confer an acidic nature to the molecule, thus classifying them as weak acids. Allyl, alkyl, and allocyclic side chains determine their pharmacological classification.

11.1.3 Pharmacology and Clinical Use

Pharmacologically and clinically, barbiturates are classified according to their duration of effect. The presence of longer and bulkier aliphatic and allocyclic side chains (Table 11.1) produces compounds that range from ultrashort-, short-, and intermediate to long-acting. Their major action is the production of sedation, hypnosis, or anesthesia through central nervous system (CNS) depression. The effect, however, depends largely on the dose, mental status of the patient or individual at the time of ingestion, duration of action of the drug, the physical environment while under the influence, and tolerance of the individual to this class of drugs. These factors determine the probability of a therapeutic or euphoric response. For instance, a 100-mg dose of secobarbital ingested in the home at bedtime to induce sleep would, most likely, only cause a mild euphoria in a habitual user at a social gathering, without significant sedation.

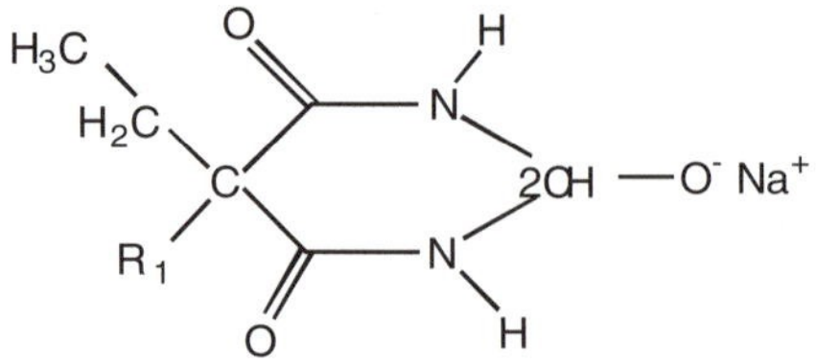

FIGURE 11.1 Structure of prototype barbiturate.

11.1.4 TOXICOKINETICS AND METABOLISM

In general, an increase in the number of carbons and bulkier side chains results in enhanced lipid solubility, with a corresponding increase in toxicity. Attachment of a methylbutyl (1-mb) and replacement of the C_2 with a sulfur group (as with thiopental) decreases its electron negativity, making it less acidic, more lipid soluble. Consequently, thiopental is an ultrashort-acting barbiturate used exclusively as a preoperative sedative/hypnotic.

As a class, the barbiturates are largely nonionic, lipid-soluble compounds, and their pK_a ranges between 7.2 and 7.9. The dissociation constants, therefore, do not account for differences in duration of action, especially with the long-acting compounds. Rapid movement into and out of the CNS appears to determine rapid onset and short duration. Conversely, the barbiturates with the slowest onset and longest duration of action contain the most polar side chains (ethyl and phenyl with phenobarbital structure, Table 11.1). Thus, the structure in Table 11.1 dictates that phenobarbital enters and leaves the CNS very slowly as compared to the more lipophilic thiopental (with intermediate pK_a). In addition, the lipid barriers to drug metabolizing enzymes lead to a slower metabolism for the more polar barbiturates, considering that phenobarbital is metabolized to the extent of 10% per day. Similarly, distribution in biological compartments, especially the CNS, is governed by lipid solubility.

Metabolism of oxybarbiturates occurs primarily in liver, whereas thiobarbiturates are also metabolized, to a limited extent, in kidney and brain. Phase I reactions introduce polar groups at the C5 position of oxybarbiturates, transforming the radicals to alcohols, ketones, and carboxylic acids. These inactive metabolites are eliminated in urine as glucuronide conjugates. Thiobarbiturates undergo desulfuration, to corresponding oxybarbiturates, and opening of the barbituric acid ring. Side chain oxidation at the C5 position is the most important biotransformation reaction leading to drug detoxification.

11.1.5 MECHANISM OF TOXICITY

CNS depression accounts for all of the toxic manifestations of barbiturate poisoning. The drugs bind to an allosteric site on the GABA-Cl⁻ ionophore complex (γ-aminobutyric acid), an inhibitory neurotransmitter, in presynaptic or postsynaptic neuronal terminals in the CNS. This complex formation prolongs the opening of the chloride channel. Ultimately, by binding to $GABA_A$ receptors, barbiturates diminish the action of facilitated neurons and enhance the action of inhibitory neurons.

TABLE 11.1
Properties of Barbiturates

Compounds[a]	R₁	Classification	Sedative/Hypnotic Dose (Total mg Daily)	Toxic Concentration (mg/dl)	t₁/₂ (h)	pKa
Barbital	ethyl	LA	100–200/300–500	6–8	–	7.8
Phenobarbital	phenyl	LA	30–90/100–200	4–6	24–140	7.2
Amobarbital	isopentyl	IA	30–150/100–200	1–3	8–42	7.8
Pentobarbital	1-mb	SA	20–150/100	0.5–1.0	16–48	7.9
Secobarbital[b]	1-mb	SA	30–200/100	0.5–1.0	20–34	7.9
Thiopental	1-mb, C₂=S	UA	3–5 mg/kg	<0.5	<1	7.4

Note: R₁ = side group substitutions corresponding to Figure 11.1; 1-mb = 1-methylbutyl; LA = long-acting, IA = intermediate-acting, SA = short-acting, UA = ultrashort-acting.

[a] Grouped according to classification.
[b] The ethyl group for secobarbital is replaced by an allyl side chain.

Barbiturates concomitantly stimulate the release of GABA at sensitive synapses. Thus, the chemicals have GABA-like effects by decreasing the activity of facilitated neurons and enhancing inhibitory GABA-ergic neurons.

Two major consequences account for the toxic manifestations:

1. Barbiturates decrease postsynaptic depolarization by acetylcholine, with ensuing postsynaptic block, resulting in smooth, skeletal, and cardiac muscle depression.
2. At higher doses, barbiturates depress medullary respiratory centers, resulting in inhibition of all three respiratory drives.

The **neurogenic drive**, important in maintaining respiratory rhythm during sleep, is initially inhibited. Interference with carotid and aortic chemoreceptors and pH homeostasis disrupts the **chemical drive**. Lastly, interruption of carotid and aortic baroreceptors results in a decreased **hypoxic drive** for respiration. Thus, with increasing depth of depression of the CNS, the dominant respiratory drive shifts to the chemical and hypoxic drives.

11.1.6 SIGNS AND SYMPTOMS OF ACUTE TOXICITY

Signs and symptoms of barbiturate poisoning are related directly to CNS and cardiovascular depression. Reactions are dose-dependent and vary from mild sedation to complete paralysis. Clinical signs and symptoms are more reliable indicators of clinical toxicity than plasma concentrations. This is especially true when CNS depression does not correlate with plasma concentrations, an indication that other CNS depressants may be involved.

At the highest doses, blockade of sympathetic ganglia triggers hypotension, bradycardia, and decreased inotropy, with consequent decreased cardiac output. In addition, inhibition of medullary vasomotor centers induces arteriolar and venous dilation, further complicating the cerebral hypoxia and cardiac depression. Respiratory acidosis results from accumulation of carbon dioxide, shifting pH balance to the formation of carbonic acid. The condition resembles alcoholic inebriation as the patient presents with hypoxic shock, rapid but shallow pulse, cold and sweaty skin (hypothermia), and either slow, or rapid, shallow breathing. Responsiveness and depth of coma are evaluated according to the guidelines for the four stages of coma (see Chapter 3).

11.1.7 CLINICAL MANAGEMENT OF ACUTE OVERDOSE

Treatment of overdose is symptomatic and follows the general guidelines adapted from the Scandinavian method for symptomatic treatment for CNS depressants. This includes maintaining adequate ventilation, keeping the patient warm, and supporting vital functions. To this end, oxygen support, forced diuresis, and administration of volume expanders has been shown to maintain blood pressure and adequate kidney perfusion and prevent circulatory collapse. If fewer than 24 h have elapsed since ingestion, gastric lavage, induction of apomorphine emesis, delivery of a saline cathartic or administration of activated charcoal, enhances elimination and decreases absorption, respectively. In particular, multidose activated charcoal (MDAC) increases the clearance and decreases the half-life of phenobarbital. Alkalinization of the urine to a pH of 7.5 to 8.0 increases clearance of long-acting barbiturates, while short- and intermediate-acting compounds are not affected by changes in urine pH.

Should renal or cardiac failure, electrolyte abnormalities, or acid-base disturbances occur, hemodialysis is recommended. Although most cases of phenobarbital overdose respond well to cardiopulmonary supportive care, severe cases will also require hemodialysis or charcoal hemoperfusion. Neither of these procedures will remove significant amounts of short- or intermediate-acting barbiturates. Through ion exchange, hemodialysis is more effective in removing long-acting barbiturates than short-acting compounds because there is less protein and lipid binding of the former. If renal and cardiac function are satisfactory, alkalinization of the urine and plasma with sodium bicarbonate promotes ionization of the acidic compounds. This maneuver hastens their excretion, provided that reabsorption and protein and lipid binding are minimized. Incorporation of CNS stimulants or vasopressors in the treatment protocol is not recommended, since mortality rates from pharmacological antagonism are as high as 40%.

Even with complete recovery, complications affect prognosis. This includes the development of pulmonary edema and bronchopneumonia, infiltration with lung abscesses, and renal shutdown.

11.1.8 TOLERANCE AND WITHDRAWAL

Pharmacodynamic tolerance (functional or adaptive) contributes to the decreased effect of barbiturates, even after a single dose. With chronic administration of gradually increasing doses, pharmacodynamic tolerance continues to develop over a period of weeks to months, as the homeostatic feedback response to depression is activated in the presence of the compounds. Interestingly, no concomitant increase in LD_{50} is observed; rather, as tolerance increases, the therapeutic index decreases.

Pharmacokinetic tolerance (drug dispositional) contributes less to the development of this phenomenon. Enhanced metabolic transformation and induction of hepatic microsomal enzymes ensues subsequent to pharmacodynamic tolerance, of which the former reaches a peak after a few days. In either situation, the effective dose of a barbiturate is increased six-fold, a rate which is primarily accounted for by the production of pharmacodynamic tolerance.

Sudden withdrawal of barbiturates from addicted individuals runs the risk of development of hallucinations, sleeplessness, vertigo, and convulsions, depending upon the degree of dependency.

11.2 BENZODIAZEPINES

11.2.1 INCIDENCE

The introduction of chlordiazepoxide in 1961 started the era of the benzodiazepines. Although this class of S/H did not render the barbiturates obsolete, the benzodiaz-

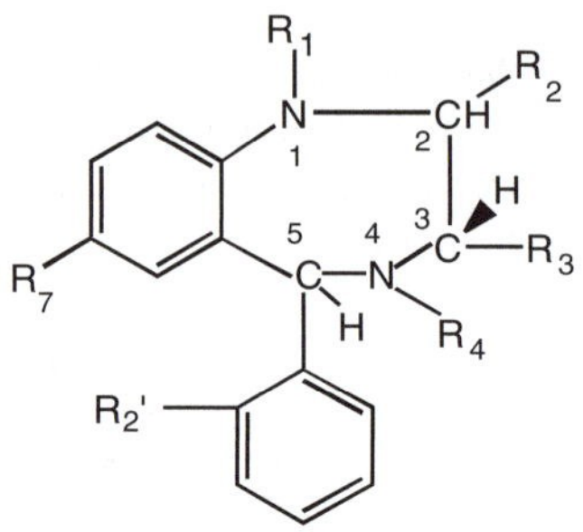

FIGURE 11.2 Structure of prototype benzodiazepine.

epines have since enjoyed wide use as S/H, anxiolytics, anticonvulsants, preanesthetic sedatives and muscle relaxants. Their increased therapeutic index, relative to
barbiturates, and lack of anesthetic properties have promoted the substitution of
benzodiazepines for barbiturates.

11.2.2 MEDICINAL CHEMISTRY

Figure 11.2 illustrates the 5-aryl-1,4-benzodiazepine structure. All the important
benzodiazepines currently in use (Table 11.2) contain a 5-aryl or 5-cyclohexenyl
moiety. The chemical nature of substituents at positions 1 and 3 varies widely. Their
half-life correlates well with their duration of action, as well as duration of toxic
manifestations. Structure-activity relationship, however, has failed to correlate the
pharmacological and toxicological profiles with the chemical structure.

11.2.3 PHARMACOLOGY AND MECHANISM OF TOXICITY

Benzodiazepines bind to all three omega receptor subtypes in the areas of the limbic
system, thalamus, and hypothalamus. Benzodiazepines bind to an allosteric site of the
α and/or β subunits of the GABA$_A$-Cl$^-$ ionophore complex. This action increases the
frequency of the opening of the chloride channels. Ultimately, the drugs enhance the
affinity of GABA for GABA$_A$ receptors and potentiate the effects of GABA throughout
the nervous system. The effects of GABA-mediated actions account for benzodiazepines' sedative/hypnotic, anticonvulsant, and skeletal muscle relaxation properties.

At high doses, benzodiazepines induce neuromuscular blockade and cause
vasodilation and hypotension (after i.v. administration). The compounds do not
significantly alter ventilation, except in patients with respiratory complications, in
the elderly population, and in the presence of alcohol or other S/H. There is also
minimal effect on cardiovascular integrity.

11.2.4 TOXICOKINETICS

With the exception of clorazepate (Table 11.2), all of the benzodiazepines are
completely absorbed, primarily due to their high nonionic/ionic ratio. Lipophilicity,
however, does not account for the variation in polarity and electron negativity
conferred by the various substituents.

TABLE 11.2
Properties of Benzodiazepines

Generic Name[a]	Proprietary Name	Classification	Sedative/Hypnotic Total Daily Dosage (mg)	Toxic Concentration	$t_{1/2}$ (h)
Alprazolam	Xanax	Anxiolytic	0.25–1.5/0.5–1.0	0.4 µg/dl	12–19
Chlordiazepoxide	Librium	Anxiolytic	5–100/25–50	3.5–10 mg/l	7–28
Clorazepate	Tranxene	Anxiolytic-S/H	3.75–22.5/7.5–15	—	30–60
Diazepam	Valium	Anxiolytic-S/H, SKR, anticonvulsant	2–40/5–10	0.5–2.0 mg/dl	20–90
Flurazepam	Dalmane	Hypnotic	—/15–30	0.25 mg/dl	24–100
Lorazepam	Ativan	Anxiolytic-S/H, anticonvulsant	0.5–3.0/2–4	0.3 µg/dl	10–20
Oxazepam	Serax	Anxiolytic-S/H	10–120/10–30	3–5 mg/l	5–10
Temazepam	Restoril	S/H	—/7.5–30	1.0 mg/l	9–12
Triazolam	Halcion	Anxiolytic-S/H	0.25–1.5/0.125–0.5	7 µg/kg (toxic dose)	2–3

Note: S/H = sedative/hypnotic; SKR = skeletal muscle relaxant.

[a] Grouped by generic name.

11.2.5 Signs and Symptoms of Acute Toxicity

Although signs and symptoms are generally nonspecific, apparent toxicity depends on the extent of intoxication. Serum toxic concentrations of benzodiazepines do not correlate well with signs and symptoms, and are generally listed as "cutoff" points (Table 11.2).

Mild toxicity is characterized by ataxia, drowsiness, and motor incoordination. Psychologically, the patient displays different degrees of paranoia or erratic behavior and is easily aroused. In moderate toxicity, the patient is aroused by verbal stimulation, although he or she may enter coma stage one or two. Patients in severe toxicity are unresponsive except to deep pain stimulation, consistent with coma stage one or two. In general, respiratory depression and hypotension are rare.

11.2.6 Clinical Management of Acute Overdose

Clinical management is symptomatic, and may also incorporate the use of a specific antidote. Flumazenil, a 1,4-imidazobenzodiazepine, is a benzodiazepine antagonist. It competitively antagonizes the binding and allosteric effects of benzodiazepines. Flumazenil completely reverses the sedative, anxiolytic, anticonvulsant, ataxic, anesthetic, comatose, and muscle relaxant effects. Administration of 0.2 to 1.0 mg i.v. has an acute onset of 1 to 3 min and a peak effect at 6 to 10 min. Routine use of flumazenil, however, must allow for the determination of concomitant drug ingestion. The presence of stimulants such as cocaine, amphetamine, or tricyclic antidepressants precludes the routine use of the antidote, since the anticonvulsant effects of a benzodiazepine may be negated by flumazenil.

11.2.7 Tolerance and Withdrawal

Cross tolerance to barbiturates and alcohol has been noted with benzodiazepines, although the withdrawal syndrome is not as severe in the former and is slower in onset (as long as 2 weeks). Interestingly, depending on the dose, flumazenil administration can precipitate acute withdrawal in benzodiazepine-addicted individuals. As with barbiturates and alcohol, benzodiazepine withdrawal signs and symptoms are similar.

11.3 MISCELLANEOUS SEDATIVE/HYPNOTICS

11.3.1 Chloral Hydrate

Although it has no analgesic effect, and more effective, less toxic drugs are available, chloral hydrate is still used therapeutically as a S/H.* Currently available in oral liquid dosage forms only, the compound is lipid soluble, and is a derivative of chloral betaine and triclofos (see structure, Figure 11.3). The long-acting metabolite of chloral hydrate, trichloroethanol, is responsible for most of its toxicity, its low

---

* The mixture of chloral hydrate and ethanol is called a *Mickey Finn* or knock-out drops. The drink was popularized as such in classic early twentieth century films for its dramatic and instantaneous hypnotic effect.

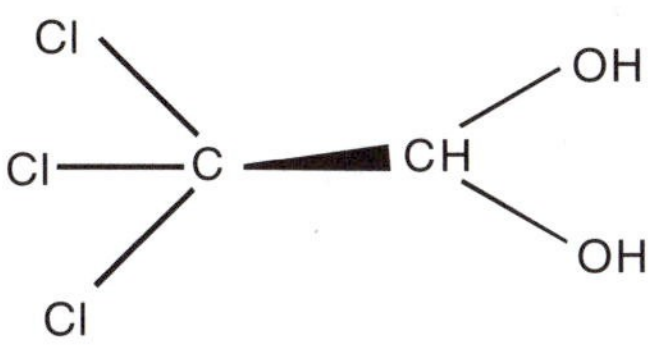

FIGURE 11.3 Structure of chloral hydrate.

therapeutic index, and its undetectable presence in plasma. Signs and symptoms of toxicity include: CNS depression, ataxia, gastrointestinal irritation, cardiovascular instability, and proteinuria. In addition, chloral hydrate significantly impairs myocardial contractility by sensitizing the myocardium to catecholamines. An increased risk of sudden death with chloral hydrate intoxication is a result of the development of arrhythmias. Beta-blockers, such as propranolol, are recommended in ameliorating chloral hydrate-induced cardiac arrhythmias. Recently, chloral hydrate has been implicated as a carcinogen, although this finding remains controversial.

11.3.2 MEPROBAMATE (MILTOWN®, EQUANIL®)

A propanediol carbamate derivative, meprobamate is still marketed as an alternative S/H to barbiturates. It enjoyed some popularity until the introduction of benzodiazepines, yet its toxicity is similar to that of the barbiturates, including the production of ataxia and coma. Chronic use of the drug has been associated with severe hematopoietic disturbances such as aplastic anemia and thrombocytopenia.

11.3.3 ZOLPIDEM TARTRATE (AMBIEN®)

Zolpidem is a nonbenzodiazepine hypnotic of the imidazopyridine class. It interacts with the GABA-BZ receptor complex and shares some of the pharmacological properties of the benzodiazepines. In contrast to the latter, zolpidem binds preferentially to the ω_1 receptor. This receptor is found primarily in the midbrain, brain stem, and thalamic regions. The selective binding to the ω_1 receptors explains the relative absence of muscle relaxation, anticonvulsant activity, and induction of deep sleep. The drug is relatively safe, as large ingestions produce mostly drowsiness. Coma and respiratory failure are rare.

11.3.4 BUSPIRONE (BUSPAR®)

Buspirone is an antianxiety agent that is not chemically or pharmacologically related to the benzodiazepines, barbiturates, or other S/H drugs. It does not exert anticonvulsant or muscle relaxant effects, nor does it interact with GABA receptors. Instead, it has high affinity for serotonin (5-HT$_{1A}$) and dopamine (D$_2$) receptors. It is indicated for the management of anxiety disorders characterized by motor tension, autonomic hyperactivity, apprehensive expectation, and vigilance and scanning (hyperattentiveness). Additive effects with ethanol are minimal. It has not been associated with the production of dependence or withdrawal, and unlike the barbiturates and benzodiazepines, buspirone is not a federally controlled substance.

11.3.5 Flunitrazepam (Rohypnol®)

Although flunitrazepam is used internationally in the treatment of insomnia and as a preanesthetic benzodiazepine, it is a U.S. federal schedule I controlled substance with no legitimate therapeutic or prescribing uses. The tablets are tasteless, odorless, relatively inexpensive, dissolve rapidly in alcohol, and are easily administered by intranasal or oral routes. Flunitrazepam has been used as a "date-rape" drug for its intoxicating and amnestic effects.* The agent causes euphoria, hallucinations, and disinhibiting effects, and has also been used to enhance heroin and cocaine euphoria. It is highly lipid soluble, with a quick onset (20 to 30 min) and a duration of up to 12 h. It affects GABA$_A$ receptors with a potency of up to ten times that of diazepam. Consequently, drowsiness, disorientation, and dizziness ("DDD"), slurred speech, and nausea can progress rapidly to amnesia, psychomotor impairment, respiratory depression and coma. Treatment is supportive, with respiratory maintenance of primary importance (ABCs). Flumazenil is used as an antidote for the respiratory depression, except in the presence of stimulants.

11.3.6 GHB (Gamma-Hydroxybutyrate)

Since its synthesis in 1960, GHB has been promoted and abused for sleep disorders (narcolepsy), as an anesthetic agent, as treatment for alcohol and opiate withdrawal, and currently, as an inducer of growth hormone (bodybuilding) and an aphrodisiac. The tasteless, odorless, liquid or gel, makes it convenient for use as a "date-rape" drug.

Pharmacologically, GHB interacts with GABA-B and GHB receptors, as well as opioid receptors, resulting in a predominant CNS depression. It has a quick onset (15–30 min) and relatively short duration (3 h). Most users of GHB report that it induces a pleasant state of relaxation and tranquility. Frequent effects are a tranquil mental state, mild euphoria, emotional warmth, well-being, and a tendency to verbalize. Ingestion of GHB in an alcoholic drink by an unsuspecting victim, however, causes hallucinations and amnesia, as well as symptoms not unlike flunitrazepam. Alcohol potentiates the depressant and adverse reactions, including dizziness, nausea, vomiting, respiratory collapse, seizures, coma, and possibly death.

At higher doses in the absence of alcohol, its toxicity outweighs the euphoric effects. Within 15 min of ingestion, the individual experiences marked agitation upon stimulation, apnea, hypoxia, and vomiting. This is followed by dose-dependent respiratory depression, bradycardia, involuntary muscle contractions, decreased cardiac output, coma, and amnesia.

As with flunitrazepam, treatment of GHB toxicity is supportive, with respiratory maintenance of primary importance (ABCs).

---

* According to the U.S. Department of Justice, "drug-facilitated rape," or acquaintance rape, is defined as the sexual assault of a woman who is incapacitated or unconscious while under the influence of a mind-altering drug and/or alcohol. The victim of a drug-facilitated sexual assault may exhibit signs of confusion, memory loss, drowsiness, impaired judgment, slurred speech, and uninhibited behavior. Suspicion of acquaintance rape is based on clinical history and emergency department presentation.

Withdrawal symptoms are significant. The addicted individual experiences profuse sweating, anxiety attacks, and increased blood pressure a few hours after the last dose. The reactions may subside after several days, depending on the depth of addiction, or may be followed by a second phase of hallucinations and altered mental state.

11.3.7 Ethchlorvynol (Placidyl®), Methaqualone (Quaalude®), Glutethimide (Doriden®), Methyprylon (Noludar®)

Historically, these compounds were associated with significant toxic potential and abuse, and their popularity in the illicit drug market soared in the 1960s. The compounds, however, are no longer available therapeutically and have not resurfaced as drugs of abuse since. Their toxicology is thoroughly discussed in review articles.

11.4 METHODS OF DETECTION

Urine screening is useful for detecting many illicit drugs except flunitrazepam, which requires specific analysis. Because of their short half-life and low concentrations, most commercially available toxicology screens are unable to detect flunitrazepam or GHB used in acquaintance rape. The most definitive detection of flunitrazepam is gas chromatography-mass spectrometry (GC-MS). Many states are developing programs to analyze for date rape drugs as part of sexual assault kits.

The immunoassays, enzyme-multiplied immunoassay technique (EMIT) and radioimmunoassay (RIA), are designed to identify unmetabolized secobarbital in the urine. Both assays will detect other commonly encountered barbiturates as well, depending on the concentration of drug present in the sample. Positive tests for phenobarbital have been noted in chronic users up to several weeks after discontinuation. Thin layer chromatography (TLC) is less sensitive than most chromatographic techniques but can demonstrate the presence of barbiturates up to 30 h. Some reliable methods used for confirmation of the barbiturates include gas chromatography with flame ionization detection after derivatization (GC/FID), GC with nitrogen phosphorus detection (GC/NPD), and GC with mass spectroscopy (GC/MS).

Benzodiazepines are generally detected as a structural class. A broad spectrum of analytical methods, including GC, HPLC, TLC, GLC/MS, RIA, and EMIT, has been reported for the analysis of the benzodiazepines. Many benzodiazepines have common metabolites; therefore, it is not always possible to determine the specific drug taken through the use of urine testing. The EMIT screening procedure rapidly recognizes oxazepam, a common and specific metabolite of many benzodiazepines. Other screening procedures, such as TLC and HPLC, are used to detect benzodiazepines in urine alone or in combination with other major drugs of abuse. RIA methods are sensitive enough for the determination of diazepam directly in microsamples of blood, plasma, and saliva, for up to 16 h following oral administration of a single 5-mg dose. Confirmation of positive results from tests performed with immunoassay or TLC may be difficult. More specific GC and GC/MS procedures may not be able to confirm the metabolites screened with TLC.

REFERENCES

SUGGESTED READINGS

Goldberg, H.L., Benzodiazepine and nonbenzodiazepine anxiolytics, *Psychopathology,* 17, 45, 1984.

Nemeroff, C.B., Anxiolytics: past, present, and future agents, *J. Clin. Psychiatry,* 64, 3, 2003.

Rossoff, I.S., *Encyclopedia of Clinical Toxicology,* Parthenon/CRC Press, Boca Raton, FL, 2002.

Schulz, M. and Schmoldt, A., Therapeutic and toxic blood concentrations of more than 500 drugs, *Pharmazie,* 52, 895, 1997.

REVIEW ARTICLES

Ashton, H., Guidelines for the rational use of benzodiazepines. When and what to use, *Drugs,* 48, 25, 1994.

Bailey, D.N., Methaqualone ingestion: evaluation of present status, *J. Anal. Toxicol.,* 5, 279, 1981.

Barbey, J.T. and Roose SP. SSRI safety in overdose, *J. Clin. Psychiatry,* 59, 42, 1998.

Beebe, D.K. and Walley, E., Substance abuse: the designer drugs, *Am. Fam. Physician,* 43, 1689, 1991.

Druid, H., Holmgren, P., and Ahlner, J., Flunitrazepam: an evaluation of use, abuse and toxicity, *Forensic Sci. Int.,* 122, 136, 2001.

Elko, C.J., Burgess, J.L., and Robertson W.O., Zolpidem-associated hallucinations and serotonin reuptake inhibition: a possible interaction, *J. Toxicol. Clin. Toxicol.,* 36, 195, 1998.

ElSohly, M.A. and Salamone, S.J., Prevalence of drugs used in cases of alleged sexual assault, *J. Anal. Toxicol.,* 23, 141, 1999.

Freese, T.E., Miotto, K., and Reback, C.J., The effects and consequences of selected club drugs, *J. Subst. Abuse Treat.,* 23, 151, 2002.

Gary, N.E. and Tresznewsky, O., Clinical aspects of drug intoxication: barbiturates and a potpourri of other sedatives, hypnotics, and tranquilizers, *Heart Lung,* 12, 122, 1983.

Giri, A.K. and Banerjee, S., Genetic toxicology of four commonly used benzodiazepines, *Mutat. Res.,* 340, 93, 1996.

Kellogg, C.K., Drugs and chemicals that act on the central nervous system: interpretation of experimental evidence, *Prog. Clin. Biol. Res.,* 163, 147, 1985.

Kosten, T.R. and O'Connor, P.G., Management of drug and alcohol withdrawal, *N. Engl. J. Med.,* 348, 1786, 2003.

Lydiard, R.B., The role of GABA in anxiety disorders, *J. Clin. Psychiatry.,* 64, 21, 2003.

Miller, N.S. and Gold, M.S., Benzodiazepines: reconsidered, *Adv. Alcohol Subst. Abuse,* 8, 67, 1990.

O'Connell, T., Kaye, L. and Plosay, J.J. III, Gamma-hydroxybutyrate (GHB): a newer drug of abuse, *Am. Fam. Physician,* 62, 2478, 2000.

Smith, K.M., Larive, L.L. and Romanelli, F., Club drugs: methylenedioxymethamphetamine, flunitrazepam, ketamine hydrochloride, and gamma-hydroxybutyrate, *Am. J. Health Syst. Pharm.,* 59, 1067, 2002.

Stewart, S.H. and Westra, H.A., Benzodiazepine side-effects: from the bench to the clinic, *Curr. Pharm. Des.,* 8, 1, 2002.

Tanaka, E., Toxicological interactions between alcohol and benzodiazepines, *J. Toxicol. Clin. Toxicol.,* 40, 69, 2002.

Traub, S.J., Nelson, L.S., Hoffman, R.S., Physostigmine as a treatment for gamma-hydroxybutyrate toxicity, *J. Toxicol. Clin. Toxicol.,* 40, 781, 2002.

12 Opioids and Derivatives

12.1 OPIOIDS

12.1.1 HISTORY AND CLASSIFICATION

There has been no greater disruption of modern civilizations than the insidious havoc brought upon them by the addictive potential of opioid compounds and their derivatives. From the introduction of opium into China in the seventeenth century, resulting in the undermining of its organized system, to the modern-day pharmaceutical production of synthetic narcotic analgesics, these compounds have infiltrated urban and rural societies alike. Today, narcotic addiction permeates all socioeconomic classes, from economically underserved communities, to affluent neighborhoods, to the U.S. armed forces. The number of emergency department (ED) visits involving heroin/morphine increased 15% in 2000, from 84,409 to 97,287, accounting for 15% of all hospital admissions related to drug use. Opioid analgesics are readily and easily available. These compounds are not necessarily obtained only through illicit drug dealing (street drugs), but their supply is also abundant through fraudulent and illegitimate prescriptions, as well as in the course of overprescribing practices. Health care professionals are also particularly vulnerable to the addictive potential of narcotics, principally due to easy accessibility.

The variety of opioid derivatives encountered in the twentieth century reflects the cyclical appearance and disappearance of individual compounds, mostly because of popularity among users and availability. In the 1980s, opioid addicts inadvertently ingested what they thought was a designer derivative of meperidine (4'-methyl-α-pyrrolidinopropiophenone, MPPP). Instead, synthesis and contamination with 1-methyl-4-phenyl-1,2,3,6-tetrahydropyridine (MPTP) lead to the development of an idiopathic Parkinson-like state in these patients. In the same decade, a new more potent form of heroin from Mexico (Black tar heroin) made its appearance, resulting in an increase in acute overdose fatalities. Simultaneously during this period, heroin usage began to wane, only to be replaced with the more versatile forms of cocaine. Despite the counter-effects of narcotic law enforcement efforts to remove or dissuade its nontherapeutic use, opioid use is still a major public health problem.

Initial narcotic ingestion is often an unpleasant experience. Patients usually complain of nausea, dizziness, and muscular weakness. With continued use, individuals build tolerance to the unpleasant adverse reactions in preference to the euphoric effects. Opioid compounds are ingested orally in tablet or capsule form, the most common method of administration (considering both therapeutic and illicit drug use). As greater tolerance develops, ingesting the same amount of drug does not produce euphoria as initially experienced, necessitating either higher doses or an alternate, more immediate method of administration. This includes rendering the tablets to a powder, or using a preformulated powder form, for nasal insufflation (*snorting*), for injection subcutaneously (*skin popping*) or intravenously (*mainlining*).

12.1.2 CLASSIFICATION

By definition opioids, as a class, exert their pharmacological effects at opioid receptors, whereas opiates are alkaloid extracts of the opium poppy. The opioids are traditionally classified according to their source, as summarized in Table 12.1. Opium, the parent crude form of the naturally-occurring compounds, is derived from the milky exudates of the unripe capsule of *Papaver somniferum L.* (opium poppy). The plant is cultivated in the Mediterranean and Middle East regions, India, and China. About two dozen alkaloids, of which morphine occupies about 10%, are formed primarily in various cells of the poppy plant and excreted into the lactiferous ducts. Depending on diurnal variations, the isolated latex undergoes alkaloid biosynthesis and metabolic destruction, which contribute to the variability in alkaloid composition of crude opium samples.* The narcotic, antispasmodic, sedative, hypnotic, and analgesic properties of the extract have been recognized for centuries. Interestingly, the numerous and very small seeds of the plant do not contain opium.

Few pharmacological and toxicological differences exist between the classes. Some pharmacokinetic properties, however, distinguish the compounds, especially among the many narcotic derivatives (listed below).

12.1.3 MEDICINAL CHEMISTRY

Table 12.1 illustrates the structure of morphine and side chains of the derivatives. The opioids are composed of six-membered saturated heterocyclic rings forming the phenanthrene nucleus (in bold) to which is attached a piperidine ring. The structure represents the prototype for all opioids except methadone and meperidine (Table 12.2). Although the more important opiate alkaloids exhibit a phenanthrene nucleus, the majority of the derivatives have the isoquinoline ring structure. Esterification of the phenolic functions, such as in the formation of diacetylmorphine, results in a compound with increased lipid solubility and increased potency and toxicity.

12.1.4 MECHANISM OF TOXICITY

The mechanism of opiate toxicity is an extension of its pharmacology and is directly related to interaction with stereospecific and saturable binding sites or receptors in the CNS and other tissues. These receptors are classified according to the empirical observations noted for the variety of opioid effects. The opioid receptors are biologically active sites of several endogenous ligands, including the two pentapeptides, methionine-enkephalin and leucine-enkephalin. Several larger polypeptides that bind to opioid receptors, such as β-endorphin, are the most potent of the endogenous opioid-like substances.** In addition, three receptor classes have been identified:

---

* In non-Western medicine, opium refers to the dried capsule from which the latex has been extracted.
** Collectively, the term *endorphin* refers to the three families of endogenous opioid peptides: the enkephalins, the dynorphins, and the β-endorphins.

TABLE 12.1

Categories, Structure (of Morphine), and Proprietary Names of Opiate Analgesics, Derivatives, and Narcotic Antagonists Currently Available

Category	Compound	Proprietary Name	3[a]	6[a]	14[a]	N17[a]	Other[d]
Naturally occurring	Morphine	Various	OH	OH	H	CH$_3$	—
	Codeine (methylmorphine)	Various	O–CH$_3$	OH	H	CH$_3$	—
Semisynthetic	Diacetylmorphine	Heroin[b]	OCO–CH$_3$	OCO–CH$_3$	H	CH$_3$	—
	Oxymorphone	Numorphan	OH	=O	OH	CH$_3$	Single bond
	Hydromorphone	Dilaudid	OH	=O	H	CH$_3$	Single bond
Synthetic	Oxycodon	Percodan,[c] Percocet,[c] Oxycontin	O–CH$_3$	=O	OH	CH$_3$	Single bond
	Levorphanol	Levo-dromoran	OH	H	H	CH$_3$	Single bond no O
	Hydrocodone	Vicodin, Lorcet, Hycodan[c]	O–CH$_3$	=O	H	CH$_3$	Single bond
Narcotic antagonists	Naloxone	Narcan	OH	=O	OH	CH$_2$CH=CH$_2$	Single bond
	Naltrexone	Trexan	OH	=O	OH	CH$_2$–Δ	Single bond
	Nalmefene	Revex	OH	=CH$_2$	OH	CH$_2$–Δ	Single bond

[a] Numbers 3, 6, 14 and 17 refer to the positions in the phenanthrene nucleus; only morphine and diacetylmorphine have the C7-C8 double bond.

[b] Street name.

[c] Component of a formulation.

[d] Other = single bond between C7-C8, no O between C4-C5.

TABLE 12.2
Categories, Structural Features, and Proprietary Names of Meperidine and Methadone Congeners Currently Available

Meperidine

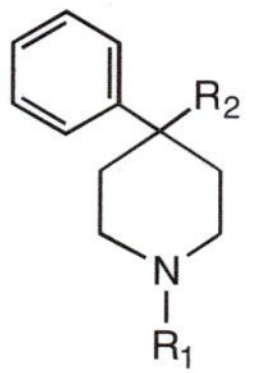

Methadone

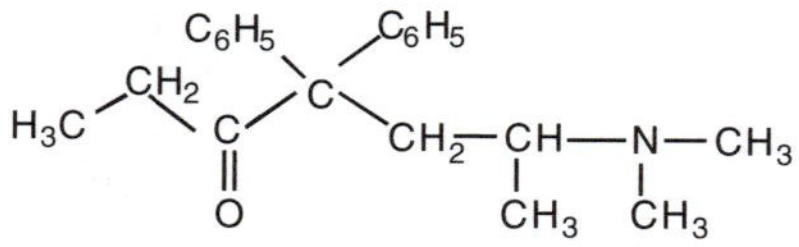

Category[a]	Compound	Proprietary Name	R1	R2
Phenylpiperidine analgesics	Meperidine	Demerol	CH_3	$COOCH_2CH_3$
	Fentanyl	Sublimaze Duragesic	CH_2CH_2–phenyl	N-(phenyl)-$COCH_2CH_3$[b]
	Diphenoxylate	Lomotil[c]	CH_2CH_2C-(phenyl)$_2$-CN	$COOCH_2CH_3$
Methadone congeners	Methadone	Dolophine	Substituted diphenyl pseudopiperidine derivative	
	Pentazocine	Talwin-NX[c]	Benzazocin derivative	
	Propoxyphene	Darvon, Darvocet-N[c]	Substituted diphenyl pseudopiperidine derivative	

[a] All synthetic compounds.
[b] Sole *para*-substitution on piperidine ring.
[c] Component of a formulation.

1. Compounds that selectively bind to the **mu-receptor (μ)** exhibit morphine-like analgesia, euphoria, respiratory depression, miosis, partial gastrointestinal (GI) inhibition, and sedative effects.
2. Narcotic antagonists such as pentazocine, nalorphine, and levorphanol appear to bind to the **kappa-receptor (κ)**, although analgesia, sedation, delusion, hallucinations (psychotomimesis), GI inhibition, and miotic effects still persist.
3. Pentazocine and nalorphine are also described as having affinity for the **delta-receptors (δ),** although this binding is primarily associated with dysphoria and mood changes (inhibition of dopamine release). The role of epsilon and zeta receptors have yet to be delineated in humans. The sigma receptor (σ), purported to have affinity for pentazocine, was once understood to represent an opioid receptor.

12.1.5 TOXICOKINETICS

Morphine is rapidly absorbed from an oral dose and from i.m. and s.c. injections. Peak plasma levels occur at 15 to 60 min and 15 min, respectively. Morphine is metabolized extensively, with only 2 to 12% excreted as the parent molecule, while 60 to 80% is excreted in the urine as the conjugated glucuronide. Heroin is rapidly biotransformed, first to monoacetylmorphine and then to morphine. Both heroin and monoacetylmorphine disappear rapidly from the blood ($t_{1/2}$ = 3 min, 5 to 10 min, respectively). Thus, morphine levels rise slowly, persist longer, and decline slowly. Codeine is extensively metabolized, primarily to the 6-glucuronide conjugate. About 10 to 15% of a dose is demethylated to form morphine and norcodeine conjugates. Therefore, codeine, norcodeine, and morphine in free and conjugated form appear in the urine after codeine ingestion.

12.1.6 SIGNS AND SYMPTOMS OF CLINICAL TOXICITY

Clinical signs and symptoms correlate with the highest concentrations of binding sites in CNS and other tissues. In particular, the limbic system (frontal and temporal cortex, amygdala, and hippocampus), thalamus, corpus striatum, hypothalamus, midbrain, and spinal cord have the highest concentrations. Analgesia appears to affect spinal ascending and descending tracts, extending up to the medullary raphe nuclei (midbrain). Effect on mood, movement, and behavior correlate with interaction with receptors in the globus pallidus (basal ganglia) and locus ceruleus, while mental confusion and euphoria (or dysphoria) alter neuronal activity in the limbic system. Hypothalamic effects are responsible for hypothermia. Miosis (pinpoint pupils) is thought to occur from μ-receptor stimulation at the Edinger-Westphal nucleus of the oculomotor nerve.

The clinical presentation of the opioid toxidrome (triad) is characterized by CNS depression (coma), miosis, and respiratory depression. Miosis is generally an encouraging sign, since it suggests that the patient is still responsive. Respiratory depression is a result of depressed brain stem and medullary respiratory centers responsible for maintenance of normal rhythm. Mu-receptor agonists depress respiration in a dose-dependent manner and can lead to respiratory arrest within minutes. Fifty percent of acute opioid overdose is accompanied by a frothy, noncardiogenic, pulmonary edema, responsible for the majority of fatalities. The condition involves loss of consciousness and hypoventilation, probably resulting from hypoxic, stress-induced, pulmonary capillary fluid leakage. Peripheral effects include bradycardia, hypotension, and decreased GI motility. Urine output also diminishes as a consequence of increased antidiuretic hormone (ADH) secretion.

12.1.7 CLINICAL MANAGEMENT OF ACUTE OVERDOSE

Maintenance of vital functions, including respiratory and cardiovascular integrity, is of paramount importance in the clinical management of acute opioid toxicity. Gastric lavage and induction of emesis are effective if treatment is instituted soon after ingestion. It is possible to reverse the respiratory depression with opioid antagonists. **Naloxone** (Narcan®) is a pure opioid antagonist available as an injectable only. A 2-mg bolus repeated every 5 min, followed by 0.4 mg every 2 to 3 min as needed (up to 24 mg total), dramatically reverses the CNS and respiratory depression (in this capacity, naloxone is also indicated in the diagnosis of suspected acute opioid overdose). Depending on the extent of narcotic overdose, a continuous infusion of naloxone may be required, especially in the presence of opioids with longer half-lives, such as propoxyphene or methadone. As respiration improves, naloxone, which has a half-life of 60 to 90 min, may be discontinued and resumed as necessary. If there is no response after 10 mg of naloxone, concomitant ingestion with other depressants is likely. It should be noted that naloxone is of little benefit in reversing noncardiogenic pulmonary edema.

    Naltrexone (Revia®) is also a pure opioid antagonist available as oral tablet dosage form only. A 50-mg dose of naltrexone blocks the pharmacological effects of opioids by competitive binding at opioid receptors. It is also indicated in the treatment of alcohol dependence. Naltrexone has been noted to induce hepatocellular injury when given in excess.

    Nalmefene (Revex®), available in 100 µg/ml and 1 mg/ml ampules, is indicated for the complete or partial reversal of natural or synthetic opioid effects. It is a 6-methylene analog of naltrexone. Nalmefene has been associated with cardiac instability, although this reaction appears to be the result of abrupt reversal of opioid toxicity.

    Several drugs have agonist activity at some receptors (κ) and antagonist activity at other (μ) receptors. Nalbuphine (Nubain®) is a potent analgesic with narcotic agonist and antagonist actions. Other mixed agonist-antagonist compounds are designated as partial agonists, such as butorphanol (Stadol®), buprenorphine (Buprenex®), and pentazocine (Talwin® and various tablet combinations). These compounds are potent analgesics and weakly antagonize the effects of opioids at the μ-receptor, while maintaining some agonist properties at the κ- and δ-receptors.

    Drug enforcement personnel and customs officials respond to different conditions of opioid overdose, especially those involving *body packers* and *body stuffers*. The drug carriers, who differ only in the apparent manner of sealing and concealing illicit drug packets, run into problems when the packets leak or burst. The overall clinical response to the situation requires rapid detection with body cavity searches and abdominal radiographs. Decontamination with activated charcoal, gastric lavage, high-dose continuous infusion with naloxone, and attention to the ABCs of emergency management of toxicity in anticipation of a developing opioid syndrome are also warranted.

12.1.8 TOLERANCE AND WITHDRAWAL

The Department of Mental Health and Substance Dependence at the World Health Organization (WHO), in collaboration with the U.S. National Institute on Drug Abuse (NIDA), defines several terms important in understanding drug abuse and the phenomena of tolerance and withdrawal. **Addiction** involves compulsive psychoactive drug use with an overwhelming involvement in the securing and using of such drugs. As described below, the withdrawal syndrome occurs as a result of sudden or abrupt discontinuation of the substance. **Compulsive drug use** involves the psychological need to procure and use drugs, often referred to as "craving." In this case, the uncontrollable drive to obtain the drugs is necessary to maintain an optimum state of well-being. **Habituation** refers to psychological dependence. **Physical (physiological) dependence** involves the need for repeated administration in order to prevent withdrawal (abstinence) syndrome. In fact, with repeated chronic dosing, seizure threshold for opiate narcotics is elevated, threatening the precipitation of seizure upon withdrawal (rebound effect). Cross-dependence occurs with all opioids, regardless of category.

The more complex phenomenon of **tolerance** requires the satisfaction of several criteria. With repeated administration, addicted individuals necessitate greater amounts of drug in order to achieve the desired effect. Conversely, the effect is markedly diminished with continued use of the same amount of drug. Since various pharmacological effects on different organ systems are not uniformly distributed, tolerance is not evenly demonstrated. While a diminished euphoric effect continues with progressive tolerance, the increasing doses threaten induction of respiratory depression. Increased metabolism, adjustment to the sedative, analgesic, and euphoric effects, are proposed as possible mechanisms for the development of tolerance — i.e., the physiological drive to achieve homeostasis.

Depending on the drug, the withdrawal syndrome is precipitated hours after the last narcotic dose with peak intensity occurring at about 72 h (Table 12.3). The intensity of the syndrome is greatest with heroin, followed by morphine, and methadone. Heroin withdrawal is characterized by acute, sudden symptoms of greater vigor while methadone withdrawal is distributed over 7 to 10 days and of lower intensity. The development of muscle spasms has come to define the syndrome, commonly known as "kicking the habit." Although the syndrome is rarely fatal, administration of an opioid at any time during withdrawal alleviates the condition.

12.1.9 CLINICAL MANAGEMENT OF ADDICTION

The NIDA publishes *The Principles of Drug Addiction Treatment — A Research Based Guide*. The Guide outlines the social and clinical approach associated with

TABLE 12.3
Characterization of the Opioid Withdrawal Syndrome

Stage	Time after Last Dose	Signs and Symptoms
Anticipatory	3–4 h	Withdrawal, fear, craving, compulsive drug seeking behavior
Early withdrawal	8–12 h	Lacrimation, sweating, listless behavior, anxiety, restlessness, stomach cramps
	12–16 h	Restless sleep, nausea, vomiting, mydriasis, anorexia, tremors, cold clammy skin, fever, chills, compulsive drug seeking behavior
	48–72 h	Peak intensity; tachycardia, hypertension, hypothermia, piloerection (goose-flesh appearance of skin, "cold turkey"), muscle spasms, continued nausea, vomiting, dehydration, compulsive drug seeking behavior, risk of cardiovascular collapse
Protracted abstinence	6 months	Stimulus-driven cravings, anorexia, fatigue, bradycardia, hypotension

drug addiction treatment in the U.S. Outpatient drug-free treatment, long- and short-term residential treatment, scientifically based counseling, psychotherapeutic and community-based programs are discussed as approaches to drug addiction treatment. Among these modalities, the risks and benefits of medical detoxification associated with the use of methadone and narcotic antagonists are presented.

12.2 SPECIFIC OPIOID DERIVATIVES

12.2.1 CODEINE

Codeine (methylmorphine) is available in combination with other ingredients as an analgesic (Tylenol with Codeine®) and as an antitussive in prescription cough, cold, antihistaminic, and expectorant formulas. The usual dosage form contains 15 to 60 mg/tablet or 10 mg/5 ml liquid. About 120 mg of codeine is equivalent to 10 mg of morphine. The compound produces the same triad of signs and symptoms with high doses, although tolerance and toxicity are less severe. Interestingly, in the 1950s and early 1960s, codeine cough and cold preparations (such as Cheracol Syrup®) could be purchased without a prescription, quantities of which were monitored with only a signature.

12.2.2 DIPHENOXYLATE

A synthetic opiate chemically related to meperidine, diphenoxylate is combined with atropine (Lomotil®) for the treatment of diarrhea. The toxicity of this combination, therefore, is primarily due to the presence of the anticholinergic. Children are especially sensitive to the effects of atropine, including production of tachycardia, flushing, hallucinations, and urinary retention. The narcotic toxicity demonstrates as miosis, respiratory depression, and in severe cases, coma.

12.2.3 FENTANYL

In the 1990s, fentanyl enjoyed increasing popularity as the narcotic of choice among illicit drug users, principally because of its enhanced potency (*China white*). At 200 times and 7000 times greater potency than morphine, α-methylfentanyl and 3-methylfentanyl also display greater potential for toxicity, respectively. The median lethal dose is about 125 μg for the former and 5 μg for the latter.* Therapeutically, fentanyl is marketed in the form of medicated patches (Duragesic Transdermal System®) for the management of chronic pain. Depending on the size of the patch and the amount of fentanyl delivered (10–40 cm² containing 2.5–20 mg total per patch), the transdermal system can release up to 200 μg/h.

12.2.4 MEPERIDINE

The first synthetic opioid (1939), meperidine is equianalgesic with morphine. In the liver, the compound is hydrolyzed to meperidinic acid and normeperidine by carboxyesterases and by N-demethylation and microsomal enzymes, respectively. Both of the metabolites are active, although they possess half of the analgesic effects and twice the neurotoxic activity. Consequently, chronic oral ingestion of meperidine tablets is associated with CNS stimulation resulting in tremors, muscle twitching, nystagmus, and convulsions. Neurotoxicity correlates directly with opioid plasma concentrations and requires several days before onset. Benzodiazepines are recommended for treatment of CNS excitation. Use of naloxone is cautioned with chronic meperidine use, since the antagonist may decrease seizure threshold (increased potential for convulsions).

12.2.5 PENTAZOCINE

Pentazocine is a benzomorphan derivative of morphine with 3- to 4-times its analgesic potency and the same addictive potential. It is presumed to exert its agonistic actions at the κ- and δ-receptors and may precipitate withdrawal symptoms in patients taking narcotic analgesics regularly. Intravenous injection of oral preparations of pentazocine and tripelenamine, an H₁-blocking antihistamine, was a common form of drug abuse.** The tablets were crushed, dissolved in tap water, heated over a flame, and injected. The combination purportedly produced an effect similar to heroin at much lower cost. Because the method of sterilization was less than optimal, and the solution contained undissolved pieces of tablet binders and fillers, addicted individuals often developed skin decubiti, abscesses, and cellulites. Continued injection resulted in serious pulmonary artery occlusion, pulmonary hypertension, and

---

* In October 2002, Russian commandos pumped an aerosol derivative of fentanyl into a Moscow theater to end a hostage crisis. All but two of 120 deaths occurred as a result of the effects of the opioid (Russian Health Ministry).

** The combination of the crushed tablets were known as *Ts and Blues, T* for Talwin® and *Blues* for the large blue color of the antihistamine tablet.

neurologic complications. As a consequence, oral pentazocine tablets were replaced with Talwin-NX® (pentazocine plus naloxone) in order to decrease this practice. The inhibitory action of naloxone on pentazocine's analgesic effect is experienced only when the tablets are crushed and injected, since naloxone is not absorbed orally.*

12.2.6 PROPOXYPHENE

A methadone analog, propoxyphene is implicated in cardiotoxicity. The parent compound and its metabolite, norpropoxyphene, cause dose-dependent widening of the QRS complex similar to tricyclic antidepressants (see Chapter 18, Figure 18.2 for an explanation of the QRS complex). This quinidine-like effect results from inhibition of cardiac fast sodium channels, causing tachydysrhythmias. In addition, propoxyphene is frequently used as the napsylate salt in combination with acetaminophen (Darvocet-N®). The unique salt form stimulates hepatic mixed function oxidase (MFO) enzymes, increasing the presence of toxic metabolites of acetaminophen. Consequently, in chronic repeated administration, it often masks acetaminophen toxicity.

12.2.7 HYDROCODONE/OXYCODONE

Hydrocodone and oxycodone are powerful μ-receptor agonists with addictive and analgesic potential equivalent to morphine and heroine, respectively.

Hydrocodone is used as an analgesic in oral dosage forms (Vicodin®, Lorcet®, Lortabs®, Tylox®) for mild to moderate pain associated with minor surgical procedures, chronic joint and muscle pain, and inflammatory conditions. It is also used as an antitussive (in Hycodan®). Consequently, its addictive potential is significant when administered chronically.

Oxycodone, in combination with aspirin or acetaminophen (Percodan®, Percocet®, respectively, 2.5-mg per tablet) has enjoyed popularity as an effective analgesic for the relief of moderate to severe pain of chronic inflammation and surgery. It is particularly useful in the alleviation of chronic pain of many cancers. In 1985, MS Contin® was introduced as a delayed-release morphine tablet, with the advantage of decreasing the frequency of dosing in patients with chronic pain. This formulation was especially convenient for elderly individuals. By 1994, morphine consumption in the U.S. had risen by 75%. Based on this success, Oxycontin® was introduced in 1995 as a delayed-release oral dosage form of the more powerful oxycodone. Revenues from Oxycontin® rose from $55 million in 1996 to $1.14 billion in 2000, at which time it became the number one opioid analgesic, with 6.5 million prescriptions in 2000. By 1995, the first cases of Oxycontin® abuse ("oxys") appeared in rural Missouri and spread throughout the rust belt states of Pennsylvania, Ohio, West Virginia, Virginia, and Appalachian Kentucky. Increasing unemployment rates in these states, the large numbers of chronically ill and disabled elderly unable to relocate, coupled with the remoteness of the regions, created an environment conducive to illicit drug distribution (the

---

* By itself, high doses of pentazocine increase plasma epinephrine concentrations, risking the development of hypertension and increased heart rate.

drug became known as "hillbilly heroin"). Economically poor, the elderly would readily sell their Oxycontin® medication to young teens offering money, producing a captive market of nontraditional drug abusers. Unlike heroin, "oxys" are regarded as legal compounds, more easily available, and with less ambiguity associated with "copping dope" on the street. The allure of the substance was not in the potency of the tablet form but in the large quantities of active ingredient immediately accessible when a 10- to 40-mg delayed release tablet is crushed, and either "snorted" or injected.

By 1998, Oxycontin® abuse had spread to suburban and urban metropolitan areas. Since 2000, several hundred fatalities due to injected Oxycontin® overdose have been reported. Its relative purity and abundance in crushed form have created an immensely desirable compound.

12.2.8 Tramadol

Tramadol is a centrally acting synthetic analog of codeine with low affinity for the μ-receptor. It is used for moderate to severe pain control. Currently, it is not on any federal controlled substance list. Much of its effects appear to be through modulation of central monoamine pathways by inhibiting reuptake of 5-hydroxytryptamine and norepinephrine. In overdose, the effects are similar to those of other opioids, with convulsions predominating in susceptible individuals.

12.2.9 Clonidine

Clonidine (Catapres®) primarily stimulates central postsynaptic α_2-receptors that inhibit neuronal activity and decrease sympathetic overtone. Clonidine shares some pharmacological properties (μ-receptors) and clinical features with the opioids. Overdose with clonidine occurs within 60- to 90-min after ingestion, producing bradycardia, hypotension, arrhythmias, CNS depression, decreased respiration, and miosis. Although the mechanism is poorly understood, it is believed to involve antagonism of the μ-receptors. Patients who demonstrate opioid-like toxicity with clonidine respond to naloxone administration, particularly the reversal of hypoventilation and CNS depression.

12.3 METHODS OF DETECTION

Opioids are detected using a radioactive or enzyme-linked immunoassay technique (EMIT, KIMS).* The principle of the assays is the reaction of morphine in an aliquot of the urine sample with its corresponding antibody. Significant cross-reactivity occurs with opioid derivatives (as well as with components of poppy seeds) because of the reaction of the antibody with the common phenanthrene structure. Radioimmunuoassays (RIAs) are also very sensitive and can detect opioids at levels of 0.5 to 10 ng/ml. RIA, however, requires tritiated (radioactive) ligands as indicators.

---

* These methods have supplanted the traditional GC-MS and TLC methods used for urine and blood screening.

Other immunoassays for specific opioid derivatives, such as fentanyl, methadone, and meperidine, are also available.

Both EMIT and the Abuscreen® RIA detect codeine and morphine in free and conjugated forms but do not distinguish between them. Based on the toxicokinetics of the opioids noted above, distinguishing morphine from heroin or codeine is difficult but clinically and forensically important. The presence of morphine alone or its conjugate can indicate either clinical morphine use or illicit morphine or heroin use (within the previous 1 to 2 days). The distinction is possible when the test is employed 2 to 4 days after the last dose. Other narcotics identified by the immunoassays for morphine include dihydrocodeine, dihydromorphine, and hydromorphone. Confirmation of positive results, and distinction between them are accomplished with TLC, HPLC, and GLC. Acid or enzyme hydrolysis of the urine sample, however, is necessary when the latter testing techniques are used, since approximately 90% of codeine and morphine are found in urine in the conjugated glucuronide form.

REFERENCES

SUGGESTED READINGS

Cone, E.J. et al., Oxycodone involvement in drug abuse deaths: a DAWN-based classification scheme applied to an oxycodone postmortem database containing over 1000 cases, *J. Anal. Toxicol.*, 27, 57, 2003.

Wax, P.M., Becker, C.E. and Curry, S.C., Unexpected "gas" casualties in Moscow: A medical toxicology perspective, *Ann. Emerg. Med.* 41, 700, 2003.

Wines, M., The Aftermath in Moscow: Post-Mortem in Moscow; Russia Names Drug in Raid, Defending Use, Foreign Desk, *New York Times,* Oct. 31, 2002.

REVIEW ARTICLES

Budd, K., Buprenorphine and the transdermal system: the ideal match in pain management, *Int. J. Clin. Pract. Suppl.* 133, 9, 2003.

Choi, Y.S. and Billings, J.A., Opioid antagonists: a review of their role in palliative care, focusing on use in opioid-related constipation, *J. Pain Symptom Manage.*, 24, 71, 2002.

Cohen, G., The 'poor man's heroin.' An Ohio surgeon helps feed a growing addiction to OxyContin, *U.S. News World Rep.*, 130, 27, 2001.

Cone, E.J. and Preston, K.L., Toxicologic aspects of heroin substitution treatment, *Ther. Drug Monit.*, 24, 193, 2002.

Cruz, R. et al., Pulmonary manifestations of inhaled street drugs. *Heart Lung*, 27, 297, 1998.

Drug Abuse Warning Network (DAWN), Substance Abuse and Mental Health Services Administration (SAMHSA), National Institute on Drug Abuse, DHHS, U.S. Public Health Service, 2000; http://www.drugabuse.gov.

Frost, D.M., Chemical dependency and the heart, *S.D.J. Med.*, 44, 149, 1991.

Green, H. et al., Methadone maintenance programs — a two-edged sword? *Am. J. Forensic Med. Pathol.*, 21, 359, 2000.

Hancock, C.M. and Burrow, M.A., OxyContin use and abuse, *Clin. J. Oncol. Nurs.* 6, 109, 2002.

Hino, Y. et al., Performance of immunoassays in screening for opioids, cannabinoids and amphetamines in post-mortem blood, *Forensic Sci. Int.*, 131, 148, 2003.

Katz, N. and Fanciullo, G.J., Role of urine toxicology testing in the management of chronic opioid therapy, *Clin. J. Pain*, 18, S76, 2002.

Kemp, P. et al., Validation of a microtiter plate ELISA for screening of postmortem blood for opioids and benzodiazepines, *J. Anal. Toxicol.*, 26, 504, 2002.

Kobayashi, H., et al., Recent progress in the neurotoxicology of natural drugs associated with dependence or addiction, their endogenous agonists and receptors, *J. Toxicol. Sci.,* 24, 1, 1999.

Latta, K.S., Ginsberg, B., and Barkin, R.L., Meperidine: a critical review, *Am. J. Ther.* 9, 53, 2002.

Lehmann, K.A., Opioids: overview on action, interaction and toxicity, *Support Care Cancer,* 5, 439, 1997.

NIDA Research Monograph 73, Urine testing for drugs of abuse, National Institute on Drug Abuse, DHHS, Public Health Service, R.L. Hawks and C.N. Chiang (eds.), 1986.

Seger, D.L., Clonidine toxicity revisited, *J. Toxicol. Clin. Toxicol.*, 40, 145, 2002.

Shipton, E.A., Tramadol — present and future, *Anaesth. Intensive Care*, 28, 363, 2000.

Stein, M.D., Medical consequences of substance abuse, *Psychiatr. Clin. North Am.* 22, 351, 1999.

Suffett, W.L., OxyContin abuse, *J. Ky. Med. Assoc.*, 99, 72, 2001.

Wang, H.E., Street drug toxicity resulting from opioids combined with anticholinergics. *Prehosp. Emerg. Care*, 6, 351, 2002.

13 Sympathomimetics

13.1 AMPHETAMINES AND AMPHETAMINE-LIKE AGENTS

13.1.1 INCIDENCE AND CLASSIFICATION

The sporadic use of amphetamines reflects the competition and availability of other drugs of abuse, the desires of the particular socioeconomic group (generation) interested in the substance, and the efforts of law enforcement to eliminate the accessibility of any particular substance of abuse. The amphetamines made their appearance for use in weight reduction and control of obesity. Their stimulant/euphoric effects improved their popularity, which eventually gave rise to common street names such as *ups, bennies, dexies,* and *speed,* among others. Today, stimulants such as methylphenidate are available as prescription drugs, due to their frequent use in the treatment of attention deficit hyperactivity disorder (ADHD). Amphetamines are approved for the treatment of short-term depression. They are not approved but are frequently exploited for reducing fatigue among truck drivers and college students.

The homeostatic regulation of central and peripheral autonomic function is mediated principally through the actions of the sympathetic nervous system (SNS) and moderated through the opposing effects of the parasympathetic system (PNS). Stimulation of the sympathetic nervous system normally occurs in response to physical activity, psychological stress, generalized allergic reactions, and situations that require a heightened response. As a result, the physiological reaction of the SNS favors functions that support vigorous physical activity and response to stressors; thus the SNS is labeled as the "fight-or-flight" response. Increases or enhancement of cardiac contraction, vasomotor tone, blood pressure, bronchial airway tone, carbohydrate and fatty acid metabolism, psychomotor activity, mood, and behavior, are physiological responses that occur following SNS stimulation. The variety of agents listed in Table 13.1 pharmacologically mimic or alter sympathetic activity. These substances were originally classified as catecholamines for their structural resemblance to OH-substituted *o*-dihydroxybenzene (catechol). Although most are clinically useful, toxicity of these compounds results from development of the adverse reactions, from abuse or overuse, and is manifested as an exaggeration of the pharmacological profiles.

The actions of the sympathomimetic amines are classified into six broad types:

1. Peripheral excitatory smooth muscle action, including effects on peripheral blood vessels
2. Peripheral inhibitory smooth muscle, including effects on the GI tract, bronchial tree, and in skeletal muscle blood vessels

TABLE 13.1

Categories, Structures, and Proprietary Names of Naturally Occurring Sympathomimetics, Amphetamines and Amphetamine-Like Stimulants Currently Available

Category	Compound	Proprietary Name	R_1[b]	R_2	R_3
Catecholamines (naturally occurring)[a]	Epinephrine	Various	OH	H	CH$_3$
	Norepinephrine	None	OH	H	H
	Dopamine	Various	H	H	H
Amphetamines and derivatives (noncatecholamines)	Amphetamine	Various	H	CH$_3$	H
	Dextroamphetamine	Dexedrine Adderal[c]	d-isomer of d,l-amphetamine		
	Ephedrine	Various	OH	CH$_3$	CH$_3$
	Methamphetamine	Desoxyn	H	CH$_3$	CH$_3$
	Diethylpropion	Tenuate	=O	CH$_3$	(C$_2$H$_5$)$_2$
	Phenylpropanolamine[d]	PPA	OH	CH$_3$	H
	Phentermine	Fastin[d]	H	(CH$_3$)$_2$	H
	Phentermine HCl	Adipex-P			
	Pemoline	Cylert	2-amino-5-phenyl-2-oxazolin-4-one		
	Phendimetrazine	Prelu-2, Bontril, Plegine,[d] Preludin[d]	3,4-dimethyl-2-phenylmorpholine		
	Methylphenidate	Ritalin	methyl α-phenyl-2-piperidine acetate		

[a] Catecholamines are normally found throughout the body and thus are classified here as naturally occurring sympathomimetics.

[b] R-substitutions refer to the positions on the ethylamine side chain.

[c] Amphetamine/dextroamphetamine combination.

[d] No longer marketed.

3. Cardiac excitatory action, resulting in increased heart rate (chronotropy) and force of contraction (inotropy)
4. Metabolic actions, resulting in stimulation of hepatic and muscle glyco-genolysis and lipolysis
5. Endocrine actions, such as modulation of the secretion of insulin, renin, and pituitary hormones
6. Central nervous system (CNS) stimulation of respiration, enhancement of psychomotor activity, and appetite suppression

Thus, the pharmacological properties of amphetamines and amphetamine-like compounds mimic the actions of the prototype agent, epinephrine.

13.1.2 MEDICINAL CHEMISTRY

Table 13.1 illustrates the β-phenethylamine parent structure of the sympathomimetic amines, consisting of a benzene ring and an ethylamine side chain. Substitutions on the aromatic ring and the side chain (R-groups) yield a variety of compounds whose pharmacological and toxicological profiles, and their relative potencies, are distinguishable from those of epinephrine.

13.1.3 PHARMACOLOGY AND CLINICAL USE

Figure 13.1 illustrates sympathetic neurons and their receptors in the SNS. Most sympathetic postganglionic neurons are adrenergic, active in synthesizing, storing, and releasing norepinephrine. Upon release, norepinephrine diffuses and binds to adrenergic receptors, alpha and beta (α_1, α_2, β_1, β_2 and β_3) on the postsynaptic membrane, resulting in chemical activation of the effector organs mentioned above. In general, stimulation of α_1 and β_1 receptors results in excitation, while activation of α_2 and β_2 receptors causes inhibition. The α_1 receptors predominate at the effector sites of peripheral vascular smooth muscle and glandular cells. Excitation of α_1 receptors results in vasoconstriction (pressor effects), pupilary dilation (mydriasis), and closing of sphincters. The α_2 receptors are present in some effector sites of visceral and vascular smooth muscle. Activation of α_2 receptors results in vasodilation and decreased insulin secretion. β_1 receptors predominate in cardiac muscle fibers and juxtaglomerular cells of kidney. Stimulation of β_1 receptors precipitates a positive cardiac inotropy and chronotropy, as well as increased renin secretion (stimulates renin-angiotensin pathway for elevating blood pressure). β_2 receptors are present primarily in respiratory smooth muscle, cardiac, skeletal muscle, and hepatic and adipose blood vessels. The net effect of binding of amphetamines to β_2 receptors is relaxation of bronchial airways, vasodilation of coronary and skeletal muscle vasculature, and glycogenolysis. Stimulation of β_3 receptors, found primarily in adipose tissue, induces a thermogenic response (heat production). This action, in combination with the central anorexic effect, explains their use in weight reduction.

Pharmacologically, amphetamines and their derivatives are indirect agonists that mimic the actions of epinephrine and norepinephrine (Table 13.1). The agents either stimulate release of, or block the reuptake of, naturally occurring sympathomimetics.

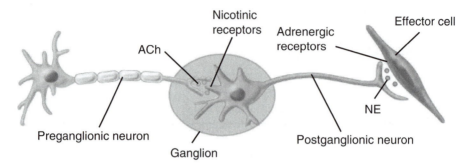

FIGURE 13.1 Sympathetic neurons and their receptors in the SNS. (From Tortora G.J. and Grabowski S.R., *Principles of Anatomy and Physiology*, 9th ed. ©2001 by John Wiley & Sons. This material is used by permission of John Wiley & Sons, Inc.)

The only approved indications for use of amphetamines and derivatives are for the treatment of attention-deficit hyperactivity disorder (ADHD), narcolepsy, and the short-term management of obesity.

13.1.4 TOXICOKINETICS

The catecholamine sympathomimetics, epinephrine, norepinephrine, and dopamine, are rapidly conjugated and oxidized in the gastrointestinal lumen and liver, rendering them ineffective when taken orally. A variety of parenteral, solubilized, and aero-solized preparations, however, are available for inhalation, intravenous, intramuscular, and intranasal administration.

Unlike the naturally occurring sympathomimetics, the amphetamine compounds are weak bases that are well absorbed orally ($pK_a \sim 10$), predominantly throughout the length of the basic environment of the small intestine.

13.1.5 EFFECTS AND MECHANISM OF TOXICITY

Amphetamine and its derivatives have powerful CNS stimulant actions (analeptic) in addition to sympathetic stimulation. Thus, the toxicity is an extension of the pharmacological properties. Table 13.2 summarizes the desirable and undesirable effects of the sympathomimetics, as well as the treatment associated with the toxicity. The therapeutic uses follow the indications outlined above, while the euphoric effects are the major reasons for psychological and physiological dependence. The psychic properties vary according to the mental state of the individual and the dose. An oral dose of 5 mg of dextroamphetamine sulfate results in the desirable feeling of alertness, wakefulness, mood elevation, and improved self-confidence that induces a sense of well-being and euphoria. Prolonged use or overdose is invariably followed by depression and fatigue (*the crash*). Treatment modalities include clinical management of signs and symptoms, especially regulating cardiovascular effects, and therapeutic intervention for the **toxic psychosis syndrome**. Although acidification of urine enhances renal elimination of amphetamines, it may worsen renal failure by exacerbating the effects of profound hyperthermia.

TABLE 13.2
Characterization of the Therapeutic, Euphoric, and Toxic Syndromes Associated with Acute Amphetamine Use or Overdose

Effects	Signs and Symptoms	Clinical Management of Acute Toxicity
Euphoric	Wakefulness, alertness, mood elevation, increased initiative and self-confidence, elation, improved motor and speech activities	Euphoric effects are overcome with S/H (benzodiazepines) or diminish with chronic use
Therapeutic	Anorexia, bronchodilation, improved cerebral circulation, improved attention span (in children with ADHD), alertness and wakefulness (for narcolepsy)	—
Neurologic	Tremors, hyperactive reflexes, seizures, convulsions, coma	Withdrawal of agent, S/H (diazepam), phenobarbital
Cardiovascular and circulatory	Headache, chilliness, palpitations; increased oxygen consumption, blood pressure, peripheral vasoconstriction; anginal pain, tachypnea, tachycardia, circulatory collapse	Withdrawal of agent or Na nitroprusside or Ca^{+2} channel blockers; digoxin, diuretics; β-blockers not recommended
Gastrointestinal	Dry mouth, metallic taste, anorexia, nausea, vomiting, diarrhea, abdominal cramps	Withdrawal of agent, S/H, or symptomatic
Renal and electrolyte disturbances	Increased blood sugar, excessive sweating, hyerkalemia, hypernatremia; renal failure	Withdrawal of agent, S/H, diuretic or symptomatic
CNS	Restlessness, dizziness, tremor, irritability, insomnia, anxiety, hyperpyrexia, mydriasis	Withdrawal of agent, S/H, or symptomatic
Toxic psychosis syndrome	Paranoid syndrome characterized by hallucinations, schizophrenic episodes, delirium, panic state, suicidal or homicidal tendencies, *parasitosis*	Self-limiting in absence of agent or phenothiazine (chlorpromazine, haloperidol), barbiturate

Note: Parasitosis refers to the irrational feeling or hallucination of worms or insects crawling on the skin; S/H = sedative/hypnotic.

In 1999, a clinical investigation sought to determine the effect of the combination of phentermine-fenfluramine ("phen-fen") on the prevalence of valvular heart disease in obese subjects enrolled in a prospective, strict weight-loss, research protocol. The "phen-fen" therapy was identified and associated with a low prevalence of, but clinically significant, aortic and mitral regurgitation, which may reflect age-related degenerative changes. This toxic finding of a frequently used stimulant forced the removal of fenfluramine (Pondimin®) from the market.

13.1.6 TOLERANCE AND WITHDRAWAL

As with many potentially addictive agents, chronic use of amphetamines leads to psychological dependence. It is not unusual for amphetamine abusers to occasionally augment their euphoria with an injection every 3 to 4 h continuously for 7 to 10 days. In addition, simultaneous administration of an opioid with amphetamine is common practice among addicts, in order to minimize the psychological withdrawal from the stimulant. In order to maximize the euphoric actions, habitual users will often ingest large quantities of antacids. The rationale for this behavior is to alkalinize the urine — i.e., maintain the basic compound in the nonionic state, force renal tubular reabsorption, and prolong the blood levels. In fact, alkalinization of urine prolongs the half-life from 7 to 8 h up to 35 h. Tolerance to the anorexic effect, as well as to the improvement of mood, is frequent but not invariable. Many patients, however, have been treated for narcolepsy for years without requiring major adjustments in dosage.

Induction of the withdrawal syndrome depends on the extent of habituation but varies between several hours to several days after discontinuation of the drug. It is characterized by prolonged sleep, lassitude, drug craving behavior, and hyperphagia. A deep depression follows interruption of prolonged or chronic use. No clear physical symptoms of withdrawal are associated with amphetamines.

13.1.7 METHODS OF DETECTION

Amphetamines and other sympathomimetics are detected using a variety of methods, depending on the sensitivity required and the sample available. Routine qualitative urine drug screening tests are commonly employed when rapid results are needed. Thin layer chromatography (TLC) with fluorescent dye staining has been used for qualitative analysis. Quantitative analysis with TLC, however, is limited due to a lack of sensitivity. RIA using tritiated ligands has sensitivities to 2.5 ng, thereby allowing for quantititative detection. HPLC analysis, with a fluorescent detector, is less common for routine screening but can detect levels of amphetamines in biological fluids to 100 fmol. Using these techniques, unchanged amphetamine has been detected in the urine up to 29 h after a single oral dose of 5 mg amphetamine.

RIA assays, such as the Roche Abuscreen®, detect only amphetamine, while Syva's EMIT (enzyme-multiplied immunoassay technique) is able to detect both amphetamine and methamphetamine. A more specific Abuscreen amphetamine assay is also available and is sometimes used as a second screen. The new Abbott TDx Drug Detection System® is reported to detect both methamphetamine and amphetamine with little or no cross-reactivity to ephedrine and phenylpropanolamine.

13.2 COCAINE

13.2.1 INCIDENCE AND OCCURRENCE

The sporadic use of cocaine during the last 50 years is a reflection of its cyclic popularity as well as availability, cost, and competition with other illicit drugs. The drug is derived from the dried leaves of the plant *Erythroxylon coca*, that appears to grow best at higher elevations (1500 to 6000 ft) in the South American countries of Peru, Bolivia, and Colombia. Historically, the ancient Incas of Peru chewed on the leaves of the plant to decrease fatigue and reduce appetite during long journeys, although it was still considered an inferior substitute for tea. Drug analysis of ancient Egyptian ruins detected the presence of cocaine and nicotine. And cocaine was sold medicinally as a brain tonic in the early 1900s (an ingredient of Coca-Cola®). Today, the illicit form of the compound is transported to the United States principally in the same manner as described for opioids (Chapter 12) — i.e., by *body packing*.* Before it arrives on the streets, the crystalline form of the drug is diluted (*cut*) with a diluent, such as lactose, mannitol, sucrose, procaine, or lidocaine. The substance is injected i.v. as a 10 to 20% solution, administered by intranasal insufflation (*snorted* as 50 to 75% powder), or burned and inhaled as the freebase (*crack* cocaine, 20% powder).**

13.2.2 Medicinal Chemistry

Coca leaves contain the alkaloids of ecgonine, tropine, and hygrine, of which only the derivatives of ecgonine are of commercial importance. Cocaine is an ester of benzoic acid and methylecgonine, the latter of which is related to the amino alcohol group found in atropine. The chemical structures of cocaine and related local anesthetics are illustrated in Figure 13.2.

13.2.3 Pharmacology and Clinical Use

Although not generally regarded as a sympathomimetic, cocaine has stimulant as well as anesthetic properties. Cocaine displays reversible CNS and peripheral actions. It blocks nerve conduction through its local anesthetic properties, primarily by inhibiting neuronal sodium permeability. It possesses local vasoconstrictor actions secondary to inhibition of local norepinephrine reuptake at adrenergic neurons. Unlike other local anesthetics, production of euphoria is due, in part, to inhibition of dopamine reuptake in central synapses. Because of its high toxicity and potential for abuse, its use is limited as a topical anesthetic/vasoconstrictor (1 to 10% solution) for surgical procedures involving the oral and nasal mucosal cavities.

13.2.4 Toxicokinetics

Cocaine is rapidly absorbed after i.v. or intranasal administration or by inhalation. Distribution depends largely on access to the systemic circulation, which is determined by protein binding and its vasoconstrictor effects, both of which limit systemic distribution. Thus, distribution of the compound after local application is diminished by its vasoconstrictor activity. This effect, however, is obviated when exposure through inhalation or i.v. routes circumvents the local effects, resulting in significant potential for systemic toxicity.

---

* Cocaine drug carriers, or *body packers*, seal and conceal illicit drug packets in body compartments either by swallowing or inserting into body orifices. As with the opioids, the packets run the risk of leaking or bursting, making the overall clinical management of these individuals of immediate attention.
** What is believed to be the last (and perhaps a forgery) of the Sherlock Holmes novels, *The Seven Percent Solution*, describes the infamous detective struggling with the addictive power of cocaine.

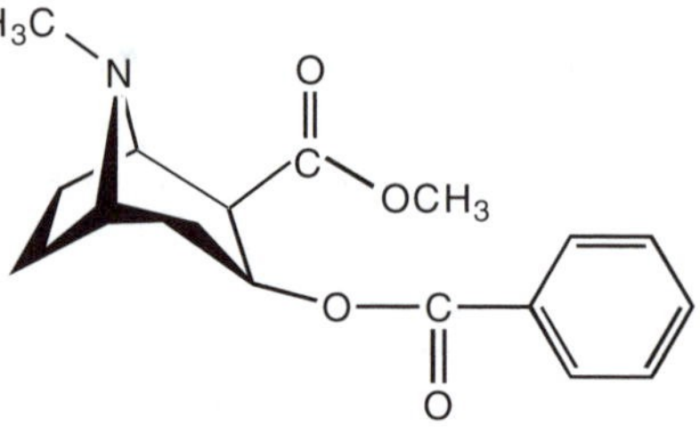

Cocaine

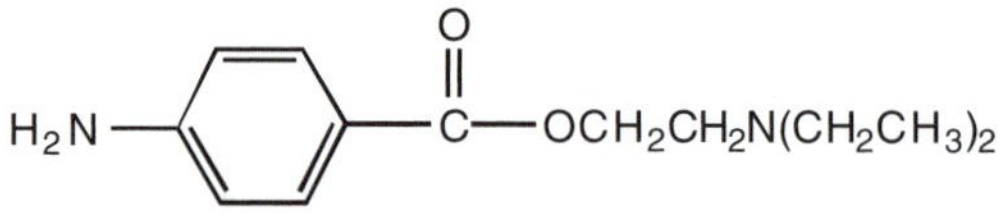

Procaine

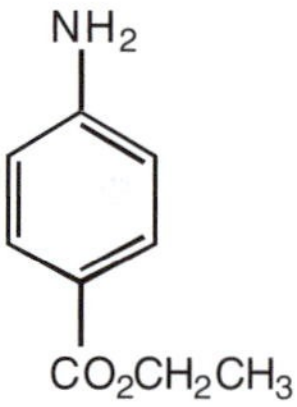

Benzocaine

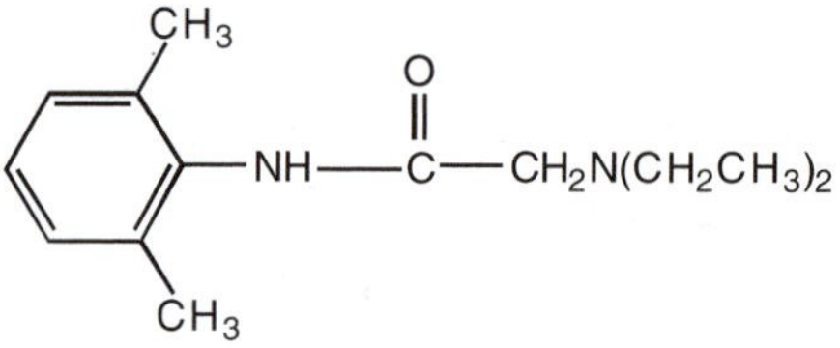

Lidocaine

FIGURE 13.2 Structure of cocaine and related local anesthetics.

13.2.5 SIGNS AND SYMPTOMS OF ACUTE TOXICITY

Central, peripheral, and parasympathetic nervous systems, as well as cardiovascular and smooth muscle, display initial signs of stimulation, followed by depression. This characteristic is presumably due to selective depression of inhibitory neurons, as well as inhibition of general neuronal activity in these areas. Initially, the stimulation mimics sympathetic activation exhibited by excitement, apprehension, nausea, vomiting, and tremors. Ensuing spasms and seizures are a result of high serum concentrations and overwhelming neuronal depression.

Its cardiovascular toxicity is evidenced by increased blood pressure and heart rate, resulting in an increase in myocardial work and oxygen demand. Thus, the drug has the potential for precipitating ventricular dysfunction and arrhythmias. Simultaneously, it induces coronary artery vasospasm as a result of sympathetic stimulation. This dual mechanism precipitates myocardial ischemia or infarction (*heart attack*). Ischemic and hemorrhagic stroke present as headaches or changes in mental status, often mistaken as psychiatric instability.

Smoking *crack cocaine* hastens episodes of asthma or chronic obstructive pulmonary disease (COPD). Mouth and pharyngeal pain, drooling, and hoarseness accompany the severe upper airway burn injury resulting from inhaling the heat from pipe smoking. In moderate toxicity, cyanosis, dyspnea, and rapid, irregular respirations ensue. Cardiogenic or noncardiogenic pulmonary edema and respiratory failure are progressive sequelae.

Other important toxic features of cocaine toxicity include the production of acute dyskinesia (*crack dancing*). This syndrome, characterized by episodes of choreoathetoid movements of the extremities, lip-smacking, and repetitive eye blinking, occurs soon after cocaine use and lasts several days. Acute renal failure, increased risk of spontaneous abortions, elevation of maternal hypertension during pregnancy, and profound hyperthermia, are significant complications of cocaine toxicity. Effects on gastrointestinal smooth muscle are not dramatic.

13.2.6 CLINICAL MANAGEMENT OF ACUTE OVERDOSE

Maintenance of airway, breathing, and circulation (ABCs) is the priority in managing patients with cocaine toxicity. Cardiovascular, neurologic, and psychiatric complications are effectively controlled with benzodiazepine administration, particularly diazepam or lorazepam. Intravenous phenobarbital is used to control cocaine-induced seizures if the benzodiazepines are inadequate. Phenytoin is not useful in cocaine-induced seizures and, since succinylcholine risks hyperkalemia and hyperthermia, a nondepolarizing neuromuscular blocker, such as pancuronium bromide, should be used in the event of intractable seizures.

13.2.7 TOLERANCE AND WITHDRAWAL

Addiction to cocaine is essentially indistinguishable from amphetamine habituation. Because of its rapid metabolism, larger doses of cocaine are required to maintain the euphoric effects in a chronic user. The development of tolerance, however, is inconsistent, and users will succumb to the toxic effects at low doses in spite of the continuous use. There is generally no cross tolerance between cocaine and sympathetic stimulants.

13.2.8 METHODS OF DETECTION

Cocaine is extensively metabolized, primarily by liver and plasma esterases, and only 1% of a dose is excreted in the urine unchanged. Approximately 70% of a dose can be recovered in the urine over a period of 3 days. About 25 to 40% of cocaine is metabolized to benzoylecgonine, the major metabolite found in the urine. About 18 to 22% is excreted as ecgonine methyl ester and 2 to 3% as ecgonine. Immunochemical techniques such as EMIT and RIA are designed to detect benzoylecgonine. Unchanged cocaine is sometimes detected by chromatographic methods for up to 24 h after a given dose, while benzoylecgonine can generally be detected by immunoassays for 24 to 48 h. The presence of cocaine and its metabolites in urine is confirmed by GLC, HPLC, and GC/MS. Benzoylecgonine can generally be detected in urine up to 2 days after cocaine use using GLC, the most specific of the chromatographic techniques.

13.3 XANTHINE DERIVATIVES

13.3.1 SOURCE AND MEDICINAL CHEMISTRY

Figure 13.3 illustrates the structures of the xanthine derivatives, caffeine, theophylline, and theobromine. The compounds contain the purine nucleus and are naturally occurring xanthine derivatives. Caffeine is the most active component of coffee and coffee beans (seeds) of *Coffea arabica,* a small evergreen shrub abundant in the tropical areas of South America, Central America, and the Middle East. It is also found in *Cola accuminata* and *Cola nitida,* tropical nuts of South America and Africa. Both caffeine and theophylline are distributed throughout the tea leaves of *Thea sinensis*, a shrub native to Japan, China, Southeast Asia, and Indonesia. *Theobroma cacao,* the 12-m cocoa plant, is indigenous to the South American, Asian, and African tropics.

13.3.2 OCCURRENCE

Because of ubiquitous occurrence, caffeine is distributed throughout coffee, tea, chocolate, and cola beverages, with coffee beans and tea leaves containing equivalent

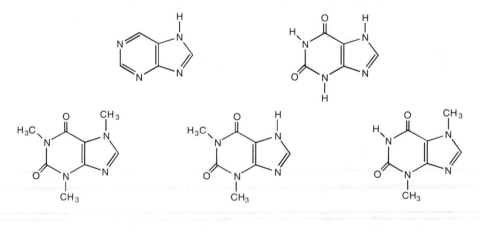

Caffeine   Purine   Theophylline   Xanthine   Theobromine

FIGURE 13.3 Structure of purine and xanthine derivatives.

amounts of the stimulant (up to 2%). Brewed coffee boasts the highest amounts of caffeine (up to 100 mg). Instant and decaffeinated coffees contain less (up to 75 and 5 mg, respectively), while a cola beverage possesses a significant dose of stimulant (up to 55 mg). A dose of 200 mg of theobromine is usually consumed in a cup of hot cocoa.

13.3.3 PHARMACOLOGY AND CLINICAL USE

The history of the use of the xanthine derivatives for their medicinal and stimulant effects dates back throughout ancient civilizations. The xanthine derivatives, particularly caffeine, exert their pharmacological actions by increasing calcium permeability in sarcoplasmic reticulum, inhibiting phosphodiesterase-promoting accumulation of cyclic AMP, and acting as competitive, nonselective antagonists of adenosine A_1 and A_{2A} receptors. Theophylline, in addition, inhibits the action of extracellular adenosine (bronchodilation effect), stimulates endogenous catecholamines (central stimulant effect), and directly promotes mobilization of intracellular calcium and β-adrenergic agonist activity (airway smooth muscle relaxation).

The predominant CNS stimulant properties of caffeine and the respiratory relaxation produced by theophylline are well documented. Caffeine stimulates cerebral activity, skeletal and cardiac muscle contraction, and general basal metabolic rate, while theophylline has less central stimulation but significant bronchial smooth muscle relaxation properties. Caffeine and theophylline enhance cardiac muscle contraction, induce coronary vasodilation, and promote diuresis. Caffeine is available in combination with ergotamine, belladonna alkaloids, or pentobarbital for the treament of migraine headaches (Wigraine® tablets, Cafergot® suppositories), for its synergistic action with ephedrine for weight loss, and as an aid for wakefulness and restoring mental alertness. In combination with sodium benzoate (injectable), caffeine is used in the treatment of drug-induced respiratory depression, and as caffeine citrate (injectable) for the short-term treatment of apnea in premature infants. Theophylline (Elixophyllin®, Theolair®, Theo-Dur® and various others) is employed in the treatment of bronchial asthma and other respiratory related disorders.

13.3.4 TOXICOKINETICS

Xanthine derivatives are well absorbed orally, reaching peak distribution within two hours. The compounds are metabolized by the liver to methylxanthine and methyluric acid derivatives. Metabolic variability among different age groups, smokers, and individuals with pathologic complications is probably due to variable levels of cytochrome P450 and N-acetyltransferase systems. The drugs are eliminated by the kidney with a half-life of 3 to 15 h in nonsmokers (4 to 5 h in adult smokers).

13.3.5 SIGNS AND SYMPTOMS AND CLINICAL MANAGEMENT OF CAFFEINE TOXICITY

The estimated LD of caffeine in humans is 5 to 10 g. Although fatalities are unlikely approaching this dose, individuals who ingest up to 10 mg/kg are at risk of developing dysrhythmias or strychnine-like seizures. More likely adverse effects of excessive caffeine intake are demonstrable as CNS stimulation, including insomnia, restlessness, sensory disturbances, and delirium. Increased skeletal muscle tension, tachycardia, premature ventricular contractions (PVCs), diarrhea, development of peptic ulcers and gastrointestinal bleeding complete the detrimental properties of acute and chronic ingestion. In addition, caffeine can neutralize the desired therapeutic effects of diuretics, antihypertensive agents, β-blockers, and sedative/hypnotics.

Myocardial tachyarrhythmias and development of seizures should be monitored in patients after an acute ingestion of 1 g or more of caffeine. A short-acting β-adrenergic blocker, such as esmolol (Brevibloc® injectable), is useful in the management of the former, while the seizures are controlled by a short-acting benzodiazepine, such as midazolam (Versed® injection).

13.3.6 SIGNS AND SYMPTOMS AND CLINICAL MANAGEMENT OF THEOPHYLLINE TOXICITY

Theophylline shares similar properties with caffeine, although its toxicity is more acute and more common; chronic toxicity, however, is unlikely. Therapeutic blood levels are strictly regulated at 10 to 20 μg/ml, but vary depending on interactions with other drugs, inaccurate dosing, accidental or intentional overdose ingestion. Seizures occur between 25 to 40 μg/ml. As with caffeine toxicity, rapid i.v. administration of theophylline is associated with headache, hypotension, dizziness, restlessness, agitation, and arrhythmias. In order to relieve the gastric irritation and nausea related with oral tablets, most theophylline preparations are available as controlled-release dosage forms.

13.3.7 TOLERANCE AND WITHDRAWAL

Caffeine withdrawal is associated with chronic use and is demonstrated abruptly within 12 to 24 h after the last dose. Initial symptoms, including headache, anxiety, fatigue, and craving behavior, last for about one week. There is demonstrated tolerance to the diuretic action and the insomnia produced with theophylline, but no tolerance develops to the CNS stimulation or bronchodilation.

13.4 OTHER SPECIFIC SYMPATHOMIMETIC AGENTS

13.4.1 STRYCHNINE

Originally labeled as an analeptic agent (stimulant), strychnine was introduced into Europe about the sixteenth century mainly for poisoning animals. Its use in medicine began about 1640, when it was found to possess CNS stimulant properties to combat depression and sleeplessness and improve respiration. It was also used as a popular gastrointestinal bitter tonic (appetite stimulant) and to increase muscle tone. Unfortunately, strychnine exhibits a narrow therapeutic index and consequently does not enjoy any favorable medicinal value. However, it is still used as a rodenticide.

Strychnine is an indole alkaloid* obtained from the dried seeds of *Nux vomica,* from the plant, *Strychnos nux-vomica,* that grows to approximately 12 m in Southeast Asia and northern Australia. It is extremely toxic as a central stimulant. Fatal poisoning in adults, especially from the ingestion of tonic tablets, results from ingesting 30 to 100 mg and, in children, from accidental ingestion of rodenticide (15-mg can be a lethal dose). Since the alkaloid is predominantly a lipophilic glycoside, it is well absorbed orally, and it is metabolized via the hepatic microsomal enzyme system.

Strychnine inhibits the postsynaptic receptor for glycine, an inhibitory neurotransmitter, allowing for the development of spinal convulsions of the tonic type (characterized as extensor thrusts). Strychnine exerts its toxic abilities by blocking postsynaptic conduction in the inhibitory spinal Renshaw motor neurons, where it interferes with ascending and descending motor tracts, resulting in convulsions of spinal cord origin.

Signs and symptoms of toxicity are similar to those seen in experimental animals. Early stages are characterized by a grimacing stiffness of the neck and face, followed by increased reflex excitability that is precipitated by sensory stimulation. Tonic convulsions (traditionally demonstrated as arched back or *opisthotonus*) are followed by coordinated extensor thrusts. Convulsions occur as full contractions of all voluntary muscles, including thoracic, abdominal, and diaphragmatic, which ultimately suppress respiration. Convulsive episodes are continuous or intermittent, with depression and sleep interspersed, depending on the depth of toxicity, and the patient is generally conscious and in pain. After several full convulsions, medullary paralysis due to hypoxia is the cause of death.

Treatment must be instituted swiftly and is aimed at preventing convulsions, maintaining ventilation, and administration of an anticonvulsant/skeletal muscle relaxant, such as diazepam. Successful treatment with diazepam (10 mg i.v., repeated as needed) depends on the following criteria: (1) the dose of poison is below the lethal dose; (2) if intervention is started soon after ingestion; and (3) if convulsions have not ensued. Gastric lavage is only indicated when the compound is suspected to be in the stomach contents and if convulsions have subsided.

13.4.2 Nicotine

Nicotine is a pyridine alkaloid (1-methyl-2(3-pyridyl) pyrrolidine) obtained from the cured and dried leaves of the tobacco plant, *Nicotiana* sp., indigenous to the southern United States and tropical South America. It is a tall annual herb introduced into Europe from the American colonies, obtained from the Native Americans.** Well before the isolation of nicotine in 1828, the finely powdered tobacco leaves were dusted on vegetable crops as an insecticide. Tobacco leaves contain from 0.6 to 9% of the alkaloid, along with other nicotinic derivatives. Although the demand for nicotine has declined recently, nicotine is the active

---

* Brucine, also an indole alkaloid in *Nux vomica*, is structurally classified as dimethoxystrychnine, and is used commercially as an alcohol denaturant.
** *Tobacco* refers to the Native American name for the "pipe" or tube used for smoking.

ingredient of commercial antismoking products and some contact insecticides (see Chapter 26).

Nicotine stimulates nicotinic receptors of all sympathetic and parasympathetic ganglia, neuromuscular junction innervating skeletal muscle, and CNS pathways (Figure 13.1). In general, nicotine toxicity is a complex syndrome whose cardiovascular toxicity varies widely between bradycardia and tachycardia. Signs and symptoms associated with nicotine overdose occur 1 to 2 h after exposure and include initial generalized stimulation, followed by predominance of parasympathetic overtone (salivation, lacrimation, urination, defecation, vomiting). Continued exposure progresses to muscular weakness, tremors, bradycardia, hypotension, and dyspnea, which if untreated, advances to convulsions and respiratory paralysis. The compound is best absorbed through inhalation, although oral absorption of nicotine-containing insecticides demonstrates severe toxicity. Mild toxicity is also observed in children who accidentally ingest the therapeutic nicotine patches (Nicoderm-CQ®), displaying symptoms of acute nicotinic syndrome (hypertension, hyperreflexia, hyperpyrexia, tremors, vomiting, and diarrhea).

Treatment of poisoning is primarily symptomatic and involves washing of the agent from the skin with water, induction of emesis if intervention starts soon after ingestion, and maintenance of vital signs.

Nicotine is a highly addictive drug. Psychological and physical tolerance develops with chronic smoking and use of tobacco products. Numerous products and programs are available to aid in smoking cessation. Abrupt withdrawal of tobacco use is associated with irritability, aggression, and depression. Changes in electroencephalographic recordings and autonomic functions are clearly demonstrated. Without some therapeutic intervention, a large percentage of attempts at stopping tobacco use results in failure.

13.4.3 EPHEDRINE

Ephedrine, an alkaloidal amine derived from the plant *Ephedra sinica*, has been used in Chinese medicine for more than five thousand years (see Chapter 21: "Herbal Remedies"). The plant is predominantly native to southeastern China as well as coastal regions of India and Pakistan. Although its effects are less pronounced, ephedrine is a long-acting orally active adrenergic sympathetic stimulant whose actions mimic epinephrine. Its principal effects are CNS stimulation, hypertension, and mydriasis. It has sustained bronchial muscle relaxation, mydriatic, and decongestant properties, making it suitable for therapeutic prescription and nonprescription use. Precautions in the use of ephedrine are similar to those outlined for the amphetamines.

Recently, continuous ephedrine use in nonprescription formulations has been associated with arrhythmias, strokes, heart attacks, and deaths, particularly when used by patients with preexisting cardiac disorders or in combination with other dietary stimulants. The Food and Drug Administration (FDA) in 1997 proposed mandating warning labels and a sharp reduction of the dose of ephedrine in herbal supplements, citing reports of 17 deaths and 800 illnesses linked to products that promise to help people lose weight, build muscle, and heighten sexual awareness.[*] In 2003, the FDA proposed plans that would sharply reduce the amount of ephedrine in dietary supplements and restrict the marketing of ephedrine-containing substances for weight loss and bodybuilding. The regulations would also require warning labels advising users of the dangers of high doses of ephedrine.

13.4.4 PHENYLPROPRANOLAMINE

Phenylpropranolamine (PPA) shares the pharmacological properties of ephedrine but causes less CNS stimulation. It is an α-agonist that can produce significant hypertension with a resultant reflex bradycardia.[**] Until 2001, PPA was found as an ingredient of numerous proprietary prescription and nonprescription formulations in combination with antihistamines, used for treatment of nasal and sinus congestion. Since then, the compound was voluntarily removed from most oral dosage forms because of its association with an increase in cerebral ischemia and strokes. The withdrawal of cold remedies and appetite suppressants from market shelves, including some that had been used for decades, came after federal regulators announced they would take steps to ban all use of the active ingredient in the products.

REFERENCES

SUGGESTED READINGS

Andrew, J. et al., Low prevalence of valvular heart disease in 226 phentermine-fenfluramine protocol subjects prospectively followed for up to 30 months, *J. Am. Coll. Cardiology*, 34, 1153, 1999.

Burros, M., F.D.A. Plans to Control Herbal Stimulant Tied to Deaths, *New York Times*, June, 1997.

Grady D., Search for Cause of Diet Pill's Risk Yields New Warning, Science Desk, *New York Times*, Jan., 1999.

Stolberg, S.G., Popular Cold Medicines Are Pulled From Market, *New York Times*, Nov., 2000.

REVIEW ARTICLES

Albertson, T.E., Derlet, R.W. and Van Hoozen, B.E., Methamphetamine and the expanding complications of amphetamines, *West. J. Med.*, 170, 214, 1999.

Albertson, T.E., Walby, W.F. and Derlet, R.W., Stimulant-induced pulmonary toxicity, *Chest*, 108, 1140, 1995.

---

[*] Until reports of adverse reactions to ephedrine began mounting, it had been the most widely used herbal ingredient in the dietary supplement industry. It was also sold as an alternative to the illicit drug, methamphetamine. Florida and New York banned ephedrine supplements after pills with such names as Herbal Ecstasy and Ultimate Xphoria promised a "natural high." The bans came when a 20-year-old student died after taking Ultimate Xphoria in 1996.

[**] This effect is also seen with phenylephrine (Neosynephrine® and various other products), an α-agonist used as a decongestant which raises blood pressure but slows heart rate.

Benowitz, N.L. and Gourlay, S.G., Cardiovascular toxicity of nicotine: implications for nicotine replacement therapy, *J. Am. Coll. Cardiol.*, 29, 1422, 1997.

Cockey, C.D., Is an ephedra ban coming? *AWHONN Lifelines,* 7, 103, 2003.

Czerwinski, W.P., Amphetamine-related disorders, *J. La. State Med. Soc.*, 150, 491, 1998.

Davidson, C. et al., Methamphetamine neurotoxicity: necrotic and apoptotic mechanisms and relevance to human abuse and treatment, *Brain Res. Rev.,* 36, 1, 2001.

Dawson, A.H. and Whyte, I.M., Therapeutic drug monitoring in drug overdose, *Br. J. Clin. Pharmacol.*, 52, 97S, 2001.

Eteng, M.U. et al., Recent advances in caffeine and theobromine toxicities: a review, *Plant Foods Hum. Nutr.*, 51, 231, 1997.

Geiger, J.D., Adverse events associated with supplements containing ephedra alkaloids, *Clin. J. Sport Med.*, 12, 263, 2002.

Gross, S.B. and Lepor, N.E., Anorexigen-related cardiopulmonary toxicity, *Rev. Cardiovasc. Med.*, 1, 80, 2000.

Gudelsky, G.A. and Yamamoto, B.K., Neuropharmacology and neurotoxicity of 3,4-methylenedioxymethamphetamine, *Methods Mol. Med.* 79, 55, 2003.

Kalman, D. et al., An acute clinical trial evaluating the cardiovascular effects of an herbal ephedra-caffeine weight loss product in healthy overweight adults, *Int. J. Obes. Relat. Metab. Disord.*, 26, 1363, 2002.

Keller, R.W., Jr. and Snyder-Keller, A., Prenatal cocaine exposure, *Ann. N. Y. Acad. Sci.*, 909, 217, 2000.

Knuepfer, M.M. and Mueller, P.J., Review of evidence for a novel model of cocaine-induced cardiovascular toxicity, *Pharmacol. Biochem. Behav.*, 63, 489, 1999.

Knuepfer, M.M., Cardiovascular disorders associated with cocaine use: myths and truths, *Pharmacol. Ther.*, 97, 181, 2003.

Kobayashi, H. et al., Recent progress in the neurotoxicology of natural drugs associated with dependence or addiction, their endogenous agonists and receptors, *J. Toxicol. Sci.* 24, 1, 1999.

Lake, C.R. et al., Adverse drug effects attributed to phenylpropanolamine: a review of 142 case reports. *Am. J. Med.,* 89, 195, 1990.

Lekskulchai, V. and Mokkhavesa, C., Evaluation of Roche Abuscreen ONLINE amphetamine immunoassay for screening of new amphetamine analogues, *J. Anal. Toxicol.*, 25, 471, 2001.

Levisky, J.A. et al., False-positive RIA for methamphetamine following ingestion of an Ephedra-derived herbal product, *J. Anal. Toxicol.* 27, 123, 2003.

Mersfelder, T.L., Phenylpropanolamine and stroke: the study, the FDA ruling, the implications, *Cleve. Clin. J. Med.*, 68, 208, 2001.

Minton, N.A. and Henry, J.A., Acute and chronic human toxicity of theophylline, *Hum. Exp. Toxicol.,* 15, 471, 1996.

Nawrot, P. et al., Effects of caffeine on human health, *Food Addit. Contam.*, 20, 1, 2003.

Shannon, M., Clinical toxicity of cocaine adulterants, *Ann. Emerg. Med.*, 17, 1243, 1988.

Shekelle, P.G. et al., Efficacy and safety of ephedra and ephedrine for weight loss and athletic performance: a meta-analysis, *JAMA,* 289, 1537, 2003.

Smolinske, S.C. et al., Cigarette and nicotine chewing gum toxicity in children, *Hum. Toxicol.*, 7, 27, 1988.

Spear, L.P. et al., Cocaine and development: a retrospective perspective, *Neurotoxicol. Teratol.*, 24, 321, 2002.

Stedeford, T. et al., Alpha1-adrenergic receptors and their significance to chemical-induced nephrotoxicity — a brief review, *Res. Commun. Mol. Pathol. Pharmacol.*, 110, 59, 2001.

Vanscheeuwijck, P.M. et al., Evaluation of the potential effects of ingredients added to cigarettes. Part 4: subchronic inhalation toxicity, *Food Chem. Toxicol.*, 40, 113, 2002.

Wolfe, S.M., MEDICINE: Ephedra — Scientific Evidence Versus Money/Politics, *Science,* 300, 437, 2003.

Zanardi, A. et al., Nicotine and neurodegeneration in ageing, *Toxicol. Lett.,* 127, 207, 2002.

14 Hallucinogenic Agents

14.1 HISTORY AND DESCRIPTION

The hallucinogens are a descriptive pharmacological class of synthetic and naturally occurring derivatives of the ergot alkaloids. These include the tryptamines, amphetamines, and related sympathomimetics. The feature that distinguishes these agents from the parent compounds is the production of hallucinations,* which are depicted as changes in perception, thought, and mood and the occurrence of dreamlike feelings. An individual who ingests hallucinogenic substances describes the effects as having a *spectator ego*, where a person experiences a bond with nature and society, a sense of overwhelming revelation and truth, and a vivid awareness of his or her surroundings. The use of hallucinogens was popularized in the 1960s by artists, musicians, writers, poets, scientists, and other celebrities (such as Timothy Leary), who aimed to enlighten the world about the benefits of the substances. The compounds were purported to improve creative abilities, foster higher levels of thinking and consciousness, and enhance perception. The hallucinogens were thus labeled as *mind expanding* drugs. In addition, they claimed to have beneficial effects in the treatment of psychiatric disorders, cancer, and alcoholism — claims that have since been proven invalid.

14.2 ERGOT ALKALOIDS

14.2.1 INCIDENCE AND OCCURRENCE

Ergot was originally derived from the dried sclerotium (resting body of fungus) of *Claviceps purpurea* (rye plant). Although preparations of the crude drug are seldom found in pharmaceutical formulas, the alkaloid derivatives are important medicinal agents derived primarily from parasitic and saprophytic alteration of the plant. Ergot produces a large number of alkaloids the most important of which are the ergotamines, ergonovines, and ergotoxine.

14.2.2 MEDICINAL CHEMISTRY

Figure 14.1 illustrates the parent structure of *d*-lysergic acid and the principal toxicologically important derivatives, ergotamine and lysergic acid diethylamide (LSD). The ergotamines, natural or semisynthetic, are all derivatives of *d*-lysergic acid.

---

* The term *hallucinogen* refers to a substance that produces visual images or auditory perceptions that may, in fact, not be real. Some have suggested that drugs that cause such distorted perceptions should be labeled *illusogens*. However, since this change has not received universal acceptance, this chapter will use the traditional terminology.

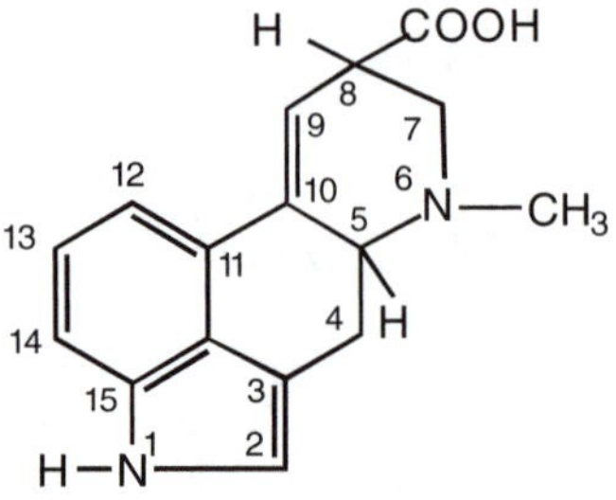

d-Lysergic acid

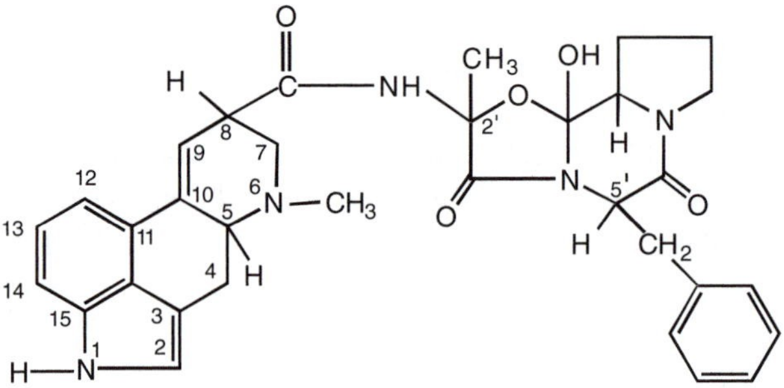

Ergotamine

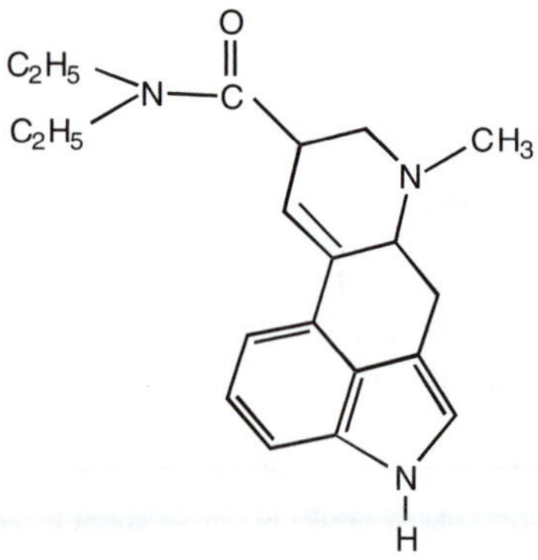

LSD (lysergic acid diethylamide)

FIGURE 14.1 Structures of *d*-lysergic acid, ergotamine, and LSD.

14.2.3 Pharmacology and Clinical Use

Ergotamine, ergonovine, and ergotoxine compounds are readily soluble in water, although their absorption rate is erratic. The ergotamine derivatives have a variety of seemingly unrelated pharmacological properties. In general, ergotamine has partial agonist or antagonist activity against trypaminergic, dopaminergic, and α-adrenergic receptors. It constricts central and peripheral blood vessels, depresses central vasomotor centers, and induces uterine contractions. For instance, methysergide (Sansert®), has no intrinsic vasoconstrictor properties in its actions against vascular headaches. Instead, it appears to block the effect of serotonin, a "headache substance" and a central neurochemical mediator, that may be involved in the production of vascular headaches. Methysergide displaces serotonin from pressor cranial arterial wall receptors during migraine headaches. Other ergot derivatives, such as methylergonovine (Methergine®), act directly on uterine smooth muscle and induce sustained contractions. Unlike the natural alkaloids, the semisynthetic dihydrogenated ergot alkaloids (ergoloid mesylates, Hydergine®) increase brain metabolism, presumably by increasing cerebral blood flow via α-adrenergic blockade, although this mechanism is contested.

Clinically, the agents are used for their oxytocin-like effect in the routine management of postpartum uterine contractions and bleeding (methylergonovine), for the prevention of vascular headaches, such as migraine or cluster headaches (dihydroergotamine, Migranal®; methysergide, Sansert®), and for the amelioration of symptoms associated with age-related mental capacity decline, as in progressive dementia and Alzheimer's dementia (dihydrogenated ergot alkaloids, Hydergine®).

14.2.4 Signs and Symptoms of Acute Toxicity

Adverse reactions occur in patients with acute ingestion of less than 5 mg of ergotamine derivatives. The most important signs and symptoms include: nausea, vomiting, neuromuscular numbness and weakness, confusion, depression, drowsiness, and convulsions. Lightheadedness, disassociation, and hallucinatory experiences reflect CNS toxicity.

14.2.5 Clinical Management of Acute Overdose

Treatment of acute overdose consists of withdrawal of the drug followed by symptomatic measures, including and not limited to, the ABCs of emergency treatment.

14.3 LYSERGIC ACID DIETHYLAMIDE (LSD)

14.3.1 Incidence and Occurrence

Lysergic acid diethylamide (LSD) does not occur naturally but is a semisynthetic preparation of d-lysergic acid (Figure 14.1, top). Discovered by A. Hoffman in 1943 during the course of experiments directed toward the synthesis of stimulants (analeptics), LSD produces opposing actions of powerful central stimulation with slight depression. Although it has no legitimate medical use today, the colorless, odorless, and tasteless compound is the most powerful psychotropic agent known, whose experimental value has proven it to be a model for psychosis.[*]

The substance is available "on the street" in liquid, powder, and microdot dosage[**] forms, with 20 to 25 µg as an effective oral dose.

14.3.2 MECHANISM OF TOXICITY

Within minutes of ingestion, an effective dose produces hallucinogenic sensations that last between 6 and 24 h. LSD produces significant pyramidal and extrapyramidal effects as a result of interaction with central 5-hydroxytryptamine (5-HT, serotonin) receptors. Specifically, the compound mimics 5-HT at 5-HT_{1A} autoreceptors on raphe nucleus cell bodies and acts as a partial or full agonist at 5-HT_{2A} and 5-HT_{2C} receptors. Selective binding to serotonin receptors accounts for the hallucinogenic and behavioral alterations associated with the substance.

14.3.3 HALLUCINOGENIC EFFECTS

The desirable effects, or in the least, the reason for intentional nontherapeutic use of the substance, vary between euphoria and dysphoria. Swift mood swings, even after a single dose within the same time period, are easily produced. The LSD *trip* is characterized predominantly by distortion in the realization of time and alteration of sensory perception, especially visual, auditory, tactile, olfactory, and gustatory. The individual experiences an intensified and altered perception of color. Objects are surrounded by halos and may leave a trail of individual afterimages when moving across a visual field. Other distortions of reality include *synesthesias*, where an auditory stimulus is perceived "visually." Normal taste, smell and touch sensations are often strange, distorted, grotesque, or uninterpretable.

The individual becomes depressed, anxious, and paranoid and may experience *ego fragmentation* or feelings of depersonalization. The latter reaction is pleasant, as the user experiences feelings of togetherness ("oneness") with the surroundings. Alternatively, the experience may be extremely uncomfortable, where the user feels a sense of loss of conscious control of thoughts and emotions and of being "out of touch" with the surroundings. In extreme cases, frightening perceptions and psychological distortions may lead to unanticipated behavior in an otherwise normal person. Such *bad trips* may be accompanied by delirium-induced self-injury or suicide.

---

[*] The seeds of *Ololiuqui* (*Rivea corymbosa*, commonly known as bindweeds or morning glories) were used as an ancient Aztec hallucinogen sporadically incorporated in Mexican religious ceremonies. The active ingredients of the seeds have been identified as ergot alkaloids, 0.05% of which include the amide and methylcarbinolamide derivatives of *d*-lysergic acid.

[**] Because of its relative potency, microgram quantities of the liquid are applied onto blotter (chromatographic or absorbent) paper and air dried. In this state, the substance is easily camouflaged and ingested by tearing and soaking the paper orally.

14.3.4 TOXICOKINETICS

Following oral ingestion of LSD, the effects are perceived within a few minutes and usually last for about 12 h. Although the cause is not clearly understood, the recurrence of *flashbacks* has been reported long after the detectable levels have disappeared. LSD is rapidly metabolized, and concentrations of the parent drug in the urine of a user do not exceed 1 to 2 ng/ml.

14.3.5 SIGNS AND SYMPTOMS OF ACUTE TOXICITY

Common adverse reactions occur within minutes after ingestion. Sympathetic stimulation results in mydriasis, hyperthermia, piloerection, tachycardia, hyperglycemia, and hypertension. Although LSD has a high therapeutic index, first time users may experience panic reactions and loss of psychological control of the immediate environment.

Flashbacks occur in 1 of 20 users. They are characterized as recurrence of the LSD experience in the **absence** of ingestion. The full range of perceptual and psychological distortions recur, including somatic and emotional hallucinations. The lack of control over the experience often leads to the development of personality changes, prolonged psychosis, neurosis, and depression. The variety, intensity, and pattern of flashbacks are unpredictable and do not rely on dose or frequency of use. The flashbacks may be triggered in unsuspecting LSD users by administration of selective serotonin reuptake inhibitors (fluoxetine, paroxetine).*

14.3.6 CLINICAL MANAGEMENT OF ACUTE OVERDOSE

Reduction of anxiety and the reassurance that a *bad trip* is due to the effects of the drug and is not permanent are important in managing LSD toxicity. Benzodiazepines are beneficial for sedation. At one time, phenothiazines were frequently used to ameliorate the psychological manifestations and perceptual distortions. The antipsychotics drugs, however, are not recommended because of the lowering of seizure thresholds. Management of symptoms of sympathetic stimulation, especially tachycardia and hyperglycemia, is also warranted.

14.3.7 TOLERANCE AND WITHDRAWAL

Chronic use of LSD is not associated with the physical and psychological tolerance or withdrawal seen with opioids or S/H, although cross-tolerance and sensitivity to mescaline and psilocybin have been reported (see below, 14.4, Tryptamine Derivatives). A return to normal functioning is common following a drug-free period.

14.3.8 METHODS OF DETECTION

Most published assays for LSD are intended for identification of the drug in illicit preparations. They do not offer the sensitivity and specificity required for detection in urine specimens. Radioimmunoassays (RIAs) for LSD appear to offer an effective means for detecting very recent drug use. However, confirmation of the presence of

---

* Prozac® and Paxil®, respectively.

LSD or its metabolites requires specific analysis. High-performance liquid chroma-tography (HPLC) combined with fluorescence detection, and capillary column gas chromatography with electron ionization mass spectrometry (GC-MS) can measure urinary concentrations as low as 0.5 ng/ml. However, neither of these assays is useful for detection of LSD in urine for more than about 12 h after ingestion.

14.4 TRYPTAMINE DERIVATIVES

14.4.1 INCIDENCE AND OCCURRENCE

Figure 14.2 illustrates the structure of tryptamine, psilocin (4-hydroxydimethyl-tryptamine), and serotonin (5-hydroxytryptamine), all of which are pharmacologi-cally and toxicologically similar.

14.4.2 MECHANISM OF TOXICITY

Ingestion of certain small mushrooms, not commonly used as food, results in hal-lucinations. The mushroom, *Psilocybe mexicana* (*food of the gods*) has been used for centuries by Mexican and Central American Indians in religious ceremonies. In 1958, A. Hoffman identified the active ingredient of the mushroom as psilocybin. As with LSD, the mechanism of toxicity is related to stimulation of sympathetic and serotonergic activity, although with less potency.

14.4.3 SIGNS AND SYMPTOMS OF ACUTE TOXICITY

The desirable pharmacological effects of psilocybin and its more active metabolite, psilocin, mimic those of LSD. A 20-mg dose of psilocin is equivalent to 100 μg of LSD. The effects, which last about 3 h, begin with anxiety and nausea, then proceed to dream-like trances and hallucinations. *Trailer* images, not unlike LSD, induce changes in color and shape perception.

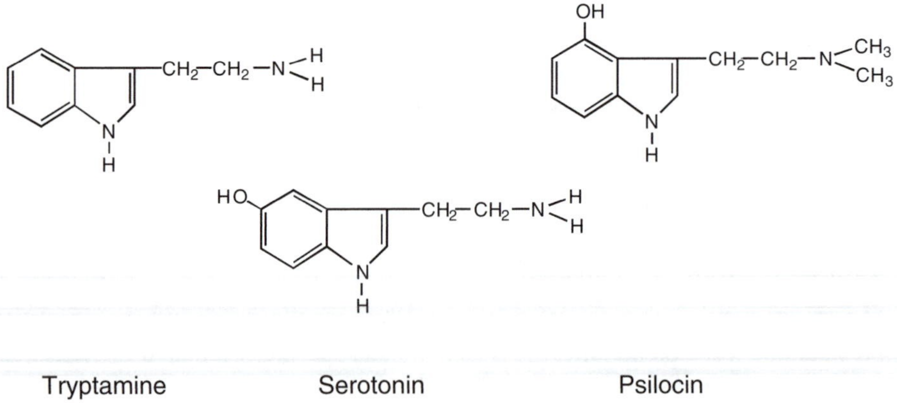

Tryptamine   Serotonin   Psilocin

FIGURE 14.2 Structures of tryptamine, serotonin (5-hydroxytryptamine), and psilocin (4-hydroxydimethyltryptamine).

Few reports of acute intoxication are available. Symptoms present within 30 to 60 min after mushroom ingestion and include agitation, hyperthermia, and possible hypotension and convulsions. Anticholinergic symptoms, such as mydriasis, blurred vision, and dizziness accompany visual disturbances.

14.4.4 CLINICAL MANAGEMENT OF ACUTE OVERDOSE

As with LSD, benzodiazepines and a cholinergic agent are useful in managing the undesirable effects of psilocybin mushroom poisoning. However, there are some special considerations surrounding the treatment of mushroom poisoning. For instance, depending on bioavailability, amount ingested, and individual susceptibility, not all persons ingesting the same meal will be symptomatic. Also, it is important to recognize that the anticholinergic effects are likely to mimic those from exposure to insecticides and may be delayed up to 6 h.

14.4.5 TOLERANCE AND WITHDRAWAL

As with LSD, chronic ingestion of psilocybin-containing mushrooms is not associated with physical and psychological tolerance or withdrawal symptoms, although cross-tolerance and sensitivity to other hallucinogens have been reported.

14.5 PHENETHYLAMINE DERIVATIVES

14.5.1 INCIDENCE AND OCCURRENCE

The synthetic hallucinogenic amphetamines are widely used among high school and college students at *rave* parties, alcoholic bars, and at events requiring endurance and alertness, such as marathon dances.

14.5.2 MEDICINAL CHEMISTRY

The β-phenethylamine derivatives are synthetic analogs of amphetamine and are illustrated in Table 14.1. Since the compounds are amphetamine-like structures, their toxicity combines the properties of stimulants with those of the hallucinogens. Compounds, such as mescaline, with a long history of abuse, and comparatively newer drugs, such as DOM (STP) and MDMA (*ecstasy*), are discussed as prototypes for this class.

14.5.3 MESCALINE

Mescaline is regarded as the first of a series of alkaloidal amine hallucinogens. The compound is derived from the dried tops of *Lophophora williamsii* (peyote or mescal buttons), from the peyote cactus. The plant is indigenous to northern Mexico and the southern United States. The plant is associated with Native American religious ceremonies. Its chief effect is the production of euphoria and hallucinations with concomitant decrease in fatigue and hunger. Ingestion of mescal buttons that contain mescaline, the most active of the peyote constituents, produces mydriasis, accom-

TABLE 14.1
Structure of the β-Phenethylamine Derivatives

Compound	Chemical Name	Common Name	2	3	4	5	R_1
					Substitutions		
Amphetamine	β-phenylisopropylamine	Speed, ups	H	H	H	H	H
Methamphetamine	β-phenylisopropylmethylamine	Meth, crank, ice, glass	H	H	H	H	CH_3
Mescaline[a]	3,4,5-trimethoxy-β-phenethylamine	Mesc, buttons	H	OCH_3	OCH_3	OCH_3	H
DOM	2,5-dimethoxy-4-methylamphetamine	STP (serenity, tranquility, peace)	OCH_3	H	CH_3	OCH_3	H
MDA	3,4-methylene-dioxyamphetamine	Harmony, love drug	H	$-O-CH_2-O-$		H	H
MDMA	3,4-methylenedioxy-methamphetamine	XTC, ecstasy, Adam	H	$-O-CH_2-O-$		H	CH_3
MDEA	3,4-methylenedioxy-ethamphetamine	Eve	H	$-O-CH_2-O-$		H	CH_2CH_3

Note: Numbered substitutions refer to the carbon positions on the phenyl ring.

[a] $CH_3 = H$ for mescaline.

panied by unusual and bizarre color perception.* Flashing lights and vivid configu-
rations characterize the initial visions, followed by dimming of colors and sleep
induction. Sensory alteration is 1000-fold less potent than LSD, but the production
of tremors, hypertension, increased heart rate, and deep tendon reflexes are significant and similar to those of the sympathomimetic amines.

Mescaline is rapidly absorbed; plasma concentrations peak at about 2 h and last
about 12 h. Other than the risk of hypertensive crisis, toxicity with mescaline is rare.

14.5.4 DOM (2,5-Dimethoxy-4-Methylamphetamine, STP)

DOM is up to 100 times more potent than mescaline. However, its effects are milder
than MDMA, which is discussed below.

14.5.5 MDMA (3,4-Methylenedioxymethamphetamine, Ecstasy)

Originally introduced as an anorexiant and popularized in the 1980s, *ecstasy* is
still promoted as a "good high, low risk" drug of abuse. The illicit substance is
available in liquid and powder forms, predominantly for oral or inhalation administration. An average dose of 100 mg produces initial symptoms similar to those
seen with amphetamine use, namely, mydriasis and hyperventilation. Unlike LSD,
individuals appear to have more control over the hallucinogenic experience, with
feelings of great affection and a desire to be with others. The individual displays
an introspective behavior, complimenting or overwhelming the euphoric effect (the
ecstatic feeling). Even with small doses, however, toxicity soon follows. Muscle
tension, especially of the neck and jaw, chills, sweating, rapid eye movement, and
a trance-like state develop. Amnesia, delirium, and erratic behavior accompany
the hypertensive crisis. The drug is responsible for several hundred deaths per
year, especially among young adults.**

Treatment of *ecstasy* toxicity is symptomatic and managed as with intoxication
with amphetamines.

14.5.6 Methods of Detection

As with amphetamines, qualitative drug screening will detect phenethylamine
derivatives in urine up to 72 h. Enzyme-linked immunoassays (ELISA) or RIA
methods are sensitive to 1000 ng/ml of urine sample. Newer synthetic derivatives,
however, may elude detection. In addition, false positives are likely in the event
of concomitant ingestion of any of the sympathomimetic amines, including popular nonprescription decongestant drugs such as ephedrine, phenylpropranolamine, and pseudoephedrine. Common adulterants that mask a positive test for
amphetamine derivatives (producing a false negative result) include bleach, bak-
ing soda, and detergents.

---

* Anhalanine is another active peyote ingredient.
** The FDA has recently approved the first study of ecstasy as a treatment for post-traumatic stress disorder
(2003).

14.6 PHENCYCLIDINE (1-PHENYLCYCLOHEXYL PIPERIDINE, PCP)

14.6.1 INCIDENCE AND OCCURRENCE

Originally marketed as an anesthetic (Sernyl®), the drug was soon identified with postanesthetic confusion and delirium. After a brief shift as an animal tranquilizer, its legitimate therapeutic use was banned, but its street popularity blossomed. Since the compound can be manufactured with ease and packaged as tablets, liquid, capsules or powder, PCP is usually sprinkled over marijuana and inhaled through smoking.*

14.6.2 TOXICOKINETICS

PCP is well absorbed following all routes of administration. Maximum plasma PCP concentrations are observed 5 to 15 min after smoking. It is a lipophilic weak base ($pK_a = 8.6$), and its volume of distribution is high ($V_d = 6.0$ l/kg). Thus, the compound is widely distributed and produces unreliable plasma concentrations. Its long half-life (several hours to days) contributes to its prolonged toxic effect, especially with chronic use.

PCP undergoes oxidation and conjugation in the body, primarily to hydroxylated metabolites. About 10% of PCP is excreted unchanged in the urine. Both parent and conjugated metabolites may be detectable in urine for several days to several weeks. Some PCP is secreted in the saliva.

14.6.3 SIGNS AND SYMPTOMS OF ACUTE TOXICITY

Toxic effects are labeled as *dissociative anesthesia*, where the patient experiences acute subjective feelings of depersonalization. Symptoms are variable and do not appear to correlate with PCP plasma concentrations. Initially, the patient exhibits excitation, paranoia, and dysphoria and may display aggressive tendencies. Disorientation, mood changes, catatonia,** and disorganized thoughts are displayed. Ataxia, impaired speech, myoclonus,*** and choreoathetoid movements**** are possible, depending on the level of exposure. Hypertension and nystagmus***** are hallmark findings with PCP toxicity. With continued toxicity or exposure to higher doses, patients develop coma of brief duration, as well as hyperthermia and risk of rhabdomyolysis. Agitation and depression are common after coma is resolved.

PCP-induced aggression and psychosis are frequently encountered and are characterized by aggressive and violent behavior of several days' duration. Recovery is

---

* Common street names vary by region and often allude to its use as a veterinary anesthetic, including *Sherman, angel dust, killer weed, snorts, PeaCe Pill,* and *embalming fluid* (named for its combination with marijuana when smoked through a formaldehyde-filled water pipe).
** A state of motor disturbance characterized by immobility with extreme muscular rigidity.
*** Muscular spasms.
**** Characterized by jerky, "tic-like" twitching (choreiform) and slow, writhing (athetoid) movements.
***** Involuntary, rhythmically oscillating movements of the eyes.

complete, although respiratory arrest, seizures, memory loss, and hallucinations are implicated in life-threatening (often fatal) self-inflicted behavior.

14.6.4 CLINICAL MANAGEMENT OF ACUTE OVERDOSE

In order to minimize aggression, patients are isolated from sensory stimuli. Supportive, symptomatic care is essential. In addition, i.v. benzodiazepines (diazepam) for seizure, along with haloperidol for agitation, are effective. Severe hypertension is treated aggressively. Urinary acidification is useless, because only a small percentage is excreted unchanged in the urine and acidification increases the risk of myoglobinuric renal failure. Psychiatric reassurance, diuretics, and hemodialysis are ineffective. Activated charcoal can be administered if ingestion is recent.

14.6.5 TOLERANCE AND WITHDRAWAL

Psychological tolerance is noted with chronic abuse of PCP and is responsible for gradual development of symptoms of paranoia, hallucinations, anxiety, and severe depression.

14.6.6 METHODS OF DETECTION

Because of its wide bioavailability, PCP concentrations vary and are an unreliable monitor for clinical effects. In fact, urine samples can remain positive for up to four weeks after ingestion in chronic users. ELISA and RIA are the methods of choice for urine drug toxicology screening. Immunochemical methods are relatively specific for PCP, its metabolites, and some of the closely related analogs. Methods for confirmation include gas-liquid chromatography with nitrogen-phosphorus detection (GLC/NPD), or gas chromatography-mass spectrometry (GC-MS). Other drugs, such as thioridazine, dextromethorphan, and chlorpromazine may show false-positive reactions in immunochemical assays for PCP.

14.7 MARIJUANA

14.7.1 INCIDENCE AND OCCURRENCE

Marijuana (Mexican cannabis, *pot*) is obtained from the dried flowering tops, seeds, and stems of the hemp plant variety of *Cannabis sativa* (Indian hemp). The plant is an annual herb indigenous to central and western Asia and is cultivated in India and other tropical and temperate regions for the fiber (manufacturing of rope) and hempseed. The oil of the hemp plant is expressed and used to make paints and soaps.* The amount of resin found in the pistil flowering tops markedly decreases as the plants are grown in more temperate regions, making the American crop of marijuana considerably less potent than the South American variety (a.k.a. *sinsemilla*, without seeds).

---

* Cannabis, the ancient Greek name for hemp, was used in China and India (*charas*) and spread to Persia (*hashish*). It was introduced into European and American botanical formularies around the seventeenth century.

The importation of crude marijuana cigarettes (*reefer, joint*) began in the 1950s and spread quickly through U.S. schools. This prompted federal and state law enforcement to start a campaign to eliminate and discourage their sale. Possession of marijuana was prohibited, and large areas of naturally growing American hemp were destroyed.[*] The effort resulted in discontinuance of the medicinal use of cannabis in the United States. Nevertheless, it is the most commonly used illegal substance in the United States and the number one cash crop, with earnings estimated at $32 billion yearly. Although a proprietary form of the active ingredient is available in capsule form as a prescription drug (dronabinol, see below), to date, grassroots efforts sporadically and periodically attempt to overturn the ban against smoking of medical marijuana.

14.7.2 MEDICINAL CHEMISTRY

Cannabis yields between 0.5 and 20% of a resin containing the major active euphoric principle, delta-9-*trans*-tetrahydrocannabinol (δ^9-THC), along with other cannabinoid constituents.

14.7.3 CLINICAL USE AND EFFECTS

Dronabinol, a synthetic form of δ^9-THC, is available in 5- and 10-mg capsules for the treatment of nausea and vomiting associated with cancer chemotherapy. It is also used as an appetite stimulant for anorexia associated with weight loss in AIDS patients. Other unlabelled uses include treatment of glaucoma and epilepsy. Non-therapeutic effects of dronabinol are identical to those of marijuana and other centrally active cannabinoids.

Smoking marijuana or oral ingestion of cannabinoids has complex central sympathomimetic effects, mediated in part by the presence of neural cannabinoid receptors. Mood changes accompany marijuana use, ranging from euphoria, depression, paranoia, and anxiety[**] to detachment. Most prominent effects are relaxation and sedation. Behavioral effects appear as loss of goal-oriented drive and short-term memory, and a vague sense of time (*temporal disintegration*). The individual is prone to spontaneous laughter, hallucinations, and delusions, although the latter are usually seen with higher doses.

Physiological symptoms involve dry mouth, stimulation of appetite, muscular incoordination, decrease of testosterone levels, urinary retention, increase in heart rate, and conjunctival injection. The last effect contributes to decreased intraocular pressure.

14.7.4 TOXICOKINETICS

An average cigarette contains about 500 to 1000 mg of the herb, each containing 1 to 2% δ^9-THC. Oral administration is almost completely absorbed (90%), while only 5 to 10% is absorbed through inhalation of marijuana smoke, primarily because of

---

[*] The herbicide paraquat was routinely sprayed on marijuana fields in northern Mexico and in the southern U.S., precipitating a syndrome of pulmonary fibrosis (see Chapter 27, "Herbicides").
[**] The aggression associated with PCP, however, is absent.

loss to pyrolysis. Inhalation results in more rapid absorption (1 to 2 min vs. 0.5 to 1 h onset for oral), with a 2- to 4-h duration. Its high lipid solubility contributes to its large volume of distribution (V_d ~10 l/kg) and long half-life ($t_{1/2}$ ~7 days). This accounts for its leakage from lipid stores and detection in plasma and urine up to 8 weeks in chronic users.

Dronabinol and δ^9-THC undergo extensive first-pass hepatic metabolism, yielding active and inactive principal metabolites, 11-hydroxy-δ^9-THC and 8,11-dihydroxy-δ^9-THC, respectively. The 9-carboxy metabolite is found principally in urine.

14.7.5 ACUTE TOXICITY AND CLINICAL MANAGEMENT

Toxic effects are an extension of the pharmacological and clinical effects. Although serious toxicity is uncommon, psychosis and dangers related to poor judgment are complications. Usually the complications result from ingestion of high doses, excessive use, poor or contaminated street quality of the substance, or when taken in combination with other S/H or hallucinogens. For instance, when marijuana is sprinkled with PCP, it produces a substance known as *superweed*, a valuable street commodity. Smoking of marijuana impairs motor skills, making driving a motor vehicle hazardous. Pneumomediastinum, characterized by over-distention and rupture, is secondary to deep inhalation of marijuana smoke.

In general, psychiatric reassurance and supportive care are adequate treatment modalities. Psychosis is transient and manageable with benzodiazepines.

14.7.6 TOLERANCE, WITHDRAWAL, AND CHRONIC EFFECTS

There is no apparent physical tolerance, and psychological tolerance is variable. Some pharmacological tolerance to the cardiovascular effects, however, are observable. The withdrawal syndrome manifests as sleep disturbances, irritability, nausea, weight loss, and restlessness.

Long-term psychological effects have suggested a sixfold increase in the incidence of schizophrenia. There is a higher incidence of mouth, throat, and lung cancer in young adults. There appears to be a decrease in sperm motility and number, and abnormal sperm morphology is associated with chronic marijuana smoking. Deleterious genetic effects, however, are debatable.

14.7.7 METHODS OF DETECTION

Cannabinoids are difficult to detect, particularly because of their high lipid solubility and low concentrations in urine and plasma. Lipid solubility increases the difficulty of separating canabinoids from the biological matrix for analysis. Qualitative drug screening, such as the labor-intensive TLC methods, will detect THC metabolites to 50 ng/ml up to several weeks post ingestion. The immunoassays (EMIT, RIA, and FIA), the preferred initial screening assays, detect the major metabolite of THC in urine (9-carboxy-THC). Some cross-reactivity occurs with many of the other glucuronide conjugated metabolites. Confirmation of positive screening tests requires the use of chromatographic techniques (GLC, HPLC, TLC, GC-MS), that are capable of separating and detecting the major metabolites. GC-MS is the most reliable confirmatory method, especially when used with electron impact (EI) and chemical ionization (CI) detector modes. Common adulterants that mask a positive test for marijuana metabolites include detergents, salt, use of diuretics, and vinegar.

14.8 MISCELLANEOUS HALLUCINOGENIC AGENTS

14.8.1 KETAMINE (*SPECIAL K*)

Ketamine is a rapid-acting general anesthetic used as a sole or supplemental anesthetic in diagnostic and surgical procedures in emergency medicine and veterinary medicine. It produces a *dissociative anesthesia* similar to that of PCP. Ketamine selectively interrupts association pathways of the brain before producing somatesthetic sensory blockade. As a drug of abuse, it is administered orally, intravenously, or by inhalation. As an acquaintance "date-rape" drug, the dissociative effect of ketamine makes it difficult for the victim to recall an account of the event.

Drug users claim that the hallucinogenic effects are superior to LSD and PCP. Low doses require 15 to 20 min onset and produce profound anesthesia with normal laryngeal-pharyngeal reflexes and respiratory stimulation. The effects of higher doses vary from the induction of pleasant dream-like states with vivid imagery and hallucinations, to delirium accompanied by confusion, excitement, and irrational behavior. Although the effect of ketamine lasts for 20 to 45 min, the duration of psychological manifestations is ordinarily a few hours, and recurrence is seen up to 24 h postoperatively. Respiratory depression, seizures, arrhythmias, and cardiac arrest are toxic sequelae.

General treatment of ketamine toxicity involves the ABCs of supportive care. The patient should be in quiet recovery with minimal stimulation. As a general anesthetic in surgical procedures, the incidence of psychological manifestations may be reduced using lower doses of ketamine with i.v. diazepam.

14.8.2 GAMMA-HYDROXYBUTYRATE (GHB)

Originally developed and used in the 1970s as an anesthetic agent and for sleep disorders, GHB is currently listed as an "orphan drug" for the treatment of narcolepsy and auxiliary symptoms of cataplexy, sleep paralysis, and hypnagogic hallucinations. It is available illegally as a colorless, odorless liquid, gel or crystalline powder, making it undetectable when combined with alcohol or other drugs. Although its use was popularized as an acquaintance date-rape drug, it is frequently used by many drug abusers. Some nicknames include: *liquid ecstasy, somatox, grievous bodily harm,* and *invigorate.* Penalties for illegal possession are similar to those of marijuana.*

---

* Interestingly, gamma-amino butyrolactone (GBL), the metabolite of GHB, is available from chemical suppliers and, when combined with sodium hydroxide, forms the active parent compound. Similarly, butyrolactone, an industrial chemical, can also be converted to GHB with similar hallucinogenic effects.

TABLE 14.2
Characterization of GHB Effects Corresponding to Dosage

Dose (mg/kg)	Signs and Symptoms
Less than 10	Drowsiness, dizziness, disorientation
10 to 20	Vomiting, rapid onset of coma, amnesia
20 to 30	Induction of REM sleep, which cycles with non-REM sleep
30 to 50	Respiratory depression, bradycardia, clonic muscle contractions, anesthesia, depressed cardiac output

GHB is an agonist for GABA-B receptors* causing CNS depression. The depression is characterized by drowsiness, dizziness, and disorientation within 15 to 30 min. Apnea and hypoxia follow larger doses. Marked agitation upon stimulation is a distinguishing feature of GHB ingestion. Table 14.2 lists the features of GHB toxicity corresponding to dosage (other depressant effects of GHB are discussed in Chapter 11, "Sedative/Hypnotics").

As with ketamine, maintenance of respiratory integrity and application of the ABCs in supportive care are crucial in overdose management. Atropine is indicated for bradycardia, while bedside suction and supplemental oxygen are necessary for maintaining a patent airway.

REFERENCES

SUGGESTED READINGS

Chamberlain, J.C., *The Analysis of Drugs in Biological Fluids*, 2nd edition, CRC Press, Inc., Boca Raton, FL., 1995.
Snyder, S.H., Faillace, L. and Hollister, L., 2,5-dimethoxy-4-methyl-amphetamine (STP): a new hallucinogenic drug, *Science,* 158, 669, 1967.

REVIEW ARTICLES

Abraham, H.D. and Aldridge, A.M., Adverse consequences of lysergic acid diethylamide, *Addiction*, 88, 1327, 1993.
Adams, I.B. and Martin. B.R., Cannabis: pharmacology and toxicology in animals and humans, *Addiction*, 91, 1585, 1996.
Ameri, A., The effects of cannabinoids on the brain, *Prog. Neurobiol.*, 58, 315, 1999.
Aniline, O. and Pitts, F.N., Jr., Phencyclidine (PCP): a review and perspectives, *Crit. Rev. Toxicol.*, 10, 145, 1982.
Bigal, M.E. and Tepper, S.J., Ergotamine and dihydroergotamine: a review, *Curr. Pain. Headache Rep.*, 7, 55, 2003.
Burgess, C., O'Donohoe, A. and Gill, M., Agony and ecstasy: a review of MDMA effects and toxicity, *Eur. Psychiatry,* 15, 287, 2000.

---

* GABA, gamma-amino butyric acid, is a naturally occurring inhibitory neurotransmitter and is discussed at length in Chapter 11.

Caldwell, J. and Sever, P.S., The biochemical pharmacology of abused drugs. I. Amphetamines, cocaine, and LSD, *Clin. Pharmacol. Ther.*, 16, 625, 1974.

Carroll, M.E., PCP and hallucinogens, *Adv. Alcohol Subst. Abuse.* 9, 167, 1990.

Deleu, D., Northway, M.G., and Hanssens, Y., Clinical pharmacokinetic and pharmacodynamic properties of drugs used in the treatment of Parkinson's disease, *Clin. Pharmacokinet.,* 41, 261, 2002.

Fraser, A.D., Coffin, L., and Worth, D., Drug and chemical metabolites in clinical toxicology investigations: the importance of ethylene glycol, methanol and cannabinoid metabolite analyses, *Clin. Biochem.*, 35, 501, 2002.

Freese, T.E., Miotto, K., and Reback, C.J., The effects and consequences of selected club drugs, *J. Subst. Abuse. Treat.*, 23, 151, 2002.

Gable, R.S., Toward a comparative overview of dependence potential and acute toxicity of psychoactive substances used nonmedically, *Am. J. Drug Alcohol Abuse.,*19, 263, 1993.

Goss, J., Designer drugs. Assess & manage patients intoxicated with ecstasy, GHB or rohypnol — the three most commonly abused designer drugs, *J. Emerg. Med. Serv.*, 26, 84, 2001.

Gudelsky, G.A., Yamamoto, B.K., Neuropharmacology and neurotoxicity of 3,4-methylenedioxymethamphetamine, *Methods Mol. Med.*, 79, 55, 2003.

Halpern, J.H. and Pope, H.G., Jr., Do hallucinogens cause residual neuropsychological toxicity? *Drug Alcohol Depend.*, 53, 247, 1999.

Hussein, H.S. and Brasel, J.M., Toxicity, metabolism, and impact of mycotoxins on humans and animals, *Toxicology,* 167, 101, 2001.

Li, J.H. and Lin, L.F., Genetic toxicology of abused drugs: a brief review, *Mutagenesis,* 13, 557, 1998.

Logan, W.J., Neurological aspects of hallucinogenic drugs, *Adv. Neurol.*, 13, 47, 1975.

Miotto, K. et al., Gamma-hydroxybutyric acid: patterns of use, effects and withdrawal, *Am. J. Addict.*, 10, 232, 2001.

Morland, J., Toxicity of drug abuse — amphetamine designer drugs (ecstasy): mental effects and consequences of single dose use, *Toxicol. Lett.,*112, 147, 2000.

Nahas, G. and Latour, C., The human toxicity of marijuana, *Med. J. Aust.*, 156, 495, 1992.

O'Connell, T., Kaye, L. and Plosay, J.J., III, Gamma-hydroxybutyrate (GHB): a newer drug of abuse, *Am. Fam. Physician,* 62, 2478, 2000.

Patel, R. and Connor, G., A review of thirty cases of rhabdomyolysis-associated acute renal failure among phencyclidine users, *J. Toxicol. Clin. Toxicol.*, 23, 547, 1985–86.

Pentney, A.R., An exploration of the history and controversies surrounding MDMA and MDA, *J. Psychoactive Drugs,* 33, 213, 2001.

Rech, R.H. and Commissaris, R.L., Neurotransmitter basis of the behavioral effects of hallucinogens, *Neurosci. Biobehav. Rev.*, 6, 521, 1982.

Rhee, D.J., Complementary and alternative medicine for glaucoma, *Surv. Ophthalmol.*, 46, 43, 2001.

Schmid, R.L., Sandler, A.N., and Katz, J., Use and efficacy of low-dose ketamine in the management of acute postoperative pain: a review of current techniques and outcomes, *Pain,* 82, 111, 1999.

Schwartz, R.H., Marijuana: a decade and a half later, still a crude drug with underappreciated toxicity, *Pediatrics,* 109, 284, 2002.

Smith, K.M., Larive, L.L., and Romanelli, F., Club drugs: methylenedioxymethamphetamine, flunitrazepam, ketamine hydrochloride, and gamma-hydroxybutyrate, *Am. J. Health Syst. Pharm.*, 59, 1067, 2002.

Smith, K.M., Drugs used in acquaintance rape, *J. Am. Pharm. Assoc. (*Wash), 39, 519, 1999.

Teter, C.J. and Guthrie, S.K., A comprehensive review of MDMA and GHB: two common club drugs, *Pharmacotherapy,* 21, 1486, 2001.

Tfelt-Hansen, P., Ergotamine, dihydroergotamine: current uses and problems, *Curr. Med. Res. Opin.,* 17, S30, 2001.

Voth, E.A. and Schwartz, R.H., Medicinal applications of delta-9-tetrahydrocannabinol and marijuana, *Ann. Intern. Med.,* 126, 791, 1997.

Zavaleta, E.G., et al., St. Anthony's fire (ergotamine induced leg ischemia) — a case report and review of the literature, *Angiology,* 52, 349, 2001.

15 Anticholinergic and Neuroleptic Drugs

15.1 INTRODUCTION TO DRUGS POSSESSING ANTICHOLINERGIC EFFECTS

A variety of chemicals, drugs, and herbal derivatives possess anticholinergic properties defined by their ability to block the neurotransmitter acetylcholine (ACh). This effect is a result of a direct interference with either of two types of cholinergic receptors — peripheral muscarinic or nicotinic receptors. Anticholinergic effects are also a consequence of adverse drug reactions (ADR), as seen with the tricyclic and phenothiazine antidepressants. In addition, many anticholinergic compounds exert their action by occupying central cholinergic receptors, thus producing alterations upon the CNS.

Autonomic neurons and their receptors govern sympathetic (SNS) and parasympathetic (PNS) activity throughout the body (see Chapter 13, Figure 13.1, for an illustration of adrenergic neurons). **Nicotinic receptors** are present in the plasma membrane of dendrites and cell bodies of both SNS and PNS postganglionic neurons, at the neuromuscular junction, and in the spinal cord. Activation of these receptors triggers postsynaptic neuronal excitation and skeletal muscle contraction. **Muscarinic receptors** are present on cell membranes of smooth and cardiac muscle and sweat glands. Activation of these receptors by acetylcholine delivers stimulation or inhibition, depending on the effector organ. Under normal circumstances, the effect of acetylcholine is transient and rapid, due to inactivation by the enzyme acetylcholinesterase. Anticholinergic agents therefore have been traditionally referred to as antimuscarinic agents or cholinergic blockers.

15.2 ANTIHISTAMINES, GASTROINTESTINAL AND ANTIPARKINSON DRUGS

15.2.1 INCIDENCE

Table 15.1 organizes representative, currently available antihistamines, gastrointestinal (GI), and antiparkinson drugs that possess anticholinergic properties, along with their most important clinical adverse effects. Antihistamines, found in cough and cold preparations, represent 5.5% of the most frequently ingested substances in children 6 years and younger. The anticholinergic properties of antiparkinson agents are therapeutically desirable. They are indicated for the adjunctive treatment of all forms of parkinsonism and are used to ameliorate the extrapyramidal symptoms (EPS) associated with traditional neuroleptic drugs. The GI agents listed were

TABLE 15.1

Categories, Representative Compounds, and Proprietary Names of Currently Available Antihistamine, Antiparkinson and Gastrointestinal Drugs Possessing Anticholinergic Properties

Category	Therapeutic Classification	Compound	Proprietary Name	Predominant Anticholinergic Effects
Antihistamines	H₁-antagonists	Brompheniramine	Dimetane	Dry mouth, mydriasis, drowsiness, dyspnea, facial flushing, sinus tachycardia
		Diphenhydramine	Benadryl	
		Dimenhydrinate	Dramamine	
		Chlorpheniramine	Chlortrimeton	
		Promethazine	Phenergan	
		Meclizine	Bonine, Antivert	
		Pyrilamine	In combination with nasal decongestants	
Antiparkinson agents	Anticholinergic[a]	Benztropine	Cogentin	Dry mouth, mydriasis, blurred vision, dyspnea, sinus tachycardia, toxic psychosis, coma, seizures, ataxia, EPS
		Trihexyphenydyl	Artane	
		Procyclidine	Kemadrin	
		Biperiden	Akineton	
Gastrointestinal anticholinergic agents	Antispasmodic	Atropine	various	Dry mouth, mydriasis, drowsiness, dyspnea, excitement, agitation, constipation, blurred vision, sinus tachycardia
		Homatropine	various	
		Belladonna alkaloids	Donnatal[b]	
		Clidinium bromide	Quarzan; Librax (with chlordiazepoxide)	
		l-Hyoscyamine	Levsin, Levsinex	
		Scopolamine	Scopace	
		Glycopyrrolate	Robinul	
		Dicyclomine	Bentyl	
		Propantheline	Pro-Banthine	

Note: Drugs such as tripelenamine have been removed from the therapeutic market.

[a] As distinguished from antidopaminergic agents.

[b] In combination with atropine, scopolamine, L-hyoscyamine, and phenobarbital.

originally developed as *spasmolytics* for the management of excessive intestinal activity associated with peptic ulcers, diarrhea, and related disorders.

15.2.2 Medicinal Chemistry, Pharmacology, and Clinical Use

Administered as tablets, capsules, liquids, and in tinctures, belladonna alkaloids are derived from the perennial herb *Belladonna* (Deadly Nightshade),[*] cultivated throughout the world. The belladonna compounds are semisynthetic derivatives from the plant's naturally occurring tropane alkaloids. Today, their usefulness as GI agents has been largely replaced by histamine-2 (H_2) blockers, such as famotidine, and proton pump inhibitors, such as omeprazole. Closely related to the belladonna derivatives are the solanaceous alkaloids, L-hyoscyamine, scopolamine, and atropine, obtained from the extremely poisonous plant species of *Hyoscyamus Linné* (*Atropa belladonna*).[**]

15.2.3 Signs and Symptoms of Acute Toxicity

In general, anticholinergic compounds exert their effects by blocking central and peripheral muscarinic and cholinergic receptors. Table 15.1 displays the most common ADRs associated with antihistamines, antiparkinson, and GI drugs. Dry mouth and mydriasis are the most common ADRs of all anticholinergic agents, as well as headache, dysuria, and dyspnea (difficulty breathing due to tightness of the chest). Increased vascular permeability and capillary perfusion is mediated by an unregulated SNS stimulation from anticholinergic activity of these compounds, and accounts for the facial and upper body flushing. Sinus tachycardia is the most sensitive sign of toxicity and may exacerbate other conduction abnormalities. Sedation is an effect common mostly to antihistamines and is mediated primarily through blocking of central H_1 receptors.

15.2.4 Clinical Management of Acute Overdose

Anticholinergic poisoning is managed by i.v. physostigmine (Antilirium®), a reversible cholinesterase inhibitor. Through its action at both central and peripheral cholinergic receptors, physostigmine reverses anticholinergic activity and ameliorates coma, delirium, and seizures that accompany severe toxicity. As discussed below, however, physostigmine is not recommended in reversing the anticholinergic actions of tricyclic and phenothiazine derivatives due to potential induction of fatal asystoles.

---

[*] In ancient Greece and Rome, the juice of the berry placed in the eyes caused mydriasis (dilation) of the pupils, thus producing a striking appearance; hence the name *Belladonna* (from the Italian, beautiful lady). The poisonous nature of the plant has been known since ancient times.

[**] Stramonium or Jimson weed (Jamestown weed, *Datura stramonium*) is indigenous to ancient Arabic lands but cultivated today throughout the world. The purple North American variety is noxious and frequently responsible for poisoning in children. It also has hallucinogenic properties, and is single-handedly accountable for quenching British troops who ingested the stramonium-laden anticholinergic seeds during Bacon's rebellion in colonial America, 1676.

Alternatively, i.v. benzodiazepines are suggested in the treatment of less critical anticholinergic CNS toxicity.

15.3 TRICYCLIC ANTIDEPRESSANTS

15.3.1 INCIDENCE

The term neuroleptic has come to replace older terminology that described the clinical effects of the major class belonging to the psychotherapeutic agents. These include the classes of compounds known as the major and minor tranquilizers, antipsychotic, antimanic, antipanic, and antidepressant drugs. Although the tricyclic antidepressants and phenothiazine derivatives possess significant anticholinergic reactions, they may still be identified with the antidepressant and antipsychotic categories, respectively. Newer atypical neuroleptic agents lack the parkinson-like effects.

The phenothiazine derivatives, chlorpromazine and promethazine, were the first neuroleptics synthesized in the 1950s and are the pharmacological prototypes for all psychoactive compounds. Because of their life-threatening toxicity and potential for inducing intentional suicide, especially in patients at increased risk for self-inflicted harm, treatment regimens are generally limited to one- or two-week supplies.

15.3.2 MEDICINAL CHEMISTRY

The neuroleptic agents are grouped by chemical classification, yet their toxicities differ based on preferential receptor activity. Table 15.2 summarizes the categories, compounds, and proprietary names of representative currently available neuroleptic agents, including the tricyclic, phenothiazine, and newer antidepressant drugs, possessing anticholinergic properties.

15.3.3 PHARMACOLOGY AND CLINICAL USE

Unlike the phenothiazines and related derivatives, tricyclic neuroleptic agents have predominantly antiserotonergic and anticholinergic activity. These central actions account for their utility as antipsychotics, particularly in producing sedation (for agitation) and in reducing hallucinations and delirium. In addition, anticholinergic and antihistaminic effects confer desirable antiemetic/antinausea properties (prochlorperazine) and antihistaminic properties (promethazine) to some agents, respectively.

15.3.4 TOXICOKINETICS

Tricyclic antidepressant drugs are rapidly absorbed with quick onset. They possess high protein binding and high volume of distribution (V_d) properties, providing for a prolonged duration of action. Their therapeutic effects, however, require 5 to 7 days before benefits are observed because of necessary depletion of neurotransmitter storage.

TABLE 15.2
Categories, Representative Compounds, and Proprietary Names of Currently Available Neuroleptic Drugs Possessing Anticholinergic Properties

Category	Neuroleptic Classification	Compound	Proprietary Name	Predominant Pharmacologic and Anticholinergic Effects
Tricyclic antidepressants	Secondary amines	Amoxapine	Asendin	Greater α-adrenergic blockade; low hypotensive, antimuscarinic, antihistaminic effects; mydriasis, ECG abnormalities; CNS depression, arrhythmias, hypothermia/hyperthermia, low EPS effects
		Desipramine	Norpramine	
		Nortriptyline	Pamelor	
		Protriptyline	Vivactyl	
	Tertiary amines	Amitriptyline	Elavil	Greater serotonergic blockade; high antimuscarinic effects, mydriasis, ECG abnormalities; CNS depression, cardiac arrhythmias, hypothermia/hyperthermia, low EPS effects
		Imipramine	Tofranil	
		Doxepin	Sinequan	
		Trimipramine	Surmontil	
	Tetracyclic	Maprotiline	various	Low α-adrenergic blockade acitivity
	Triazopyridine	Trazodone	Desyrel	
	Aminoketone	Bupropion	Wellbutrin	Four-fold increased risk of seizure (0.4%)
Phenothiazine antipsychotics	Aliphatic	Chlorpromazine	Thorazine	Significant EPS, sedative, CNS & hypotensive effects
	Piperidine	Thioridazine	Mellaril	Significant sedative & CNS effects, low EPS, moderate hypotensive effects
	Piperazine	Perphenazine	Trilafon	Significant EPS & CNS effects, low sedative, low hypotensive effects
		Fluphenazine	Prolixin	
		Trifluoperazine	Stelazine	
		Promethazine[a]	Phenergan	
		Prochlorperazine[b]	Compazine	

(continued)

TABLE 15.2 (CONTINUED)
Categories, Representative Compounds, and Proprietary Names of Currently Available Neuroleptic Drugs Possessing Anticholinergic Properties

Category	Neuroleptic Classification	Compound	Proprietary Name	Predominant Pharmacologic and Anticholinergic Effects
Phenylbutyl-piperidines	Butyrophenone	Haloperidol	Haldol	Significant EPS & sedative, low hypotensive effects
	Diphenylbutyl-piperidine	Pimozide	Orap	
Thioxanthines	Thioxanthines[c]	Thiothixene	Navane	Moderate EPS, sedative & hypotensive effects
Newer atypical neuroleptics	Dibenzodiazepine	Clozapine	Clozaril	Sedation, repiratory depression or coma with O.D.; low EPS events; low frequency of arrhythmias, hypotension, seizures, NMS; significant blood dyskrasias (agranulocytosis)
		Olanzapine	Zyprexa	Less incidence of blood dyskrasias but similar EPS and adverse effects as clozapine
	Benzisoxazole	Risperidone	Risperdal	Less incidence of blood dyskrasias but similar EPS and adverse effects as clozapine
	Dibenzothiazepine	Quetiapine	Seroquel	

Note: EPS = extrapyramidal symptoms

[a] Promethazine is used predominantly as a cough suppressant.
[b] Prochlorperazine is used as an antiemetic/antinausea drug.
[c] Chlorprothixene (Taractan) no longer marketed.

15.3.5 SIGNS AND SYMPTOMS AND MECHANISM OF ACUTE TOXICITY

Table 15.2 outlines the most significant toxicologic effects of tricyclic neuroleptic drug ingestion. CNS depression, seizures, and cardiac arrhythmias are generally observed with acute overdose, while anticholinergic and some extrapyramidal symptoms (EPS) are common ADRs. Table 15.3 describes EPS associated with tricyclic and phenothiazine drugs.

Neuroleptic-induced hypotension occurs as a result of peripheral α-receptor (adrenergic) blockade associated with the tricyclics. Decreased cardiac output and circulatory collapse are potentially life threatening.

TABLE 15.3
Characterization of the Extrapyramidal Symtoms (EPS) Associated with Neuroleptic Agents

Syndrome	Signs and Symptoms	Clinical Management
Acute dystonic reactions	Oculogyric crisis (upward gaze paralysis); muscular spasms of neck (torticolis), back (opisthotonos), tortipelvis (abdominal wall)	Anticholinergics or benzodiazepines; antihistamine (diphenhydramine); dosage reduction or discontinuation
Akathisia	Motor restlessness and discomfort, inability to sit still	Anticholinergics or benzodiazepines; dosage reduction or discontinuation
Parkinsonism (akinesia)	Bradykinesia, shuffling gait, resting tremor ("pill rolling movements"), "masked face," perioral tremors ("rabbit syndrome")	Anticholinergics or benzodiazepines; antihistamine (diphenhydramine); dosage reduction or discontinuation
Tardive dyskinesia (older males) & tardive dystonia (younger males)	Choreoathetoid movements: involuntary, repetitive, spasmodic movements of face, tongue, lips (chorea); slow, writhing, involuntary movements of fingers and hands (athetoid); may occur after years of neuroleptic therapy and are irreversible	Dosage reduction or discontinuation; clozapine as alternative; and/or botulinuum toxin, tetrabenzaine, or reserpine
Neuroleptic malignant syndrome (NMS)	Catatonia, muscle ("lead pipe") rigidity, stupor, hyperpyrexia, altered mental status, autonomic instability	For hyperpyrexia, benzodiazepines and rapid physical cooling; bromocryptine (DA agonist), dantrolene (for muscle rigidity); anticholinergics not recommended; withdraw neuroleptics for minimum of 14-days; clozapine as alternative

Although therapeutic and toxic doses of tricyclic compounds vary with the individual agents, death from neuroleptic overdose is rare and is usually a consequence of multiple drug ingestion. Some adverse reactions, however, are life threatening, require emergency intervention, and are difficult to treat. Neuroleptic-induced arrhythmias are a consequence of the quinidine-like myocardial depressant action of the compounds. Tricyclic agents decrease atrioventricular (AV) conduction. They induce vagal blockade, widening of the QRS interval, and prolongation of the QT interval. Plasma concentrations of 100 µg/dl approach toxic levels.

CNS depression, agitation, delirium, confusion, and disorientation are frequent consequences of neuroleptic administration. In addition, abnormal tendon reflexes, hypothermia or hyperthermia, and myoclonus (spastic skeletal muscle contraction), contribute to central dystonias. Loss of short-term memory, seizures, and respiratory depression are complications.

Anticholinergic blockade results in typical mydriasis with concomitant blurred vision, vasodilation (aggravating the hypotension), urinary retention, constipation, and dyspnea (resulting from lower bronchial secretions). In general, tertiary amines have greater antimuscarinic potency than secondary amines, tetracyclics or triazopyridines, of which amitriptyline is the most potent of the class (Table 15.2).

15.3.6 CLINICAL MANAGEMENT OF ACUTE OVERDOSE

Cardiovascular and respiratory functions are monitored for 12 h up to 6 days, because of the prolonged reactions of tricyclics. Treatment with i.v. fluids and vasopressors, such as norepinephrine or phenylephrine, is necessary for reversing neuroleptic-induced hypotension. Quinidine-like effects, especially ventricular dysrhythmias, are managed with lidocaine, while a widening QRS complex requires sodium bicarbonate. Class 1A antidysrhythmics, such as quinidine, procainamide, and disopyramide, should be avoided, as these compounds may aggravate AV conduction.

Ventilatory support is required in patients experiencing significant respiratory depression. Anticonvulsants, such as diazepam and phenobarbital, are beneficial for seizure management. Unlike in the treatment of anticholinergic overdose, physostigmine is not recommended for tricyclic toxicity, due to potential induction of fatal asystoles. Hemodialysis and hemoperfusion are also not useful because of the high V_d and high protein binding with tricyclics.

15.3.7 TOLERANCE AND WITHDRAWAL

Tolerance to the anticholinergic effects, such as dry mouth and tachycardia, tends to develop with continued use of tricyclics. Occasionally, patients will show physical or psychic dependence on the antidepressant effects. It is important to note, however, that decades of evidence suggest that prolonged use of tricyclic therapy is not associated with tolerance to its desirable effects.

15.4 PHENOTHIAZINE, PHENYLBUTYLPIPERIDINE, AND THIOXANTHINE ANTIPSYCHOTICS

15.4.1 CLASSIFICATION AND INDICATIONS

Formerly known as the major tranquilizers, the antipsychotic neuroleptics and related agents are grouped into several classes (Table 15.2). The drugs are indicated for the management of manifestations of psychotic disorders, as antiemetics, cough suppressants, and antivertigo agents. They are also effective in the treatment of phencyclidine (PCP)-induced psychosis, migraine headaches, and for acute agitation in the elderly, although these are unlabeled indications. As with the tricyclics, overdose is rarely fatal.

15.4.2 PHARMACOLOGY AND CLINICAL USE

Antipsychotic agents exert their actions primarily by antagonizing dopamine receptors. Varying degrees of selective dopamine blockade are seen in the cerebral limbic system and basal ganglia and along cortical dopamine tracts. Physiologically, these central pathways are associated with skeletal movement (nigrostriatal tracts), hallucinations and delusions (mesolimbic), psychosis (mesocortical), and prolactin release (tuberoinfundibular).

15.4.3 TOXICOKINETICS

Different colors and shapes of antipsychotics resemble small chocolate candies, which contributes to accidental ingestion by children. In addition, adult psychiatric patients intentionally or inadvertently combine antipsychotic medications with other S/H, alcohol, or antidepressants, thus precipitating additive or synergistic effects.

15.4.4 MECHANISM AND SIGNS AND SYMPTOMS OF ACUTE TOXICITY

Affinities of antipsychotic agents for nondopaminergic sites, such as cholinergic, α_1-adrenergic, and histaminic receptors, explain the varied ADRs produced.

As summarized in Table 15.2, phenothiazine, phenylbutylpiperidine, and thioxanthine derivatives display moderate to significant CNS reactions including sedation, muscle relaxation, and lowering of the seizure threshold. The latter sensitizes the individual to convulsions. In particular, antipsychotic drugs depress the reticular activating system (RAS) responsible for stimulating wakefulness (consciousness) and eliciting arousal reflexes. Unlike the barbiturates, these agents induce comatose-like states of consciousness that are more readily seen in children. Antimuscarinic and antihistaminic effects, such as mydriasis, dry mouth, tachycardia, and decreased gastrointestinal activity, further complicate their toxic profiles. Influence on hypothalamic nuclei is responsible for vasodilation, orthostatic hypotension, and hypothermia or hyperthermia. In addition, as with the tricyclics, α-adrenergic blockade contributes to hypotension. Quinidine-like cardiovascular AV block precipitates potentially fatal ventricular arrhythmias and cardiac arrest.

EPS signs and symptoms develop when an imbalance between antidopaminergic (greater) and anticholinergic activity is created. In general, higher-potency phenothiazines are more likely to produce EPS than lower-potency tricyclic antidepressants or the newer neuroleptics. Table 15.3 summarizes EPS reactions, signs and symptoms, and treatment management associated with antipsychotic agents. Prolonged antipsychotic therapy, idiosyncratic reactions, or toxic overdose can precipitate any or most of the syndromes. In general, the more overwhelming the antidopaminergic properties, the greater the severity of EPS reactions.

Acute dystonic reactions appear in 95% of patients, predominantly young males, within 4 days of initiation of therapy or as dosage increases. In contrast, *akathisia* affects mostly elderly patients in early treatment (first 60 days) and subsides with lower dosage. *Parkinsonism* develops within 10 weeks of therapy and affects 90% of patients, although it is reversible at lower doses. The risk of developing a *tardive disorder*, and the likelihood that it will become irreversible, increases as the duration of treatment and the total cumulative dose of neuroleptic drugs administered increases. As a neuroleptic agent is withdrawn, dopamine activity increases and tardive dyskinesia emerges. The effect is probably due to upregulation of dopamine receptors in the corpus striatum, especially with chronic neuroleptic treatment. *Neuroleptic malignant syndrome (NMS)* is a potentially fatal idiosyncratic complication occurring in 2% of patients on antipsychotic therapy. It is an extreme EPS reaction resulting from excessive antidopaminergic activity. Precipitating factors include abrupt withdrawal of anti-Parkinson dopamine agonist drugs (L-dopa) or anticholinergic medication, or rapid increase in the dose of neuroleptics. Meningitis and anticholinergic poisoning mimic NMS and must be ruled out.

15.4.5 CLINICAL MANAGEMENT OF ACUTE OVERDOSE

As with tricyclic toxicity, cardiovascular and respiratory adverse effects with antipsychotics are monitored for 12 h, up to 6 days. Treatment for reversing neuroleptic-induced hypotension and quinidine-like effects, especially ventricular dysrhythmias, is similarly managed with lidocaine and sodium bicarbonate, as needed. Convulsions or hyperactivity is controlled with pentobarbital or diazepam.

Although ostensibly dangerous, extrapyramidal adverse effects are not fatal[*] and are best treated with anticholinergics or benzodiazepines. Several days of treatment are necessary to reverse acute dystonic reactions. Prophylactic anticholinergic therapy is useful in prevention of EPS. In severe situations, consideration should be given to discontinuation of the neuroleptic, since dystonic reactions usually subside within 24 to 48 h after drug cessation. In contrast, tardive dyskinesia is difficult to manage, especially if symptoms appear at doses where the neuroleptic is therapeutically effective. Drug discontinuation and substitution with

---

[*] Antipsychotic agents have therapeutic indexes (TI). For instance, the TI for chlorpromazine extends up to 5000 mg (adult daily average dose range = 30 to 800 mg, with 100 mg daily as an average daily effective dose); for haloperidol, the TI is up to 30 mg (adult daily average dose range = 1 to 15 mg, with 2 mg as an average daily effective dose).

an atypical neuroleptic, such as clozapine, is usually considered, as these agents have a lower incidence of EPS. Clozapine may also be effective in reversing phenothiazine-induced tardive dyskinesia.

15.4.6 TOLERANCE AND WITHDRAWAL

As with the tricyclic antidepressants, tolerance to the anticholinergic effects develops with continued use of antipsychotic agents. Occasionally, patients will show physical or psychic dependence with the antidepressant effects. Prolonged use of antipsychotic therapy is not associated with tolerance to the desirable effects.

15.5 METHODS OF DETECTION

RIAs using radiolabeled tritiated ligands are used for the analysis of neuroleptics and some antihistamines. Although sensitivity is generally below 1 ng/ml, urine drug screening is not routinely performed.

REFERENCES

SUGGESTED READINGS

Dyer, K.S., Anticholinergic poisoning, in *Toxicology Secrets*, Ling, L.J. et al., Eds., Hanley & Belfus, Inc., Philadelphia, 2001, chap. 10.
Gossel, T.A. and Bricker, J.D., Anticholinergics, phenothiazines, and tricyclic antidepressants, in *Principles of Clinical Toxicology*, 3rd ed., Raven Press, New York, 1994, chap. 15.

REVIEW ARTICLES

Berchou, R.C., Maximizing the benefit of pharmacotherapy in Parkinson's disease, *Pharmacotherapy*, 20, 33S, 2000.
Catterson, M.L. and Martin, R.L., Anticholinergic toxicity masquerading as neuroleptic malignant syndrome: a case report and review, *Ann. Clin. Psychiatry*, 6, 267, 1994.
Geddes, J.R. et al., SSRIs versus other antidepressants for depressive disorder, *Cochrane Database Syst. Rev.*, 2, CD001851, 2000.
Gill, H.S., DeVane, C.L., and Risch, S.C., Extrapyramidal symptoms associated with cyclic antidepressant treatment: a review of the literature and consolidating hypotheses, *J. Clin. Psychopharmacol.*, 17, 377, 1997.
Gumnick, J.F. and Nemeroff, C.B., Problems with currently available antidepressants, *J. Clin. Psychiatry*, 61, 5, 2000.
Henry, J.A., Epidemiology and relative toxicity of antidepressant drugs in overdose, *Drug Saf.*, 16, 374, 1997.
Henry, J.A., Toxicity of antidepressants: comparisons with fluoxetine, *Int. Clin. Psychopharmacol.*, 6, 22, 1992.
Knight, M.E. and Roberts, R.J., Phenothiazine and butyrophenone intoxication in children, *Pediatr. Clin. North Am.*, 33, 299, 1986.
Lane, R.M., SSRI-induced extrapyramidal side-effects and akathisia: implications for treatment, *J. Psychopharmacol.*, 12, 192, 1998.

Lejoyeux, M. and Ades, J., Antidepressant discontinuation: a review of the literature, *J. Clin. Psychiatry.*, 58, 11, 1997.

Liebelt, E.L. and Shannon, M.W., Small doses, big problems: a selected review of highly toxic common medications, *Pediatr. Emerg. Care,* 9, 292, 1993.

Mitchell, P.B., Therapeutic drug monitoring of psychotropic medications, *Br. J. Clin. Pharmacol.*, 49, 303, 2000.

Sachdev, P.S., The current status of tardive dyskinesia, *Aust. N. Z. J. Psychiatry,* 34, 355, 2000.

Sarko, J., Antidepressants, old and new. A review of their adverse effects and toxicity in overdose, *Emerg. Med. Clin. North Am.,* 18, 637, 2000.

Stahl, S.M., Selecting an antidepressant by using mechanism of action to enhance efficacy and avoid side effects, *J. Clin. Psychiatry.* 59, 23, 1998.

Tune, L.E., Anticholinergic effects of medication in elderly patients, *J. Clin. Psychiatry.* 62, 11, 2001.

Vanderhoff, B.T. and Mosser, K.H., Jimson weed toxicity: management of anticholinergic plant ingestion, *Am. Fam. Physician,* 46, 526, 1992.

Wolfe, R.M., Antidepressant withdrawal reactions, *Am. Fam. Physician,* 56, 455, 1997.

16 Acetaminophen, Salicylates, and Nonsteroidal Anti-Inflammatory Drugs (NSAIDs)

16.1 HISTORY AND DESCRIPTION

Acetaminophen, salicylates (aspirin), and nonsteroidal anti-inflammatory agents are found alone and in combination with other analgesic/antipyretic* compounds, in hundreds of over-the-counter (OTC) and prescription formulas. As such, these agents are routinely reported as products responsible for acute and chronic overdose, with acetaminophen accounting for the most poisoning cases within this category. Packaging laws and public service education campaigns have reduced the frequency of accidental poisoning, especially in children and teenagers. Because the drugs are available OTC, however, it suggests that these agents are innocuous, although they are marketed with clearly marked warnings and suggestions for use.

In general, analgesic, antipyretic, and anti-inflammatory agents are used in the *household* management of nonnarcotic relief of mild to moderate pain, for inflammation associated with a variety of rheumatic conditions, and for reduction of fever.

16.2 ACETAMINOPHEN (N-ACETYL-PARA-AMINOPHENOL, APAP, PARACETAMOL)

16.2.1 INCIDENCE

Poisoning cases with APAP exceed those of all other agents in this category (five-times greater incidence than with aspirin). It is the most common drug involved in overdose, registering approximately 60% of all analgesic exposures, and the second most common cause of liver failure in the U.S. The U.S. Food and Drug Administration (FDA) reports that over 56,000 emergency room visits per year are due to acetaminophen OD, resulting in about 100 deaths each year. One fourth of these visits are intentional. Due to lack of hospital reporting, the numbers may greatly underestimate the extent of the problem.

---

* Mild to moderate pain relief and fever-reducing properties, respectively.

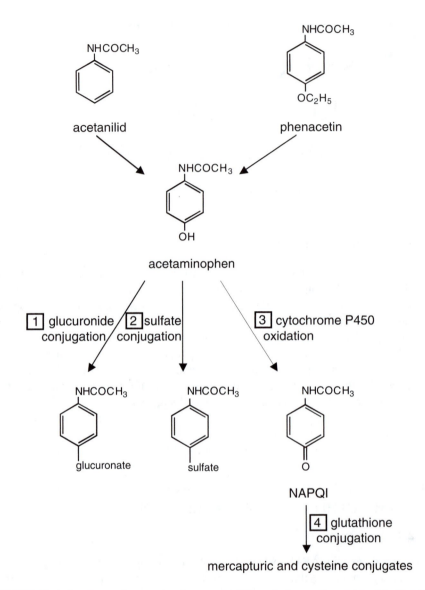

FIGURE 16.1 Structure of acetaminophen, acetanilid, and phenacetin, and metabolic pathways.

16.2.2 MEDICINAL CHEMISTRY AND PHARMACOLOGY

Acetaminophen is the major hydroxylation metabolite of two potent analgesic parent compounds, acetanilid and phenacetin (Figure 16.1). The antipyretic activity of the molecules resides in the aminobenzene structure.

APAP reduces fever by a direct action on the heat regulating centers in the hypothalamus, dissipating heat via vasodilation and increased sweating. Analgesic and antipyretic properties are equivalent to that of aspirin. Its inhibition of central prostaglandin synthetase is more effective than its peripheral action, rendering it a weak anti-inflammatory agent compared to aspirin. The site and mechanism of its analgesic action is, to this day, unclear.

16.2.3 CLINICAL USE

APAP is recommended as an analgesic/antipyretic in the presence of aspirin allergy, in patients that demonstrate blood coagulation disorders, in children, and in patients who receive oral anticoagulants or who demonstrate upper gastrointestinal disease. It is useful in a variety of arthritic and rheumatic conditions, including musculo-skeletal disorders, headache, and other minor pain, and for the management of fever associated with bacterial and viral infections.

16.2.4 METABOLISM AND MECHANISM OF TOXICITY

Acetaminophen is rapidly absorbed from the gastrointestinal tract and uniformly distributed, with peak plasma levels achieved by 0.5 to 2.0 h. Hepatic glucuronide and sulfate conjugation (Reactions 1 and 2, Figure 16.1) produce the inactive cor-responding conjugates, which account for 95% of metabolism and elimination in urine. In addition, at therapeutic acute doses, the remaining 4 to 5% of the product is detoxified and eliminated in the minor cytochrome P450 oxidase pathway (Reac-tion 3). The result is the production of the reactive intermediate, N-acetyl-*p*-benzo-quinoneimine (NAPQI) metabolite. Further conjugation by cellular glutathione results in the production of mercapturic acid and cysteine conjugates (Reaction 4). With chronic use or with large doses,[*] the glucuronide and sulfate conjugation metabolic routes (1 and 2) are saturated, and more importantly, glutathione stores are depleted (4). This leaves the cytochrome P450 oxidase pathway (Reaction 3) to accumulate toxic NAPQI metabolite. Binding of NAPQI to hepatocyte membranes and sulfhydril proteins accounts for the hepatotoxic sequelae.

16.2.5 SIGNS AND SYMPTOMS OF ACUTE TOXICITY

In general, delayed acute toxicity is manifested by the lack of apparent initial signs and symptoms for about 24 h, after which symptoms may appear quickly. However, the potential for latent permanent hepatic failure and death exists, even with the progression to an apparent recovery stage. Table 16.1 outlines the stages of acetami-nophen toxicity.

Initial symptoms are nonspecific, and a careful history and an acetaminophen plasma level should be performed so that impending toxicity is not missed. This

---

[*] Over a 24-h period, not more than 4 g or 90 mg/kg total is recommended in adults and children, respectively. In addition, the recommended length of therapy should not exceed beyond 10 days for adults or 5 days for children, or not more than 3 days for fever (adults and children). Interestingly, children are more tolerant to acetaminophen-induced hepatotoxicity, perhaps due to an increase in glutathione turn-over. Potential hepatotoxicity of APAP may be increased in chronic alcoholics, in malnutrition, and in HIV patients. Large doses or prolonged administration of hepatic microsomal enzyme inducers such as phenytoin, barbiturates, isoniazid, and rifampin, also increase hepatotoxic risk.

TABLE 16.1
Stages of Acetaminophen Toxicity

Stage	Time Postingestion (h)	APAP Plasma Concentration (mg/dl)[a]	Signs and Symptoms	Laboratory Findings
1	4	≥ 150	Anorexia, nausea, vomiting, pallor, diaphoresis, malaise, confusion, hypotension, arrhythmias	Hepatic transaminases (AST, ALT) rising
	8	≥ 75		
	12	≥ 35		
	24	≥ 5		
2	24–72	≥ 1 (at 72 h)	Clinical improvement, right upper quadrant pain, renal function deterioration	Transaminases peaking; bilirubin & PT elevated
3	72–96	≥ 1	Hepatic centrilobular necrosis: jaundice, coagulopathy, encephalopathy (coma); reappearance of nausea & vomiting, arrythmias, acute renal failure, death	Peak levels of AST (20,000 U/ml) & ALT
4	4–14 days	≥ 1	Resolution of hepatic dysfunction and recovery if liver damage is reversible	Return to baseline levels

Note: AST = aspartate aminotransferase, ALT = alanine aminotransferase, PT= prothrombin time; other laboratory tests include blood urea nitrogen (BUN), creatinine, electrolytes, and blood glucose.

[a] Based on Rumack-Matthew nomogram; the current practice in the U.S. is to treat all patients who have acetaminophen levels above these values as at "possible risk" for toxicity; the nomogram assumes that absorption of a single overdose is complete by 4 h and that the half-life, based on elimination toxicokinetics, is 4 h.

affords the patient the opportunity of early treatment and prevention of potential irreversible hepatic damage. A quiescent recovery period (Stage 2) is characterized by clinical improvement after 24 to 72 h postingestion. Treatment at this stage is generally based on laboratory findings and acetaminophen plasma levels. Liver function tests are monitored throughout the critical periods until complete recovery is ensured. It is important to note that acetaminophen plasma levels based on the Rumack-Matthew nomogram are intended for single acute overdose and do not apply in suspected toxicity with chronic or prolonged ingestion of therapeutic doses. Monitoring of these patients involves the same criteria as noted in Table 16.1, especially the determination of drug concentrations every 2 to 4 h to establish baseline toxicity criteria. Continued observation and repeat levels are warranted.

16.2.6 CLINICAL MANAGEMENT OF ACUTE OVERDOSE

Early treatment and careful evaluation of clinical history leading to the emergency event is paramount in treatment. Activated charcoal is beneficial if administered to an individual who presents within 1 to 2 h postingestion. An acetaminophen level obtained 4 h later determines follow-up treatment with the antidote. At 8 h postingestion, activated charcoal, emetics, or gastric lavage are not necessary.

N-acetylcysteine (NAC, Mucomyst®, Figure 16.2) is the antidote for acetaminophen poisoning. In its conversion to cysteine, NAC restores glutathione reserves by providing sulfhydril donors for the eventual detoxification of NAPQI. In addition, NAC increases sulfate conjugation, thereby preventing excess NAPQI production. NAC also acts as an antioxidant, enhancing oxygen utilization; this effect may be of benefit in patients with fulminant hepatic failure.

NAC is administered as a 10 or 20% solution for oral administration or through nasogastric instillation. It should be delivered within 8 h of ingestion and whenever a potentially toxic acetaminophen concentration is measured above the toxic level. Protection against hepatotoxicity is 100% within 8 h of APAP ingestion. Efficacy decreases, however, when administered beyond 8 h, although NAC therapy may be beneficial even 36 h postingestion.

Currently, the protocol is 140 mg/kg oral loading dose followed by 17 doses of 70 mg/kg every 4 h, for a total of 1330 mg/kg over 72 h. The dose is continuous over the 72 h until the acetaminophen assay reveals a nontoxic level. If the patient vomits the loading or maintenance dose within 1 h of administration, the dose is repeated. Antiemetics, such as metoclopramide (Reglan®), may be helpful in retaining the NAC. Among the possible adverse effects associated with large doses of NAC are hypersensitivity, gastrointestinal disturbances, urticaria, pruritis, angioedema, bronchospasm, tachycardia, and hypotension. Most of the serious reactions are ascribed to i.v. administration.

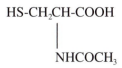

FIGURE 16.2 Formula for N-acetylcysteine.

16.3 SALICYLATES AND ACETYLSALICYLIC ACID (ASPIRIN, ASA)

16.3.1 INCIDENCE AND CLINICAL USE

Prompted, in part, by the search for effective substitutes for quinine, early British researchers at the end of the nineteenth century synthesized and identified sodium salicylate for use as an antipyretic (for the treatment of rheumatic fever) and analgesic (for the treatment of gout). By 1915, the inception of the aspirin tablet established ASA as the most popular compound of the times. Today, salicylates and related analgesics are major sources of pediatric drug product poisoning in the U.S. Although accidental poisoning in children has decreased with improved packaging safety requirements, aspirin and salicylate toxicity continue to be problems, primarily because of the increased risk to children with fevers. At a pediatric toxic dose level of 150 to 200 mg/kg, as little as ten to twelve adult 325-mg tablets of aspirin produce mild toxicity in an average 5-year-old (20-kg) child.

Aspirin and salicylic acid products are the active ingredients of hundreds of therapeutic prescription and OTC products. ASA products are used as analgesics, antipyretics, anti-inflammatory (arthritis) agents, and in cough/cold, antihistamine, and decongestant formulations. Oil of wintergreen (betula oil) is an older product traditionally used as an analgesic liniment for the relief of sore muscles and stiff joints. It is a methyl salicylate concentrate (530 mg/ml) that produces severe toxicity in children with a 5-ml dose.[*] Finally, aspirin has shown some success as an antiplatelet agent in patients with thromboembolic disease, although this is an unofficial indication.

Consequently, the ubiquitous nature of aspirin products and ready availability has created the impression that aspirin is generally innocuous, which further contributes to the compound's persistent appearance in poisoning events.

16.3.2 TOXICOKINETICS

Salicylates are rapidly and completely absorbed, but distributed unevenly throughout body tissues after oral use.[**] Metabolism follows first-order kinetics (dose dependent) to form oxidized and conjugated metabolites. Renal clearance accounts for most of the compound's elimination and is enhanced from 2% to more than 80% as pH, and ionization, increase.

16.3.3 MECHANISM OF TOXICITY

Table 16.2 summarizes the mechanisms, metabolic consequences, and clinical pathology of acute aspirin toxicity. The primary result of high serum concentrations of salicylic acid is interference with acid-base balance. The stability of serum pH

---

[*] Pepto-Bismol®, an antacid and antidiarrheal preparation, contains 262-mg of bismuth subsalicylate per 15 ml (one tablespoonful or one-half ounce), or about 130 mg total salicylate. The recommended 8-ounce dose contains the equivalent of 6 to 7, 325-mg tablets of adult aspirin.

[**] Aspirin is partially hydrolyzed to salicylic acid during absorption and distributed unevenly to all body fluids and tissues. V_d = 0.15–0.20 l/kg, which is equivalent to the extracellular space.

TABLE 16.2
Pathology and Mechanism of ASA Toxicity

Mechanism of Toxicity	Pathological Consequence	Metabolic Compensation	Signs and Symptoms
Elevated ASA serum concentration (acidic substance)	Decreases serum pH	Contributes to metabolic acidosis; alters platelet function (hypoprothrombinemia)	Increases bleeding time
Stimulation of medullary respiratory center	Hyperventilation	Decreases plasma PCO_2 with respiratory alkalosis	Tachypnea, pulmonary edema, tachycardia, dehydration
Renal compensation for respiratory alkalosis	Kidneys excrete more bicarbonate ions; retain more hydrogen ions	Contributes to compensatory metabolic acidosis; CNS toxicity	Irritability, restlessness, tinnitus, dehydration, seizures, coma
Inhibition of Kreb's cycle enzymes	Accumulation of organic acids (oxaloacetate)	Contributes to metabolic acidosis and lactic acidosis	Gastric irritation, nausea, vomiting
Oxidative uncoupling of electron transport chain	Prevents combination of phosphate with ADP	Decreases formation of ATP, enhanced glycolysis, lactic acid, pyruvic acid; contributes to metabolic acidosis	Hyperthermia, tachycardia, dehydration, cardiovascular collapse, hypoglycemia
	Increases peripheral demand for glucose	Stimulates lipid metabolism, releases fatty acids, contributes to metabolic acidosis	

(7.4) depends on the maintenance of a delicate ratio of bicarbonate ion to carbonic acid (HCO_3^-/H_2CO_3:20/1).[*] As salicylic acid levels rise and pH decreases, the medullary respiratory center is stimulated, resulting in an increase in ventilatory rate (hyperventilation). With a rise in respirations per minute, the victim expels more CO_2, and the equilibrium equation for the bicarbonate buffering system shifts to the left ($\uparrow$ [HCO_3^-]), causing a temporary but significant response from the renal compensatory mechanisms. In turn, the kidneys compensate for the higher HCO_3^- concentration by retaining H^+ and eliminating HCO_3^-, causing a decrease in serum pH and a *compensatory* metabolic acidosis.

The toxicity associated with oxidative uncoupling of the electron transport chain (Figure 16.3) is similar to that seen with cyanide and 2,3-dinitrophenol poisoning.

---

[*] This ratio is predicated on the physiological attempt to maintain a neutral pH. It is the kidneys' responsibility, in part, to accomplish this through reabsorption of filtered bicarbonate and/or hydrogen ions. This equilibrium is, thus, appropriately represented according to the following equation: $H_2O + CO_2 \leftrightarrow H_2CO_3 \leftrightarrow H^+ + HCO_3^-$.

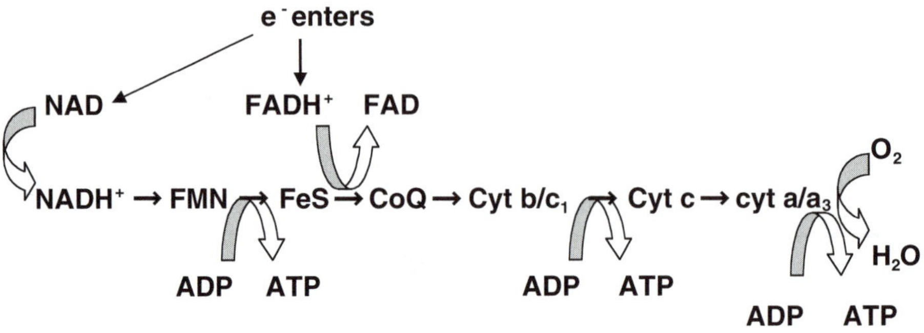

FIGURE 16.3 Electron transport and oxidative phosphorylation.

Salicylates reduce the effective shuttling of $NADH^+$ into the electron transport chain, preventing a number of adenosine triphosphate-dependent (ATP) reactions. As fewer ATPs are produced, glycolysis is enhanced but is less efficient, triggering an increase in lipid metabolism, and releasing excessive free fatty acids and ketones. In addition, oxygen consumption and glucose utilization are increased from the uncoupling effect, resulting in excess body heat production.

16.3.4 SIGNS AND SYMPTOMS OF ACUTE TOXICITY

Onset of symptoms is usually 1 to 2 h, but may be delayed 4 to 6 h due to absorption of sustained-release preparations or the formation of gastric concretions. Severity of symptoms peaks between 12 and 24 h. At low doses, elimination half-life is constant at 3 to 4 h and follows first-order kinetics (dose-**dependent**). With higher doses, or with chronic ingestion, elimination half-life shifts from first-order to zero-order kinetics (dose-**independent**), as metabolic enzymes become saturated, thus contributing to the severity of chronic, low-dose toxicity.

More severe ASA toxicity, especially the development of metabolic acidosis, is associated with chronic ingestion and with children under 5 years old. The progression is dose-related. Although a single large dose of aspirin results in signs and symptoms described in Table 16.2, death is more likely in patients with chronic poisoning and is usually a result of pulmonary or cerebral edema. In fact, the ability of ASA to traverse the blood-brain barrier is delayed due to its highly polar nature. Consequently, chronic ingestion affords the polar molecule more time for serum levels to equilibrate with CNS concentrations. Interestingly, unlike acetaminophen concentrations, ASA blood levels (Done nomogram) do not correlate well with acute or chronic signs and symptoms. Treatment decisions therefore rely on empirical observations and clinical laboratory function tests.

16.3.5 CLINICAL MANAGEMENT OF TOXICITY

Although serum salicylate concentrations are not dependable for guiding treatment, the change in serum concentrations — i.e., a drop of 10% every 3 to 4 h — is a good indicator of recovery. In addition, lack of symptoms 6 h after ingestion is associated with mild to moderate (less than severe) complications. In general, serum salicylate levels are used as a gauge for moderate (50 mg/dl), severe (75 mg/dl), and potentially lethal (100 mg/dl) poisoning. Complete clinical laboratory tests, especially for blood glucose, serum electrolytes (determination of the anion gap),[*] and liver function, are important in calculating the risk of metabolic acidosis.

Administration of emetics is not totally useful, as vomiting will not remove all stomach contents or sustained-release preparations. Activated charcoal and cathartics are recommended to effectively bind salicylates and to prevent intestinal obstruction due to concretions, respectively. Sodium bicarbonate administration enhances ASA elimination by alkalinizing the urine (maintains the salicylic acid as a polar molecule) while simultaneously reversing metabolic acidosis. Other supportive measures include correcting the dehydration, maintaining kidney function (forcing fluids), rectifying electrolyte imbalance (especially potassium for hypokalemia that may result from bicarbonate infusion), and instituting supportive measures for hyperthermia, seizure control, and pulmonary edema. Since death is possible from chronic (or severe acute) toxicity, cardiovascular collapse, seizures, hyperthermia, and pulmonary edema are closely attended.

Specific antidotes are not available for salicylate poisoning.

16.4 NONSTEROIDAL ANTI-INFLAMMATORY DRUGS (NSAIDS)

16.4.1 History and Description

The search for potent anti-inflammatory agents similar to aspirin led to the discovery of phenylbutazone in 1949, a synthetic analog and solubilizing agent for aminopyrine. It was initially used as an anti-inflammatory agent and subsequently for its analgesic and antipyretic actions. Because of the serious adverse hematologic reactions associated with phenylbutazone (agranulocytosis), the search for safer drugs with anti-inflammatory properties began. The acetic acid derivatives, including indomethacin, were introduced for the treatment of rheumatoid arthritis and related disorders. Several groups of aspirin-like drugs soon followed, many with significant advantages over aspirin, but with a variety of accompanying ADRs.

16.4.2 Classification, Pharmacology, and Clinical Use

Table 16.3 lists selected and currently available NSAIDs. NSAIDs exhibit antipyretic, analgesic, and anti-inflammatory activities, resulting from inhibition of prostaglandin synthesis. In particular, NSAIDS inhibit cyclooxygenase (COX), an enzyme that catalyzes the synthesis of prostaglandins from arachidonic acid (Figure 16.4). Two COX isoenzymes are present mainly in platelets, endothelial cells, gastrointestinal tract, and kidney. The selective functions of the enzymes, and their general inhibition by the NSAIDs, explain in part, the toxic effects of

---

[*] See Chapter 3, "Therapeutic Monitoring of Adverse Drug Reactions," for discussion of metabolic acidosis and determination of anion gap.

TABLE 16.3
Representative and Currently Available Anti-Inflammatory Drugs

Classification	Compound	Proprietary Name	Enzyme Inhibition[a]	Major Toxic Effect[b]
Indole and indene acetic acids	Indomethacin Sulindac	Indocin Clinoril	Selective for COX-1	High incidence of peptic ulcers; CNS depression; hypersensitivity reactions; blood dyskrasias
Heteroaryl acetic acids	Tolmetin Diclofenac Ketorolac	Tolectin Voltaren Toradol	Slightly selective for COX-1	High incidence of peptic ulcers; blood dyskrasias; hypersensitivity
Arylpropionic acetic acids	Ibuprofen Naproxen Flurbiprofen Ketoprofen Oxaprozin	Motrin, Advil Naprosyn, Aleve Ansaid Orudis Daypro	Slightly selective for COX-1	Gastric irritation, hepatic function impairment
Anthranilic acids	Mefenamic acid Meclofenamate	Ponstel various	Slightly selective for COX-1	Gastric irritation, peptic ulcers, hepatic function impairment
Enolic acids	Piroxicam Meloxicam Phenylbutazone[c]	Feldene Mobic Butalzolidin	Selective for COX-1	High incidence of peptic ulcers; hypersensitivity
Alkanones	Nabumetone	Relafen	Slightly selective for COX-2	High incidence of peptic ulcers
Pyranocarboxylic acid	Etodolac	Lodine	Selective for COX-2	High incidence of peptic ulcers; hypersensitivity
COX-2 inhibitors	Celecoxib Rofecoxib Valdecoxib	Celebrex Vioxx Bextra	Selective for COX-2	Gastric irritation; hypersensitivity

[a] Action of anti-inflammatory drugs generally involves inhibition of both COX-1 and COX-2 enzymes — predominant inhibition of either enzymes is noted.

[b] Although major toxic reactions are listed categorically, some agents within the specific groups may preferentially display one or more of the toxic effects.

[c] No longer available, principally because of high incidence of blood dyskrasias.

the compounds. COX-1 isoenzyme activity produces prostaglandins that are important in maintaining platelet aggregation, regulation of kidney and gastric blood flow, and gastric mucus secretion. The COX-2 isoenzyme is expressed during pain and inflammation. While most NSAIDs nonselectively inhibit both enzymes, preferential inhibition of either contributes to both beneficial and

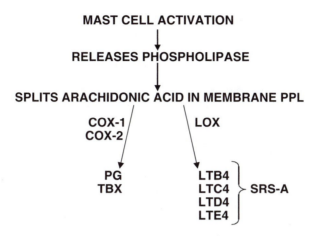

FIGURE 16.4 Schematic outline of synthesis of endoperoxides (mediators of inflammation) from arachidonic acid, as a mechanism of the effector phase of type I antibody-mediated reactions. PPL = phospholipid; COX-1,-2 = cyclooxygenase isoenzymes types 1 and 2; LOX = lipooxygenase; PG = prostaglandin; TBX = thromboxane; LT = leukotriene subclasses; SRS-A = slow reactive substance type A.

adverse effects. Inhibition of COX-1 has antiplatelet activity, an effect which may be of benefit in prevention of cardiovascular disease. However, removal of the protective gastric mucosal secretory action exposes the stomach lining to GI toxicity. The newer COX-2 inhibitors avoid GI upset associated with nonselective or selective COX-1 inhibitors. However, the antiplatelet activity and myocardial protective effects are precluded with the COX-2 inhibitors.

NSAIDs are indicated in the treatment of patients with osteoarthritis, rheumatoid arthritis, and arthritic conditions in patients with high risk of gastric or duodenal ulcers. Other indications include concomitant therapy with other arthritic treatments, mild-to-moderate pain of minor surgical procedures, and primary dysmenorrhea. Guidelines to assist in selecting the appropriate agent are mostly empirical and based on experience, occurrence of ADRs, convenience, and cost. Major adverse reactions that limit NSAID usefulness are listed in Table 16.3. Other than the adverse reactions common to most of the NSAIDs, the highest incidence of ADRs includes: GI disturbances (gastritis, heartburn); cardiovascular (hypertension, peripheral edema); CNS (dizziness, psychic disturbances); dermatologic (rash); hematologic (decreased hemoglobin and hemtaocrit); hepatic (elevated liver enzymes); renal (urinary tract infection); and, respiratory disturbances (dyspnea and upper respiratory infection). Concomitant use with salicylates is not recommended.

16.4.3 SIGNS AND SYMPTOMS OF ACUTE TOXICITY

Most overdose exposures of NSAIDs are asymptomatic or produce a self-limiting (24-h) lethargy. Nausea, vomiting, drowsiness, and potential renal ischemia and renal failure are possible, however, as a result of decrease in renal prostaglandin. Some consequences involve gastric erosion, CNS toxicity, and hemorrhage, although this toxicity requires up to 20 times the therapeutic blood concentrations.

16.4.4 CLINICAL MANAGEMENT OF ACUTE OVERDOSE

The ABCs of supportive care are generally warranted. Gastric lavage and administration of emetics are of benefit, as well as forced oral fluids and renal function tests.

16.5 METHODS OF DETECTION

Salicylates, acidic compounds, and acetaminophen, a neutral compound, are routinely monitored in suspected poisoning or cases involving toxicity. The methods of choice for both drugs include a urine screening color test and HPLC. In addition, testing for acetaminophen is also routinely performed if codeine, oxycodone, hydrocodone, or propoxyphene are detected on initial urine screening. Tables 3.7 and 3.8 (Chapter 3) show the schematic approach to testing of salicylates and APAP in biological specimens.

REFERENCES

SUGGESTED READINGS

Johnson, A.G., Seidemann, P. and Day, R.O., NSAID-related adverse drug interactions with clinical relevance. An update, *Int. J. Clin. Pharmacol. Ther.*, 32, 509, 1994.
Roberts, L.J., II and Morrow, J.D., Analgesic-antipyretic and anti-inflammatory agents and drugs employed in the treatment of gout, in *Goodman & Gilman's The Pharmacological Basis of Therapeutics*, 10th ed., Hardman, J., Limbird, L., and Gilman, A., Eds., McGraw-Hill, New York, 2001, chap. 27.

REVIEW ARTICLES

Aronson, M.D., Nonsteroidal anti-inflammatory drugs, traditional opioids, and tramadol: contrasting therapies for the treatment of chronic pain, *Clin. Ther.*, 19, 420, 1997.
Bolesta, S. and Haber, S.L., Hepatotoxicity associated with chronic acetaminophen administration in patients without risk factors, *Ann. Pharmacother.*, 36, 331, 2002.
Chu, J., Wang, R.Y., and Hill, N.S., Update in clinical toxicology, *Am. J. Respir. Crit. Care. Med.*, 166, 9, 2002.
Cranswick, N. and Coghlan, D., Paracetamol efficacy and safety in children: the first 40 years, *Am. J. Ther.*, 7, 135, 2000.
Dawson, A.H. and Whyte, I.M., Therapeutic drug monitoring in drug overdose, *Br. J. Clin. Pharmacol.*, 52, 97S, 2001.
Ishihara, K. and Szerlip, H.M., Anion gap acidosis, *Semin. Nephrol.*, 18, 83, 1998.
Johnson, A.G., Seideman, P. and Day, R.O., Adverse drug interactions with nonsteroidal anti-inflammatory drugs (NSAIDs). Recognition, management and avoidance, *Drug Saf.*, 8, 99, 1993.
Karsh, J., Adverse reactions and interactions with aspirin. Considerations in the treatment of the elderly patient, *Drug Saf.*, 5, 317, 1990.

Lane, J.E. et al., Chronic acetaminophen toxicity: a case report and review of the literature, *J. Emerg. Med.,* 23, 253, 2002.

Plaisance, K.I., Toxicities of drugs used in the management of fever, *Clin. Infect. Dis.,* 31, S219, 2000.

Prescott, L.F., Paracetamol: past, present, and future, *Am. J. Ther.,* 7, 143, 2000.

Riordan, S.M. and Williams, R., Alcohol exposure and paracetamol-induced hepatotoxicity, *Addict. Biol.,* 7, 191, 2002.

Sallis, R.E., Management of salicylate toxicity, *Am. Fam. Physician.,* 39, 265, 1989.

Sheen, C.L. et al., Paracetamol toxicity: epidemiology, prevention and costs to the health-care system, *Q.J.M.,* 95, 609, 2002.

Stein, R.B. and Hanauer, S.B., Comparative tolerability of treatments for inflammatory bowel disease, *Drug Saf.,* 23, 429, 2000.

Vane, J.R. and Botting, R.M., Anti-inflammatory drugs and their mechanism of action, *Inflamm. Res.,* 47, S78, 1998.

17 Steroids

17.1 THE ENDOCRINE SYSTEM

The endocrine, or ductless, glands secrete metabolically active chemical mediators into the vascular circulation, which in turn, are distributed to all organs.* These hormones function as chemical mediators between endocrine glands and specific effector organs, regulating metabolic processes and physiological growth and development. In contrast to the neurochemicals of the nervous system, endocrine hormones affect all body cells, require longer onset of action, have prolonged duration, and are delivered systemically rather than locally in response to nerve impulses.

17.2 NEUROENDOCRINE PHYSIOLOGY

17.2.1 DESCRIPTION

The endocrine system is a conglomeration of many organs working interdependently and follows a complex series of feedback reactions. Normal endocrine function depends on cyclical events with stimuli originating both externally and internally. The goal of the endocrine organs, in coordination with the nervous system, is to maintain homeostasis, or equilibrium, throughout the body. The nervous system stimulates or inhibits the release of hormones in coordination with the endocrine glands, thus forming a communicating network of signals in response to physiological requirements. This pathway allows the neuroendocrine superstructure to regulate growth and development in growing humans while maintaining physiological homeostasis in adults.

The hypothalamic-pituitary system, through auto-feedback somatosensory control centers, regulates secretion of hormones in response to physiological, emotional, or physical stress.** The hypothalamus synthesizes and secretes at least nine different hormones. The hormones travel from the hypothalamus down the hypothalamo-hypophyseal portal system or neuronal tracts, to the anterior pituitary (adenohypophysis) or posterior pituitary (neurohypophysis), respectively. The hormones stimulate the respective areas of the pituitary gland to release any of seven distinct hormones that, in turn, will respond to the initial stimulus in an attempt to counteract or balance that force. This negative or positive feedback system ultimately regulates virtually all aspects of homeostasis, growth, development, and metabolism.

---

* In some instances, mixed glands, such as pancreas and liver, also serve exocrine functions since they secrete chemical mediators into the lumen of organs through duct systems.
** It is important to note that the term physiological stress implies the existence of normal stimuli (nonpathologic) that challenge the maintenance of homeostasis. These stressors include conditions such as cold, exercise, pain, tiredness, and hunger, as well as daily routine emotional and behavioral pressures.

Disorders of the endocrine system are expressed in the form of excessive (hyperfunction) or diminished (hypofunction) activity. In general, disorders develop as a result of lack of hypothalamic-pituitary secretory control, or because of inadequate or dysfunctional hormone receptors. The categories of agents described below have therapeutic usefulness in alleviating or correcting endocrine imbalances. In addition, estrogens and progestins are clinically useful drugs for the prevention of fertilization and implantation. The ubiquitous illicit use of androgens and anabolic steroids, however, taken in doses beyond their therapeutic value for nontherapeutic reasons, has contributed to an array of chronic toxic syndromes previously unrecognized in routine treatment.

17.3 ANABOLIC-ANDROGENIC STEROIDS

17.3.1 DEFINITION AND INCIDENCE

Androgens are hormones that stimulate the development and activity of accessory male sex organs (primary sex characteristics), and encourage the development of male sex characteristics (secondary sex characteristics). Androgens prevent changes in the latter that follow a decrease in the hormone levels, such as with castration. *Anabolic steroids* are familiar as synthetic derivatives of the androgens that promote skeletal muscle growth (anabolic effect) and development of male sex characteristics (androgenic effect). Since its discovery in 1935, testosterone, the principal male androgen, and its numerous derivatives, have been used as important components of treatment of endocrine-related disorders. As the knowledge about the compound's ability to facilitate the growth of skeletal muscle in laboratory animals was understood, testosterone and related agents were incorporated into the lifestyle of bodybuilders, weight lifters, and other athletes, professional or otherwise. Since the 1950s, athletes have ingested anabolic-androgenic steroids* to increase muscle size, reduce body fat, and to improve general performance in sports. Today, steroid abuse is widespread and rising, especially among adolescents. About 3% of eighth to twelfth graders have taken anabolic steroids at least once in their lives, representing a significant increase from the last reports in 1991. Among adults, hundreds of thousands are estimated to use anabolic steroids at least once a year. The abuse is higher among males but growing rapidly among young females.

Individuals who have experienced physical or sexual abuse cite that their reason for abusing steroids is to increase their muscle size to protect themselves. Some adolescents abuse steroids as part of a pattern of high-risk behaviors. Finally, muscle dysmorphia is a behavioral syndrome characterized by a distorted, unrealistic image of one's body. Men and women with the condition use steroids in an attempt to overcome their perception of inadequate physical appearance.

---

* The term *steroids* will be subsequently used in this chapter to refer collectively to the androgenic-anabolic steroid compounds.

17.3.2 PHARMACOLOGY AND CLINICAL USE

Table 17.1 shows the structure of testosterone and lists some commonly abused steroids. More than 100 different steroids have been developed and, with the exception of the dietary supplements, are classified as federal C-III controlled substances under the Anabolic Steroids Act of 1990. Dietary supplements, such as dehydroepiandrosterone (DHEA) and androstenedione (Andro) are not controlled substances and can be purchased legally without a prescription. Interestingly, these agents are not food products but are converted to testosterone, although the quantities available for conversion are probably insufficient to produce the desirable anabolic effects. Their adverse reactions and their potential for toxicity, however, remain to be determined.

Testosterone is produced and secreted by the interstitial cells (Leydig cells) of the testes. The compound is converted at effector organs to dihydrotestosterone, which then binds to target cytosolic protein receptors. The effects of testosterone include growth and maturation of male sex organs (prostate, seminal vesicles, penis, scrotum), development of male hair distribution, laryngeal enlargement, and alterations in body musculature and fat distribution. Androgens increase protein anabolism.

Androgenic steroids are indicated for a variety of endocrine disorders, including the treatment of hypogonadism, delayed puberty in males, and metastatic cancer in females. Androgens stimulate adolescent growth and precipitate termination of linear growth by fusion of skeletal epiphyseal growth centers. Exogenous androgen administration inhibits endogenous testosterone release through a pituitary luteinizing hormone (LH) feedback pathway.

Anabolic steroids are closely related to testosterone and have high anabolic, low androgenic properties. These compounds are indicated for the treatment of certain types of anemia, hereditary angioedema, and metastatic breast cancer. Anabolic steroids promote tissue-building and reverse tissue-depleting processes.

17.3.3 ADVERSE REACTIONS

Anabolic-androgenic steroids affect many organ systems as a result of suppression of normal endocrine function, as well as their direct actions on target cell processes. Steroids cause serious disturbances of growth and sexual development in children and suppress gonadotropic functions of the pituitary. In particular, virilization is the most common undesirable side effect, especially in women and prepubertal males.

Table 17.1 summarizes the potential adverse reactions exhibited with prolonged,* illicit use of steroids. In addition to the side effects noted in Table 17.1, females may experience irreversible virilization and clitoral enlargement. Females may also develop other sexual characteristics generally associated with male development, such as hirsutism (increased body hair growth) and deepening of the voice. Menstrual irregularities, male pattern baldness, acne, and changes in libido are reversible.

---

* As often or as little as several months of frequent use is regarded as prolonged treatment with steroids and may result in noted reversible and irreversible changes.

TABLE 17.1
Structure of Testosterone and Classification of Selected, Commonly Used Androgenic-Anabolic Testosterone Derivatives

Testosterone

Classification[a]	Compound	Proprietary Name	ADRs
Oral steroids	Oxymethalone Oxandrolone Methadrostenolone Stanozolol	Anadrol-50 Oxandrin Dianabol Winstrol	CNS: headache, anxiety, depression, paresthesias; Dermatologic: acne, male pattern baldness, hirsutism; GI: nausea, hepatocellular neoplasms, abnormal liver function tests, cholestatic jaundice; GU: frequent & prolonged erections, gynecomastia, oligospermia; Metabolic: electrolyte imbalance, increased serum cholesterol
Injectables	Nandrolone decanoate Nandrolone phenpropionate Testosterone cypionate Boldenone undecylenate	Deca-Durabolin Durabolin Depo-testosterone Equipoise	Same as for oral steroids plus pain & inflammation at injection site, seborrhea
Transdermal	Testosterone transdermal system	Testoderm, Androderm	Same as for oral steroids plus CNS: pain, dizziness, vertigo; Dermatologic: itching, erythema, burning, pruritis, blisters at site of application; GU: prostate disorders
Implants	Testosterone pellets	Testopel	Same as for oral steroids plus pain & inflammation at injection site
Topical	Testosterone gel	Androgel 1%	Same as for oral steroids plus CV: hypertension, peripheral edema; CNS: asthenia, emotional instability; Dermatologic: application site reactions; GI: none; GU: impaired urination, prostate disorders; Metabolic: abnormal clinical lab tests

Note: ADRs = adverse drug reactions, CV = cardiovascular, CNS = central nervous system, GI = gastrointestinal, GU = genitourinary.

[a] The oral steroids and the nandrolone derivatives are further classified as high anabolic-low androgenic steroids, although the dissociation of these activities varies; the remaining compounds have predominantly androgenic properties.

More severe warnings associated with steroid use include the development of *peliosis hepatis*, a liver condition characterized by replacement of liver cells with blood-filled cysts. The condition is reversible upon discontinuation of drug use. *Peliosis hepatis* usually presents with minimal, unrecognized hepatic dysfunction, until life-threatening liver failure or intra-abdominal hemorrhage occurs. Similarly, benign, androgen-dependent hepatic tumors have been noted. These vascularized tumors are relatively uncommon neoplastic occurrences in humans in the absence of steroid use. With continuous steroid drug abuse, the tumors develop undetected until life-threatening intra-abdominal hemorrhage ensues. Increased risk of atherosclerosis and coronary artery disease are associated with continued use of steroids, resulting from blood lipid changes (decreased high density lipoproteins).

In addition, steroid abusers often share contaminated needles or use steroid preparations manufactured illegally under nonsterile conditions. Such practices predispose persons to viral and bacterial infections such as bacterial endocarditis, HIV, and hepatitis B.

Serious consequences of steroid administration in children and teenagers include premature epiphyseal maturation and closure, without compensatory gain in linear growth. The result is a disproportionate advancement in bone maturation and termination of the growth process. This effect may continue up to 6 months following cessation of therapeutic regimens. Ingestion or dermal contact with anabolic-androgenic steroids is contraindicated during pregnancy (category X) because of potential fetal masculinization.

In general, the ability of these agents to improve athletic performance is questionable. For body builders and weight lifters, the motivation to use steroids relies primarily on the increased muscle mass and decreased muscle recovery and healing time experienced with steroid regimens. The regimens most often used include *stacking, pyramiding,* and *cycling.** The goal of the regimens is to minimize side effects and drug detection while maintaining peak performance.

17.3.4 Addiction and Withdrawal Syndrome

An addiction syndrome is now recognized with long-term use, especially among bodybuilders, weight lifters, and professional athletes. The syndrome is characterized by physical, behavioral, and psychological changes (especially aggressiveness). The condition is not unlike the addictive and withdrawal behavior, drug craving, and signs and symptoms described for opioids, cocaine, and alcohol. Depression is the most dangerous of the withdrawal symptoms, because of its association with suicidal tendencies. If left untreated, the condition persists for a year or more after discontinuation. Concomitant drug use, such as ingestion of diuretics to counteract sodium and fluid retention (nonprescription, or thiazide and loop diuretics), often indicates chronic abuse.

---

* *Stacking* refers to the concurrent and simultaneous use of two or more agents, while varying the dosage and dosage forms over a period of 6 to 18 weeks; *pyramiding* is similar to stacking but involves the use of a single agent; *cycling* requires the scheduling of a drug-free period so that peak performance and undetectable levels will coincide with an upcoming event.

17.3.5 TREATMENT OF THE CONSEQUENCES OF CHRONIC STEROID USE

Behavioral, supportive, and educational programs are indicated to prevent and manage the growing adolescent problem of steroid abuse. Medications used for treating steroid withdrawal aim at restoring hormonal balance, while others target specific withdrawal symptoms. Recommendations include antidepressants for depression and analgesics for headaches, muscle pain, and joint pain.

17.4 ESTROGEN AND PROGESTINS

17.4.1 PHYSIOLOGY

Estrogens are secreted by the developing ovarian follicular cells as cholesterol derivatives in response to follicle-stimulating hormone (FSH) and luteinizing hormone (LH). FSH and LH are synthesized and released from the anterior pituitary in response to gonadotropin-releasing hormone (GnRH) secreted by the hypothalamus. This feedback system, balanced upon the circulating levels of estrogens and progestins, maintains the rhythm of the normal monthly reproductive cycle.

The three principal estrogens in female plasma* are 17-β-estradiol, estrone, and estriol. Physiologically, estrogens promote development and maintenance of female reproductive structures, including the vagina, uterus, fallopian tubes, and mammary glands. Estrogens are necessary for maturation of secondary female sex characteristics.** As with testosterone, estrogens work in conjunction with human growth hormone (hGH) to increase protein anabolism for muscle and bone growth. This action indirectly contributes to shaping of the skeleton and epiphyses of the long bones that allow for pubertal growth spurt and termination. Estrogens' involvement in lowering coronary heart disease in females under 50 years old is attributable to their ability to decrease blood cholesterol.

Progesterone, the principal progestin, is secreted by the corpus luteum after ovulation (about day 14 of a typical menstrual cycle). It acts synergistically with estrogen to repair, stimulate proliferation, and prepare the endometrium for implantation of the fertilized ovum. Consequently, it encourages the transformation of proliferative endometrium into secretory endometrium. Progesterone maintains pregnancy once implantation occurs, preventing spontaneous uterine smooth muscle contractions. Increased levels of estrogen and/or progesterone inhibit secretion of GnRH and LH through the negative feedback pathway, which is the basis of the pharmacological activity of oral contraceptives (OCs, see below). Table 17.2 summarizes the uses, proprietary names, and structures of the estrogens and progestins.

---

* It is important to note that estradiol also circulates in human male plasma and is usually undetectable, since most of the free precursor is used to synthesize testosterone.

** The characteristics include distribution of adipose tissue in the breasts, hips, abdomen, and mons pubis, and development of a broad pelvis, all of which prepare for pregnancy. In addition, estrogens regulate voice pitch and hair growth pattern peculiar to females.

17.4.2 PHARMACOLOGY AND CLINICAL USE

Estrogens are most commonly used in combination with progestins as OCs or as replacement therapy in postmenopausal women. Concerning the latter, estrogens are indicated for vasomotor symptoms associated with menopause — i.e., for the relief of signs and symptoms associated with decline of ovarian function. Symptoms include hot flushes, variable periods of amenorrhea, endometrial atrophy, and decrease of myometrial and vaginal epithelial mass. Estrogen replacement therapy is of value for treatment of atrophic vaginitis, and for the prevention of osteoporosis in postmenopausal women. Estrogens are also indicated as palliative therapy of advanced prostatic carcinoma in men and breast cancer in women. Unlike the anabolic-androgenic steroids, estrogen or progestins do not demonstrate illicit abuse potential.

The principal clinical uses of progestational agents are mostly related to the maintenance of pregnancy or regulation of the second half of the menstrual cycle. Progestins are indicated for amenorrhea, abnormal uterine bleeding, endometriosis,[*] AIDS wasting syndrome (appetite enhancement), infertility, and for breast or endometrial carcinoma.

For the prevention of pregnancy, oral and injectable contraceptives contain estrogen/progesterone combinations or progesterone alone. In addition, the combinations are used for emergency contraception, long-term (1- and 3-month) contraception, and in the treatment of acne vulgaris in females 15 years of age or older.[**]

17.4.3 CLINICAL TOXICITY OF PROLONGED ESTROGEN AND/OR PROGESTIN ADMINISTRATION

Decades of clinical use of estrogens, progestins, and combinations has resulted in the accumulation of a vast amount of data related to adverse reactions of this class of substances, summarized in Table 17.2. In particular, use of estrogens in replacement therapy is associated with an increased risk of endometrial carcinoma in postmenopausal women. In fact, recent studies report that routine replacement therapy may not be as beneficial for the prevention of osteoporosis as previously believed. In addition, long-term estrogen ingestion produces a variety of unwarranted metabolic, endocrine, and hematologic effects. Similarly, progestins are accompanied by serious metabolic side effects. Progestins have been associated with congenital anomalies because of unnecessary use during the first trimester of pregnancy for the prevention of habitual or threatened abortions. Finally, the most significant deleterious effects of continuous use of OCs appear to be the elevated risk of cardiovascular (CV) adverse reactions. The risk from CV mortality increases about tenfold when OCs are used concomitantly with cigarette smoking and increasing age (over 35). In general, women who use OCs should refrain from smoking.

---

[*] An abnormal gynecologic condition characterized by ectopic growth and function of endometrial tissue. Serious consequences occur when abnormal growth interferes with pelvic organs.

[**] Interestingly, OCs are not associated with an increase in the risk of developing breast or cervical cancer. In fact, there may be a protective effect, as users appear half as likely to develop ovarian and endometrial cancer as women who have never used OCs.

TABLE 17.2
Structure, Classification, and Properties of Selected, Commonly Used Estrogen and Progesterone Derivatives

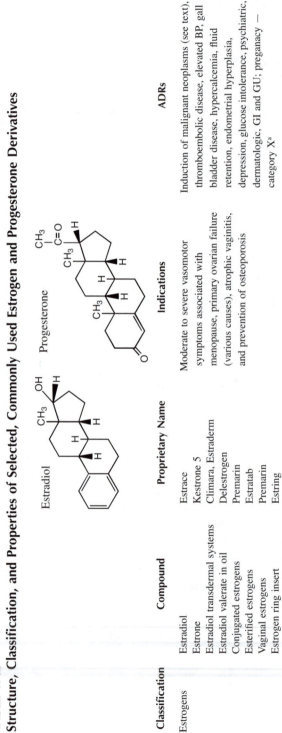

Estradiol   Progesterone

Classification	Compound	Proprietary Name	Indications	ADRs
Estrogens	Estradiol	Estrace	Moderate to severe vasomotor symptoms associated with menopause, primary ovarian failure (various causes), atrophic vaginitis, and prevention of osteoporosis	Induction of malignant neoplasms (see text), thromboembolic disease, elevated BP, gall bladder disease, hypercalcemia, fluid retention, endometrial hyperplasia, depression, glucose intolerance, psychiatric, dermatologic, GI and GU; preganacy — category X[a]
	Estrone	Kestrone 5		
	Estradiol transdermal systems	Climara, Estraderm		
	Estradiol valerate in oil	Delestrogen		
	Conjugated estrogens	Premarin		
	Esterified estrogens	Estratab		
	Vaginal estrogens	Premarin		
	Estrogen ring insert	Estring		

Progestins	Progesterone — Prometrium, Progesterone in Oil, Progesterone Gel; Medroxyprogesterone — Provera; Norethindrone — Aygestin; Megestrol — Megace	Amenorrhea, abnormal uterine bleeding, AIDS wasting syndrome, infertility, endometriosis; gel is used to support embryo implantation; megestrol is used in the palliative treatment of advanced breast or endometrial carcinoma	Congenital anomalies when administered during first 4-months of pregnancy, ophthalmic effects; rest of ADRs similar to estrogens
Combinations	Estrogen/progesterone tablets and patches — Prempro, Premphase	As with individual components above	As above
	Alesse, Ovral and various others	Oral contraceptives	As above

Note: BP = blood pressure, GI = gastrointestinal, GU = genitourinary.

[a] Category X = should not be used during pregnancy.

REFERENCES

Suggested Readings

Graham, S. and Kennedy, M., Recent developments in the toxicology of anabolic steroids, *Drug. Saf.*, 5, 458, 1990.

Simon, J.A., Safety of estrogen/androgen regimens, *J. Reprod. Med.*, 46, 281, 2001.

Review Articles

Crandall, C., Combination treatment of osteoporosis: a clinical review, *J. Womens Health Gend. Based Med.*, 11, 211, 2002.

Dossing, M. and Sonne, J., Drug-induced hepatic disorders. Incidence, management and avoidance, *Drug Saf.*, 9, 441, 1993.

Hoyer, P.B., Reproductive toxicology: current and future directions, *Biochem. Pharmacol.*, 62, 1557, 2001.

Jordan, A., Toxicology of progestogens of implantable contraceptives for women, *Contraception*, 65, 3, 2002.

Lane, J.R. and Connor, J.D., The influence of endogenous and exogenous sex hormones in adolescents with attention to oral contraceptives and anabolic steroids, *J. Adolesc. Health.*, 15, 630, 1994.

Lukas, S.E., Current perspectives on anabolic-androgenic steroid abuse, *Trends Pharmacol. Sci.*, 14, 61, 1993.

NIDA Research Report Series, Anabolic Steroid Abuse, National Institute on Drug Abuse, DHHS, Public Health Service, 2000, http://www.drugabuse.gov.

OH, W.K., Secondary hormonal therapies in the treatment of prostate cancer, *Urology*, 60, 87, 2002.

Simon, J.A., Safety of estrogen/androgen regimens, *J. Reprod. Med.*, 46, 281, 2001.

Sullivan, M.L. et al., The cardiac toxicity of anabolic steroids, *Prog. Cardiovasc. Dis.*, 41, 1, 1998.

18 Cardiovascular Drugs

Yunbo Li and Zhuoxiao Cao

18.1 INTRODUCTION

Despite some recent declines, cardiovascular disease (CVD) remains a leading cause of death in the human population. In the U.S., more than 60 million people have CVD, including coronary heart disease, congestive heart failure, hypertension, stroke, and congenital CV defects. CVD is responsible for nearly one million deaths (about 40% of total deaths) annually in the U.S. CVD is typically progressive, and patients with CVD usually require years of therapy and extensive health care. As such, the costs to society are prodigious. For example, the total cost of CVD in 2003 alone in the U.S. was estimated to be more than $350 billion. As the population ages and the costs rise, this annual estimate is expected to increase. Although the above statistical data are intimidating, important advances in the understanding of the initiation and progression of CVD have emerged, and effective therapies continue to evolve as mechanisms are better defined.

CVD is the number one killer of the human population, which is also indicative of the vital functions of the CV system. Included within functions of the CV system are (1) cardiac pumping ability, including the rhythmic nature of the electrical signals, force of contraction, and magnitude of the discharge pressure; (2) integrity of the vasculature, including muscular tone and structural integrity of vessel walls, and the tight regulation of blood pressure; and (3) blood volume and composition, including water and electrolyte balance, lipid composition, and capabilities of clot formation and lysis. These functions are compromised, to varying extents, in CVD, which can be modified therapeutically or prophylactically with a number of drugs. The proper use of the CV drugs has greatly reduced the mortality and morbidity caused by CVD. On the other hand, many CV drugs have the potential to cause toxicity, particularly when used inappropriately or in overdoses. As such, a greater understanding of the clinical toxicology of CV drugs will contribute to our ability to effectively manage CVD. This chapter will discuss the clinical toxicology of commonly used CV drugs.

18.2 REVIEW OF CV PHYSIOLOGY

18.2.1 AN OVERVIEW OF THE CV SYSTEM

A clear grasp of the normal anatomy and physiology of the CV system provides the basis for understanding the effects (both pharmacological and toxicological effects) of drugs on this vital system. Blood flows through a network of blood vessels that extend between the heart and peripheral tissues. These blood vessels can be subdivided into (1) a pulmonary circuit, which transports blood to and from the gas exchange surfaces of the lungs, and (2) a systemic circuit, which carries blood to and from the rest of the body. Each circuit begins and ends at the heart, and blood travels through these circuits in sequence. For example, venous blood returning to the heart from the systemic circuit must complete the pulmonary circuit to become oxygenated before reentering the systemic circuit.

18.2.2 Physiology of the Heart

The main purpose of the heart is to pump blood to the lungs and the systemic arteries so as to provide oxygen and nutrients to all the tissues of the body. The heart consists of four muscular chambers: the right and left atria and the right and left ventricles. Venous blood from the systemic circulation enters the right atrium and right ventricle, from which it is then pumped into the lungs to become oxygenated. The left atrium and ventricle then receive the oxygenated blood via pulmonary veins and eject it to the systemic circulation via the aorta. In addition, the heart receives the oxygenated blood from the coronary arteries, which begin at the root of the aorta.

18.2.2.1 Electrophysiology

Each cardiac contraction cycle consists of an orchestrated series of events that lead to the blood pumping action of the heart. The normal electrophysiological properties of the cardiac muscles contribute to the coordinated action of the atria and ventricles. Two types of cardiac muscle cells are involved in a normal heart beat: (1) contractile cells, which produce the contractions that pump blood, and (2) specialized muscle cells of the conducting system that control and coordinate the activities of the contractile muscle cells. The functionality of the heart, including conductivity and contractibility of cardiac muscle cells resides at the tightly regulated membrane transport of various ions, which in turn forms the basis of an action potential. In contractile cardiac muscle cells, an action potential results in increased levels of cytosolic Ca^{2+}, leading to muscle contraction. A typical action potential in contractile cardiac muscle cells consists of 4 characteristic phases (Figure 18.1). The membrane potential in a resting cell is normally about −90 mV (Phase 4). When an action potential is initiated, voltage-gated Na^+ channels open, leading to a rapid influx of Na^+, which depolarizes the cell from approximately −90 mV to greater than 0 mV, giving rise to the upstroke of the action potential. The initial, brief, and rapid repolarization that occurs immediately following phase 0 is produced by the closure of the Na^+ channels and the opening of the voltage-gated transient outward K^+ channels (Phase 1). During Phase 1, the voltage-gated Ca^{2+} channels open and Ca^{2+} begins a slower but prolonged inward influx at about −30 to −40 mV, giving rise to Ca^{2+} current. As the K^+ current dissipates, Ca^{2+} continues to enter the cell, resulting in a plateau appearance of Phase 2. Final repolarization (Phase 3) of the cell results from the closure of Ca^{2+} channels, and the K^+ efflux through K^+ channels. The resting potential (Phase 4) is then restored. Following the action potential, the normalization of the Na^+ and K^+ concentration gradients is achieved via the action of sarcolemma Na^+-K^+-ATPase. In addition, Ca^{2+} needs to be extruded from the cell or sequestered into intracellular stores, primarily through the sarcoplasmic reticulum (SR).

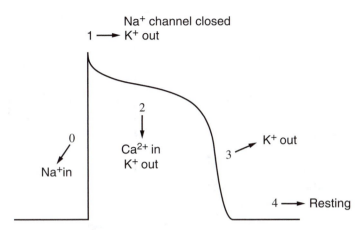

FIGURE 18.1 An action potential in contractile cardiac muscle cells.

The appearance of an action potential in the cardiac muscle cell membrane is coupled by a muscle contraction. This process occurs in two steps: (1) Ca^{2+} entering the cell during Phase 3 of the action potential provides roughly 20% of the Ca^{2+} required for a contraction; (2) the influx of extracellular Ca^{2+} is the trigger for the release of additional Ca^{2+} from the SR (i.e., Ca^{2+}-induced Ca^{2+} release). As a result, the muscle cell contraction continues until Phase 3 ends. The intracellular Ca^{2+} then is sequestered by the SR or pumped out of the cell, leading to muscle relaxation.

18.2.2.2 The Conducting System

The cardiac conducting system is a network of specialized cardiac muscle cells that initiates and distributes electrical impulses. The conducting system consists of (1) the sinoatrial (SA) node, located in the wall of the right atrium, (2) the atrioventricular (AV) node, located at the junction between the atria and ventricles, and (3) the conducting cells, which interconnect the two nodes and distribute the contractile stimulus throughout the myocardium. Conducting cells in the atria are found in the internodal pathways, which distribute the contractile stimulus to atrial muscle cells as the impulse travels from the SA node to the AV node. The ventricular conducting cells include those in the AV bundle and the bundle branches as well as the Purkinje fibers, which distribute the stimulus to the ventricular myocardium. The cells in the conducting system share an important feature: they cannot maintain a stable resting potential. Each time repolarization occurs, the membrane potential again gradually drifts toward a threshold. The rate of spontaneous depolarization varies in the different portions of the conducting system. It is fastest at the SA node, which establishes the heart rate. As such, the SA node is also known as the cardiac pacemaker.

18.2.2.3 Electrocardiography

The electrical activities occurring in the heart are powerful enough to be detected by electrodes placed on the body surface. A recording of these electrical activities

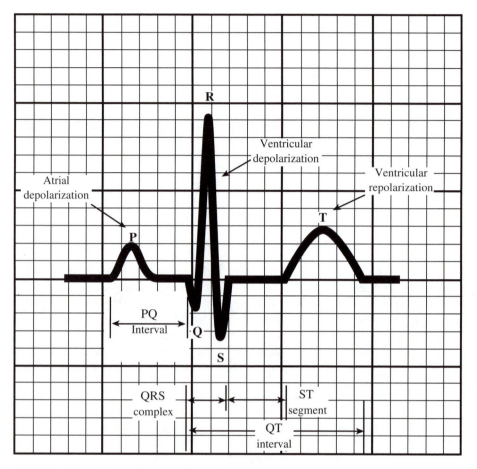

FIGURE 18.2 A typical electrocardiograph.

constitutes an electrocardiogram (ECG) (Figure 18.2). A typical ECG has the following components: (1) the small P wave, which results from the depolarization of the atria, (2) the QRS complex, which appears as the ventricles depolarize, and (3) the small T wave, which indicates ventricular repolarization. ECG is an important tool for diagnosis of cardiac dysfunction. ECG analysis is particularly useful in detecting and diagnosing cardiac arrhythmias. The cardiac toxicity of therapeutic agents, especially CV drugs, is often reflected by changes in ECG.

18.3 DIGITALIS GLYCOSIDES

Digitalis glycosides (DGs) have played a prominent role in the therapy of congestive heart failure since William Withering codified their use in his late eighteenth century monograph on the efficacy of the leaves of the common foxglove plant (*Digitalis purpurea*). Despite their widespread acceptance into medical practice in the ensuing

200 years, both the efficacy and the safety of this class of drugs continue to be a topic of debate.

18.3.1 MEDICINAL CHEMISTRY

DGs possess a common molecular motif, a steroid nucleus containing an unsaturated lactone at the C17 position and one or more glycoside residues at C3 position. Digitoxin differs from digoxin only by the absence of a hydroxyl group at C12, which makes digitoxin more lipophilic than digoxin. Although digitoxin and ouabain are still available, digoxin is the most widely prescribed drug of this class in the U.S., due to the ready availability of techniques for measuring its levels in serum, flexibility in routes of its administration, and its intermediate duration of action.

18.3.2 PHARMACOLOGY AND CLINICAL USE

DGs have been widely used for more than two centuries as therapeutic agents of congestive heart failure. The beneficial effects of these drugs appear to be derived from a positive inotropic effect on failing myocardium and efficacy in controlling the ventricular rate response to atrial fibrillation. DGs at therapeutic doses selectively bind and partially inhibit the intrinsic membrane protein Na^+-K^+-ATPase. This partial inhibition of the Na^+-K^+-ATPase leads to an increase in the intracellular Na^+ concentration, which is sufficient to reduce Ca^{2+} extrusion via the Na^+/Ca^{2+} exchange system in the sarcolemma. The resulting increase in cytosolic and, hence, sarcoplasmic Ca^{2+} concentrations, enhances the force of cardiac muscle contraction. While the direct inhibition of the Na^+-K^+-ATPase is the principal mechanism of action for the positive inotropic effects of DGs, it was recently recognized that DGs are also able to modulate sympathetic nerve system activity, an additional mechanism contributing to their efficacy in the treatment of patients with heart failure.

18.3.3 TOXICOKINETICS

Absorption of DGs occurs in the gastrointestinal (GI) tract. Because digoxin is more polar than digitoxin, GI absorption of digoxin is less rapid and less complete than that of digitoxin. DGs bind to plasma proteins, especially albumin. Substances that are highly protein bound may thus displace DGs from albumin and increase the levels of free DGs in blood. This may potentially increase their toxicity. Once absorbed into the circulation, DGs are widely distributed throughout the body, with the highest concentrations in muscular tissues. For instance, the concentrations of DGs in the myocardium are about 30 times higher than those in blood. DGs are mainly metabolized in the liver. In addition, gut flora may also metabolize digoxin to inactive products. Routes of elimination include urinary and bile excretion. The half-life of digoxin is about 36 h, whereas that of digitoxin is 5 to 7 days. Enterohepatic circulation occurs for digitoxin, which may be partially responsible for its long half-life. Because liver and kidneys are crucially involved in the metabolism and excretion of DGs, the half-life of DGs may be significantly prolonged with an increased likelihood of intoxication in patients with impaired renal and hepatic function.

18.3.4 CLINICAL MANIFESTATIONS OF TOXICITY

DG poisoning may be acute or chronic. Acute poisoning most frequently occurs in adults following a suicidal ingestion of a large dose. It may also result from unintentional ingestion in children. Chronic poisoning is more common, and typically develops in patients receiving DGs for therapeutic purposes. The incidence and severity of DG toxicity have been substantially reduced in the past two decades due partially to the development of alternative drugs for the treatment of heart failure, as well as to the improved management of DG intoxication. In spite of the decreased incidence, intoxication from DGs still remains common.

Manifestations of DG toxicity involve the CV, the central nervous system (CNS), and the GI tract. The hallmark of cardiac toxicity is an increased automaticity coupled with concomitant conduction delay. Although no single dysrhythmia is always present, certain aberrations such as frequent premature ventricular beats, bradyrhythmias, paroxysmal atrial tachycardia with block, junctional tachycardia, and bidirectional ventricular tachycardia are common. DG toxicity is also manifest as dysfunction of CNS, including delirium, fatigue, malaise, confusion, dizziness, abnormal dreams, blurred or yellow vision, and halos. Disturbances of color vision are frequently reported — a relatively specific sign of digoxin intoxication. GI disturbances in DG intoxication may include anorexia, nausea, vomiting, and abdominal pain.

18.3.5 MECHANISMS OF TOXICITY

The toxic effects of DGs are at least partially the extensions of their pharmacological actions. The electrophysiological effects of DGs are due to their direct actions on cardiac contractile and conducting cells (i.e., inhibition of sarcolemmal Na^+-K^+-ATPase) and indirect effects on the autonomic nervous system. At therapeutic, nontoxic doses, digoxin increases the vagal tone and decreases the sympathetic activity, resulting in decreased automaticity, primarily in SA and AV nodes. At higher concentrations of digoxin, the above effects may progress to cause bradycardia, prolongation of AV conduction, or heart block. In addition, DGs, especially digoxin at toxic doses, can increase both intracellular Ca^{2+} loading and sympathetic nerve system activity, leading to atrial and ventricular dysrhythmias, including the life-threatening ventricular fibrillation. At toxic concentrations, DGs may cause vasoconstriction as a result of increased intracellular Ca^{2+} in smooth muscle of the vessel wall. CNS toxicity of DGs appears to be related to the inactivation of Na^+-K^+-ATPase, resulting in altered ionic transport across excitable neuronal membranes with consequent membrane irritability and instability.

18.3.6 METHODS OF DETECTION

Detection of the serum levels of DGs is of critical importance for the diagnosis of DG intoxication. Drug-specific radioimmunoassays are the most widely used methods for detecting DGs in serum. Enzyme and fluorescence polarization immunoassays are also available.

18.3.7 CLINICAL MANAGEMENT OF INTOXICATION

Successful management of DG intoxication depends on early recognition. Treatment depends on the clinical conditions rather than serum drug levels. Management varies from temporary withdrawal of the medication, general supportive care, and proper treatment of the DG-induced cardiac arrhythmias, to administration of digoxin-specific Fab fragments (i.e., Digibind®) for life-threatening CV compromise.

18.4 BETA-ADRENERGIC RECEPTOR ANTAGONISTS

18.4.1 β–ADRENERGIC RECEPTOR SYSTEM

β-Adrenergic receptors are members of the superfamily of G-protein-coupled receptors. There are at least three β-adrenergic receptor subtypes: (1) β1, found in heart and coronary blood vessels predominantly, but also present in liver, kidney, and adipose tissues; (2) β2, found in lungs, muscle tissue, and most other sympathetic target organs; and (3) β3, located primarily in adipose tissue. Upon β-receptor stimulation, the G-protein undergoes a conformational change that activates adenylyl cyclase, leading to increased levels of intracellular cAMP. cAMP stimulates protein kinase A, which phosphorylates Ca^{2+} channels, leading to Ca^{2+} entry into the cell. Ca^{2+} entry into the cell triggers additional Ca^{2+} release from the SR. Stimulation of β1 receptors results in increased chronotropy and inotropy in the heart, as well as increased renin secretion by the kidneys. Stimulation of β2 receptors leads to relaxation of smooth muscle cells in blood vessels and bronchial tree. Activation of β3 receptors appears to be involved in the increased metabolism of lipid. In view of the relatively specific actions mediated by each β receptor subtype, selective modulation of these subtypes by pharmacological agents has proven to be of clinical significance.

18.4.2 PHARMACOLOGY AND CLINICAL USE

β-Adrenergic receptor antagonists, also called β-blockers, have received enormous clinical attention because of their efficacy in the treatment of a broad spectrum of illnesses. CV applications include hypertension, ischemic heart disease, congestive heart failure, and certain arrhythmias. Non-CV uses include the treatment of essential tremor, pheochromocytoma, glaucoma, anxiety, and migraine headaches. Due to their broad clinical applications and availability, β-blocker overdoses and intoxications are commonly encountered.

Currently, three classes of β-blockers are available for clinical uses: (1) nonselective β-blockers, including propranolol, nadolol, timolol, pindolol, and labetalol; (2) selective β1-blockers, such as metoprolol, atenolol, esmolol, acebutolol, and bisoprolol, and (3) β-blockers with vasodilating activity, including carvedilol, bucindolol, and nebivolol.

18.4.3 CLINICAL MANIFESTATIONS OF TOXICITY

The β-blocker overdoses mainly cause deleterious effects on the CV system, CNS, and lungs. The CV compromise may present as bradycardia, conduction delay, and decreased cardiac contractibility with systemic hypotension. The manifestations of CNS toxicity in severe intoxication may include psychosis, depressed consciousness, and seizures. Another major toxic effect of β-adrenergic antagonists is exerted by blockage of the β2 receptors in bronchial smooth muscle. β2 receptors are critical for promoting bronchodilation in patients with bronchospastic disease, such as asthma. β-blockers may thus cause a life-threatening bronchoconstriction in such patients. Other unusual manifestations of β-blocker intoxication may include acidosis and hypoglycemia.

18.4.4 Mechanisms of Toxicity

It is generally believed that the principal mechanism of CV toxicity of β-blockers involves excessive blockage of β receptor signaling (i.e., diminishing cAMP production), leading to decreased metabolic, chronotropic, and inotropic effects of physiological catecholamines. Other possible mechanisms may also be involved in the manifestations of CV toxicity. For example, β-blockers have been suggested to cause cardiotoxicity through disruption of ion transport and homeostasis in cardiac muscle cells. In addition, cardiac toxicity may result from the direct effects of β-blockers on the CNS. The mechanism underlying β-blocker-induced CNS toxicity is unclear, but may be associated with cellular hypoxia resulting from suppressed cardiac output or direct neuronal toxicity.

18.4.5 Clinical Management of Intoxication

The goal of clinical management of β-blocker intoxication is to restore perfusion to critical organ systems by improving myocardial contractility or increasing heart rate, or both. General measures may include supportive care and gastrointestinal decontamination. Pharmacotherapy may include the use of glucagon, β-adrenergic receptor tagonists, phosphodiesterase inhibitors, and atropine. Glucagon has become the first-line therapy for β-blocker intoxication. It enhances cardiac performance by increasing intracellular cAMP through action on a distinct glucagon receptor on cardiac muscle cells. Thus, glucagon bypasses the blocked β-receptors to restore suppressed cardiac function.

18.5 CALCIUM CHANNEL ANTAGONISTS

It was observed four decades ago that the effects of certain phenylalkylamines, such as phenylamine and verapamil, on isolated cardiac muscle preparations, were indistinguishable from the effects of Ca^{2+} removal. The effect of these drugs, which is similar to Ca^{2+} depletion, diminished the contractile force without affecting the action potential, thus inducing excitation-contraction uncoupling. Verapamil and phenylamines, together with a number of other drugs that inhibit excitation-contraction coupling, have been designated Ca^{2+} antagonists. The major action of these drugs is to diminish the inward movement of Ca^{2+} through the L-type voltage-dependent Ca^{2+} channels located in sarcolemma. As such, these drugs are also termed Ca^{2+} channel blockers. So far, ten Ca^{2+} channel antagonists have been approved for clinical use in the U.S. They are classified into four chemical classes (Table 18.1).

TABLE 18.1
Classification of Ca^{2+} Channel
Antagonists

Chemical Class	Drug
Phenylalkylamines	Verapamil
Benzothiazepines	Diltiazem
Dihydropyridines	Amlodipine
	Felodipine
	Isradipine
	Nicardipine
	Nifedipine
	Nimodipine
	Nisoldipine
Diarylaminopropylamine esters	Bepridil

18.5.1 PHARMACOLOGY AND CLINICAL USE

Ca^{2+} channel antagonists affect the contractility of both smooth and cardiac muscle cells. At least three distinct mechanisms have been suggested to lead to increased levels of cytosolic Ca^{2+} and the subsequent contraction of smooth muscle: (1) extracellular Ca^{2+} influx through voltage-sensitive Ca^{2+} channels in response to the depolarization of the membrane; (2) second messenger- (i.e., inositol triphosphate) mediated release of a Ca^{2+} from the SR; and (3) influx of extracellular Ca^{2+} via receptor-operated Ca^{2+} channels in response to receptor occupancy. Ca^{2+} channel antagonists inhibit the voltage-dependent Ca^{2+} channels in vascular smooth muscle cells at much lower concentrations than those required to interfere with the release of intracellular Ca^{2+} from the SR or to block receptor-operated Ca^{2+} channels.

All of the Ca^{2+} channel antagonists are capable of inducing relaxation of vascular smooth muscle, leading to vasodilation. As stated earlier, the contraction of cardiac muscle is dependent on the influx of extracellular Ca^{2+} through the L-type channels, and the subsequent Ca^{2+}-induced Ca^{2+} release from the SR. Thus, Ca^{2+} channel antagonists exert a negative inotropic effect on myocardium. Although this is true of all classes of Ca^{2+} channel antagonists, the greater degree of peripheral vasodilation seen with the dihydropyridines is accompanied by a sufficient baroreflex-mediated increase in sympathetic activity to overcome the negative inotropic effect. In the SA and AV nodes, depolarization is largely dependent on the influx of extracellular Ca^{2+} through the L-type channels. Therefore, Ca^{2+} channel antagonists have the potential to depress the rate of sinus node pacemaker and slow AV conduction. In addition, all approved Ca^{2+} channel antagonists are able to decrease coronary vascular resistance and thereby increase coronary blood flow. In view of the above pharmacological effects, Ca^{2+} channel antagonists are efficacious in the treatment of various types of CV disorders, including hypertension, angina pectoris, myocardial infarction, and cardiac arrhythmias.

18.5.2 Clinical Manifestations of Toxicity

The most common toxic effects caused by the Ca^{2+} channel antagonists, particularly the dihydropyridines, are due to excessive vasodilation. These effects may be manifest as dizziness, hypotension, headache, flushing, digital dysesthesia, and nausea. Patients may also experience constipation, peripheral edema, coughing, wheezing, and pulmonary edema. At therapeutic and moderate toxic doses, dihydropyridines are well recognized to produce reflex increases in heart rate with an increase in left ventricular stroke volume, leading to an increase in cardiac output. With severe overdoses that result in dramatic Ca^{2+} channel blockage, all Ca^{2+} channel antagonists exert a negative inotropic effect with depressed cardiac contraction, conduction blockage, hypotension, and shock. Other overdose effects may present as metabolic acidosis with hyperglycemia. The mechanism of hyperglycemia is likely related to the suppressive effect by Ca^{2+} channel antagonists on pancreatic β cell insulin release coupled with whole-body insulin resistance.

18.5.3 Clinical Management of Intoxication

In the management of intoxication, early recognition is critical. Calcium channel antagonists are frequently prescribed, and the potential for serious morbidity and mortality with overdoses is significant. Ingestion of these agents should be suspected in any patient who presents in an overdose situation with unexplained hypotension and conduction abnormalities. The general management of intoxication of Ca^{2+} channel antagonists includes three major objectives: (1) providing supportive care, (2) decreasing drug absorption, and (3) augmenting myocardial function with cardiotonic agents. Because there is no specific antidote, decontamination of the GI tract via the use of activated charcoal is crucial. Intravenous injection of calcium salts is the first-line treatment of Ca^{2+} channel antagonist overdoses. Other cardiotonic drugs may include glucagon, atropine, and catecholamines.

18.6 ANGIOTENSIN-CONVERTING ENZYME (ACE) INHIBITORS

18.6.1 Pharmacology and Clinical Use

The ACE inhibitors work by blocking ACE, thereby decreasing the formation of angiotensin II, a potent vessel pressor, which is critically involved in raising systemic blood pressure. As such, ACE inhibitors are commonly used in the treatment of hypertension. These drugs are also efficacious in the treatment of congestive heart failure, left ventricular systolic dysfunction, acute myocardial infarction, and chronic renal disease. At present, 12 ACE inhibitors are approved (11 marketed) for use in the U.S. They include benazepril, captopril, enalapril, enalaprilat, fosinopril sodium, lisinopril, moexipril, perinopril, quinapril, ramipril and trandolapril.

18.6.2 Clinical Manifestations of Toxicity

Serious toxic effects caused by ACE inhibitors are rare, and in general, these drugs are well tolerated. Overdoses have been reported with some ACE inhibitors.

Hypotension is the most common manifestation in patients with ACE inhibitor overdoses. Adverse effects reported at therapeutic doses include first-dose hypotension, headache, cough, hyperkalemia, dermatitis, renal dysfunction, and angioedema. The drugs may also cause adverse fetal effects; thus, this class of drugs is contraindicated in pregnancy. Other rare toxic effects include neutropenia, bone marrow suppression, and hepatotoxicity. Some adverse effects (e.g., hypotension, hyperkalemia, and headache) of ACE inhibitors are predictable on the basis of the fundamental pharmacology of this class of drugs. However, other effects are idiosyncratic in nature, and the mechanisms remain largely unknown.

18.6.3 CLINICAL MANAGEMENT OF INTOXICATION

Supportive care constitutes the primary treatment of patients with ACE intoxication. In drug overdoses, activated charcoal may be used to enhance its elimination from the GI tract. Hypertension should be treated with standard procedures. Angioedema may rapidly obstruct the airway, which can be life threatening and must be treated aggressively.

18.7 VASODILATORS

The direct vasodilators, including hydralazine, minoxidil, diazoxide, and nitroprusside represent another class of antihypertensive drugs. These drugs produce vascular smooth muscle relaxation independent of innervation or known pharmacological receptors. In view of their direct vasodilating activities, these drugs are also used in the management of other CV diseases, such as angina pectoris, congestive heart failure, and peripheral vascular disease. Hydralazine, minoxidil, and diazoxide cause arterial vasodilation, whereas nitroprusside is able to induce both arterial and venous vasodilation.

18.7.1 PHARMACOLOGY AND CLINICAL USE

Hydralazine was one of the first orally active antihypertensive drugs to be marketed in the U.S. It appears to activate guanylate cyclase, leading to increased cGMP in arterial vascular smooth muscle to cause vasorelaxation. Formation of cGMP results in decreased levels of cytosolic Ca^{2+} in smooth muscle. Minoxidil needs to undergo biotransformation in the liver to produce the active N-O sulfate metabolite. Minoxidil sulfate is able to activate the ATP-sensitive K^+ channels, thus producing vasodilation by hyperpolarizing arterial smooth muscle cells. The drug has proven to be efficacious in patients with the most severe and drug-resistant forms of hypertension. Similar to minoxidil, diazoxide causes vasodilation via activation of ATP-sensitive K^+ channels. This drug is clinically used in the treatment of hypertensive emergencies. Nitroprusside is metabolized by the vessel wall to form nitric oxide. Nitric oxide then activates guanylyl cyclase, resulting in increased levels of cGMP and subsequent vasodilation. Nitroprusside is used mainly in the treatment of hypertensive emergencies, but it can also be useful in situations when short-term reduction of cardiac preload and/or afterload is desired.

18.7.2 CLINICAL MANIFESTATIONS OF TOXICITY

Two types of adverse effects have been observed with hydralazine intoxication: (1) toxic effects due to the extensions of the pharmacological effects of the drug, including hypotension, headache, nausea, flushing, palpitation, dizziness, tachycardia, and angina pectoris. Tachycardia and angina pectoris result from the baroreflex-induced stimulation of the sympathetic nervous system; and (2) toxic effects resulting from autoimmune reactions, including lupus syndrome, vasculitis, serum sickness, hemolytic anemia, and rapidly progressive glomerulonephritis. Among the autoimmune reactions, lupus syndrome is the most common. The mechanisms underlying these reactions are not clear, but hydralazine has been reported to induce overexpression of lymphocyte function-associated antigen 1 (LFA-1) and T cell autoreactivity.

The clinical manifestations of minoxidil intoxication may include (1) fluid and salt retention, (2) CV compromise, and (3) hypertrichosis. The most common toxic effects of minoxidil are hypotension, tachycardia and lethargy. Tachycardia is caused by the baroreceptor-mediated increase of the sympathetic tone. Hypertrichosis occurs in all patients who receive minoxidil for an extended period of time and is probably a consequence of K^+ channel activation induced by this drug. The opening of intracellular K^+ channels is an important mechanism regulating hair growth.

The most common manifestations of diazoxide intoxication are myocardial ischemia, salt and water retention, and hyperglycemia. Myocardial ischemia may be precipitated or aggravated by diazoxide, and it results from the reflex adrenergic stimulation of the heart and from the increased flow of blood to nonischemic regions. Hyperglycemia appears to result from its inhibition of the secretion of insulin from pancreatic β cells.

The short-term toxic effects of nitroprusside are caused by excessive vasodilation and the ensuing hypotension. Toxicity may also result from the conversion of nitroprusside to cyanide and thiocyanate. Cyanide blocks the ability of cells to utilize oxygen and to generate ATP through oxidative phosphorylation (see Chapter 23, "Gases"). The organ systems most commonly affected by cyanide poisoning are those most sensitive to hypoxia, i.e., the heart and brain. One of the earliest and most consistent manifestations in patients with nitroprusside-induced cyanide poisoning is the development of an anion gap metabolic acidosis. Early nitroprusside-induced cyanide poisoning frequently presents as unexplained sinus tachycardia. Sinus bradycardia may also develop as the myocardium becomes more hypoxic. Pump failure, asystole, or ventricular dysrhythmias may be the CV terminal events. Cyanide-induced CNS dysfunction is initially manifested as restlessness and agitation and may progress to convulsion. Encephalopathy, coma, and cerebral death often occur simultaneously with the terminal CV event.

18.7.3 CLINICAL MANAGEMENT OF INTOXICATION

The management of the vasodilator intoxication includes the general supportive care and correction of hypotension and cardiac arrhythmias. Ca^{2+} channel antagonists and β-adrenergic receptor antagonists may be useful in the treatment of myocardial ischemia caused by the vasodilators. Discontinuation of the nitroprusside infusion is the first step in the management of suspected cyanide poisoning. The patient should also be placed on oxygen supplementation. In all cases, sodium thiosulfate should be given immediately to enhance transulfuration of cyanide to thiocyanate, which is much less toxic. In severe cases, the administration of sodium nitrite is indicated.

18.8 ANTIARRHYTHMIC DRUGS

18.8.1 CLASSIFICATION, PHARMACOLOGY, AND CLINICAL USE

A number of drugs with diverse structures have been used clinically in the treatment of cardiac arrhythmias. One way to classify antiarrhythmic drugs is based on the mechanisms of action derived primarily from experimental studies. This scheme classifies drugs that depress myocardial Na^+ channels into class I, those that have sympatholytic activities into class II, those that prolong action potential duration and refractoriness into class III, and those that are Ca^{2+} channel antagonists into class IV. Drugs in classes II and IV were covered earlier in this chapter. Based on the degree of Na^+ channel blockage, drugs in class I are further classified into three subclasses: IA, IB, and IC.

The pharmacology and clinical use of drugs in classes I and III are summarized in Table 18.2.

18.8.2 CLINICAL MANIFESTATIONS OF TOXICITY

18.8.2.1 Class IA Drugs

Drugs in class IA category include quinidine, procainamide, and disopyramide. These drugs have a low toxic-to-therapeutic ratio, and their use is associated with a number of serious adverse effects during long term therapy and life-threatening sequelae following acute overdoses. The most severe manifestation of intoxication of type IA drugs is CV compromise. Sinus tachycardia with Q-Tc prolongation is seen in mild intoxication. In severe overdosage, almost any type of cardiac arrhythmia can occur, including increased Q-Tc and QRS intervals, bundle branch blockage, polymorphic ventricular tachycardia (torsade de pointes) and the fatal ventricular fibrillation. Hypotension usually develops in severe cases. It is caused by depressed myocardial contractility via the Na^+ channel blockage and peripheral vasodilation. Vasodilation results primarily from the K^+ channel blocking activity of these drugs. Type IA drug intoxication also leads to CNS symptoms, such as lethargy, confusion, coma, respiratory depression, and seizure. Quinidine intoxication causes cinchonism, a symptom complex that includes headache, tinnitus, vertigo, and blurred vision. Disopyramide also has strong anticholinergic activity, which manifests as precipitation of glaucoma, constipation, dry mouth, and urinary retention. Other toxic effects also develop in patients using type IA drugs at therapeutic doses. For example, diarrhea is the most common adverse effect during quinidine therapy. "Quinidine syncope" (a transient loss of consciousness due to paroxysmal ventricular tachycardia, frequently of the torsade de pointes type) may occur with therapeutic dosing, often in the first few days of therapy. A number of immunological

TABLE 18.2
Pharmacological Effects and Clinical Uses of Classes I and III Antiarrhythmic Drugs

Drug	Pharmacological Effects	Major Clinical Use
IA	Blockage of both Na$^+$ and K$^+$ channels	Maintenance of sinus rhythm in patients with atrial flutter or fibrillation
Disopyramide	Depression of rapid action potential upstroke	
Procainamide	Decrease of conduction velocity	Prevention of ventricular tachycardia or fibrillation
Quinidine	Prolongation of repolarization	
IB	Weak blockage of Na$^+$ channels	Ventricular arrhythmias
Lidocaine	Depression of rapid action potential upstroke in abnormal tissues	Tocainide is rarely used due to severe toxicity
Mexiletine		
Moricizine	Enhancement of repolarization	
Tocainide		
IC	Strong blockage of Na$^+$ channels	Maintenance of sinus rhythm in patients with supraventricular arrhythmias, such as atrial fibrillation
Flecainide	Marked depression of rapid action potential upstroke	
Propafenone	Little or no effects on K$^+$ channels Little or no effects on repolarization	
III	Blockage of K$^+$ channels	Ventricular tachyarrhythmias
Amiodarone	Little or no effects on Na$^+$ channels	
Bretylium	Depression of repolarization	
Sotalol	Sotalol is also a β-adrenergic receptor blocker	

reactions can occur during quinidine therapy, including thrombobocytopenia, hepatitis, bone marrow suppression, and a lupus syndrome. Long-term therapy with procainamide may also cause a lupus syndrome. The mechanisms underlying the above adverse immunological effects remain unclear.

18.8.2.2 Class IB Drugs

In severe intoxication with class IB drugs, the cardiac manifestations are similar to those of class IA drugs. CNS toxicity is more common and may be manifest as confusion, coma, or seizure. Nystagmus is an early sign of lidocaine toxicity. Tremor and nausea are the major dose-related adverse effects of mexiletine and tocainide.

Tocainide is rarely used due to its potential to cause fatal bone marrow aplasia and severe pulmonary interstitial fibrosis.

18.8.2.3 Class IC Drugs

Drugs in this class have much in common with agents in class IA. The toxicity of the Na^+-blocking activity of these drugs will be manifest as prolonged QRS and Q-Tc intervals, hypotension, and bradycardia. The prominent clinical presentations in severe overdoses include coma, respiratory depression, and seizure.

18.8.2.4 Class III Drugs

Although K^+-channel blocking action is the common property of agents in this class, the toxicity of these drugs cannot be explained by K^+ blockage alone. For example, in addition to its K^+-channel blocking effect, sotalol also has a marked β-adenergic receptor antagonist activity, which explains most of the CV compromise in overdosage. Sotalol intoxication may cause Q-Tc prolongation, bradycardia, and hypotension. Coma, respiratory depression, seizure, and ventricular dysrhythmia (torsade de pointes) occur in severe sotalol overdoses.

Bretylium is only available in intravenous form, and its intoxication is usually iatrogenic. In addition to its ability to prolong action potential by blocking K^+ channels, bretylium exhibits an initial stimulation of norepinephrine release from sympathetic neurons, leading to a transient increase in blood pressure and heart rate. Later, the drug reduces the release of norepinephrine, causing hypotension and bradycardia. In fact, hypotension is a common problem during bretylium therapy.

Amiodarone toxicity following acute overdose is rare, because poor bioavailability and a large volume of distribution limit the peak serum concentration. Acute toxicity may include hypotension due to vasodilation and depression of myocardial performance. Chronic intoxication with amiodarone represents an important clinical problem. The most severe toxic effect during chronic therapy is pulmonary fibrosis, a condition for which there is currently no effective treatment and for which patient prognosis is poor. The exact mechanisms by which amiodarone induces pulmonary fibrosis are currently unknown. Other toxic effects during long-term use of amiodarone include Q-Tc prolongation, bradycardia, corneal microdeposits, hepatitis, thyroid abnormalities, neuromuscular symptoms, and photosensitivity.

18.8.3 Clinical Management of Intoxication

The general clinical management of intoxication of classes I and III antiarrhythmic drugs include the following: (1) supportive care, early cardiac monitoring with intravenous access, and airway management; (2) GI decontamination with activated charcoal; and (3) specific treatment of cardiac arrhythmias, hypotension, coma, seizure, and other severe disorders. Attention to airway management in patients with lethargy, coma, or respiratory depression is important. For most antiarrhythmic drugs, aggressive GI decontamination is most useful early after ingestion. The slow absorption of amiodarone allows for late GI decontamination in cases of significant ingestion. Sodium bicarbonate has been shown to be efficacious in the treatment of the cardiotoxic effects of classes IA and IC drugs. Hypotension, seizure, and cardiac arrhythmia should be treated with routine pharmacological interventions.

REFERENCES

SUGGESTED READINGS

Brody, T.M., Larner, J., and Minneman, K.P., *Human Pharmacology*, 3rd ed., Mosby-Year Book, Inc., St. Louis, 1998, chap. 15 and 18.
Ford, M.D. et al., *Clinical Toxicology*, W.B. Saunders, Philadelphia, 2001, chap. 41, 42, 43, and 44.
Harsman, J.G. and Limbird, L.E., *Goodman & Gilman's The Pharmacological Basis of Therapeutics*, 10th ed., McGraw-Hill, New York, 2001, chap. 32, 33, 34, and 35.
Martini, F.H., The heart, in *Fundamentals of Anatomy and Physiology*, 4th ed., Prentice Hall, Upper Saddle River, NJ, 1998, chap. 20.

REVIEW ARTICLES

Bara, V., Digoxin overdose: clinical features and management, *Emerg. Nurse*, 9, 16, 2001.
Bristow, M.R., β-Adrenergic receptor blockade in chronic heart failure, *Circulation*, 101, 558, 2000.
Connolly, S.J., Evidence-based analysis of amiodarone efficacy and safety, *Circulation*, 100, 2025, 1999.
Dansette, P.M. et al. Drug-induced immunotoxicity, *Eur. J. Drug Metab. Pharmacokinet.*, 23, 443, 1998.
Hauptman, P.J. and Kelly, R.A., Digitalis, *Circulation*, 99, 1265, 1999.
Hofer, C.A., Smith, J.K., and Tenholder, M.F., Verapamil intoxication: a literature review of overdoses and discussion of therapeutic options, *Am. J. Med.*, 95, 431, 1993.
Kerns, W., Kline, J., and Ford, M.D., Beta-blocker and calcium channel blocker toxicity, *Emerg. Med. Clin. North Am.*, 12, 365, 1994.
Kjeldsen, K., Nørgaard, A., and Gheorghiade, M., Myocardial Na,K-ATPase: the molecular basis for the hemodynamic effect of digoxin therapy in congestive heart failure, *Cardiovas. Res.*, 55, 710, 2002.
Kolecki, P.F. and Curry, S.C., Poisoning by sodium channel blocking agents, *Crit. Care Clin.*, 13, 829, 1997.
Lip, G.Y. and Ferner, R.E., Poisoning with anti-hypertensive drugs: angiotensin converting enzyme inhibitors, *J. Hum. Hypertens.*, 9, 711, 1995.
Pentel, P.R. and Salerno, D.M., Cardiac drug toxicity: digitalis glycosides and calcium-channel and beta-blocking agents, *Med. J. Aust.*, 152, 88, 1990.
Sangha, S., Uber, P.A., and Mehra, M.R., Difficult cases in heart failure: amiodarone lung injury: another heart failure mimic? *Congest. Heart Fail.*, 8, 93, 2002.

19 Antineoplastic Agents

19.1 DESCRIPTION

Antineoplastic agents, traditionally referred to as chemotherapeutic agents, are used therapeutically in the treatment of cancer.* The drugs include a wide variety of diverse chemicals whose mechanisms of action are targeted toward arresting aberrant cell proliferation generally associated with cancerous cell growth. Although the concept that chemical agents could interfere with cell proliferation was known by about the turn of the twentieth century, it was not until the end of World War I that the biological and chemical actions of alkylating agents, such as the nitrogen mustards, were understood. By the end of World War II, the conviction that such drugs could be used in the treatment of cancer prompted the search for antineoplastic drugs that would forever impact the therapeutic intervention of neoplastic disease.

19.2 REVIEW OF THE CELL CYCLE

It is somewhat ironic that most antineoplastic agents used in cancer chemotherapy are also carcinogenic, mutagenic, or teratogenic. In fact, the adverse reactions and toxicities associated with these substances often limit their usefulness and complicate the course of treatment. Consequently, a better understanding of the toxicology and pharmacology depends on the drugs' influence on cell cycle kinetics, which in turn explains the adverse reactions and mechanisms of action, respectively.

Figure 19.1 illustrates the four successive phases of the cell cycle. Normal, proliferating somatic cells spend the majority of their existence in interphase. Cells also perform most of their maintenance functions in interphase. As a cell prepares to divide, it enters the G_1 *phase*, the period between mitosis (*M phase*) and DNA synthesis (*S phase*). The G_1 *phase* lasts from several hours to days and is characterized by synthesis of cell organelles and centriole replication (the G_0 *phase* represents a resting stage, or subphase of G_1). The *S phase* begins when DNA synthesis starts and the chromosomes have replicated. The G_2 *phase* starts when DNA replication is complete and the content of the nucleus has doubled. The G_2 *phase* ends when mitosis starts. The extended part of interphase then continues in the *M phase* with the stages of cell division — namely,

---

* Cancer is a general term referring to the uncontrolled growth of cells or tissue, characterized by the formation of a neoplasm, i.e., a new mass of cells or tissue (tumor). Cancers are classified according to their cellular origin and their benign or malignant state of histogenic differentiation. In general, benign tumors are designated by attaching the suffix -*oma* to the cell of origin (fibroma is a tumor of fibrous origin, adenomas and papillomas are of benign epithelial origin). Malignant tumors are classified according to their germ cell layers and organ of derivation. Malignant tumor nomenclature follows that of benign tumors with some exceptions: carcinoma (neoplasm of epithelial cell origin); sarcoma (tumor of mesenchymal — connective tissue — and endothelial cell origin), melanoma (melanocyte origin), lymphoma (lymphoid tissue origin), leukemia (hematopoietic cell origin), and tumors arising from the nervous system.

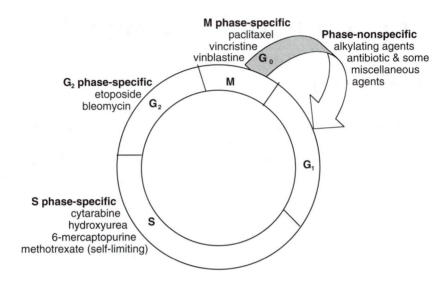

FIGURE 19.1 The four successive phases of the cell cycle.

prophase, metaphase, anaphase, and telophase. During this time the *M phase* begins with mitosis (nuclear division) and ends with cytokinesis (cytoplasmic) division. Cell division terminates with the completion of cytokinesis.

Antineoplastic agents suppress proliferation of neoplasms through interaction at one or more phases of cell replication. *Cell cycle specific agents,* some of which are indicated in Figure 19.1, interfere with at least one specific phase of cellular replication. *Cell cycle nonspecific agents* act on both proliferating and resting cells.

19.3 ANTIMETABOLITES

19.3.1 PHARMACOLOGY AND CLINICAL USE

Antimetabolites alter normal cellular functions by substituting for components within key metabolic processes. An agent may be incorporated as a substrate, or may inhibit the normal functioning of an enzyme. The net effect of interference with cellular biochemical reactions is disruption of nucleic acid synthesis. Thus, antimetabolites are effective on rapidly proliferating cells mostly during the *S phase* (DNA synthesis phase) of nucleic acid synthesis. Consequently, they are indicated for the induction and maintenance of remission of leukemias, metastatic breast cancer, colon, rectal, stomach, and pancreatic carcinomas. Antimetabolites, alone and in combination, are also used in the management of other proliferative disorders such as psoriasis and rheumatoid arthritis (methotrexate).

19.3.2 ACUTE TOXICITY

The toxic effects of the antimetabolites are related to their mechanisms of action and are summarized in Table 19.1. The most common, and potentially serious, adverse

TABLE 19.1
Classification of Selected Antimetabolite Antineoplastic Agents
and Predominant Adverse Drug Reactions (ADRs)

Category	Nonproprietary Name	Predominant Target of Inhibition	Predominant ADRs
Folic acid analogs	Methotrexate (MTX)	Dihydrofolate reductase	CNS, GI, GU,
Purine analogs	6-TG, 6-MP	Purine ring synthesis	dermatologic,
Pyrimidine analogs	5-FU	TMP synthesis	hematologic,
	Cytarabine	DNA synthesis	metabolic toxicity
Substituted urea	Hydroxyurea	Ribonucleotide reductase	

Note: 6-TG = 6-thioguanine, 6-MP = 6-mercaptopurine, 5-FU = 5-flurouracil, CV = cardiovascular, CNS = central nervous system, GI = gastrointestinal, GU = genitourinary, TMP = thymidine monophosphate.

reactions involve organ system toxicity. The toxicities are seen at any dose and include GI (nausea, vomiting, diarrhea), dermatologic (alopecia), hematologic (bone marrow suppression), metabolic (hepatotoxicity), and CNS (headaches, blurred vision) effects.

Extravasation* occurs with any of the parenterally administered antimetabolites. Prevention of extravasation requires optimum administration technique. However, should it occur, several steps are required to alleviate the situation, including discontinuation of the medication, administration of an antidote where appropriate, and surgical debridement with skin grafting. The antibiotic antineoplastics are generally associated with severe, local, necrotic (vesicant) reactions.

19.3.3 CLINICAL MANAGEMENT OF ACUTE OVERDOSE

Leucovorin (citrovorum factor, folinic acid) is a specific antidote for methotrexate (MTX) overdose, especially as a therapeutic modality — i.e., in order to overcome the resistance to MTX, an antifolate drug, high doses are administered concomitantly with leucovorin. This *rescue procedure* permits the intracellular accumulation of MTX in concentrations sufficient to inactivate dihydrofolate reductase, while diminishing hematologic toxicity. The combination is effectively used, along with other chemotherapeutic agents, in patients with nonmetastatic osteosarcoma.

19.4 ALKYLATING AGENTS

19.4.1 PHARMACOLOGY AND CLINICAL USE

Alkylating agents are strong electrophiles that form highly reactive carbonium ions. They replace hydrogen atoms with alkyl radicals, resulting in cross-linking and

---

*Treatment schedules with some antineoplastic agents are generally prolonged and continuous. Consequently, the i.v. fluid containing the medication may leak into interstitial tissue at the site of administration, causing complications ranging from painful erythematous swelling to deep necrotic injury of underlying skin.

abnormal base-pairing in nuclear DNA. These radicals also covalently bind to sulfhydryl, phosphate, and amine groups, inhibiting cellular metabolic processes that terminate reactions in proliferating and stationary cells. The net effect is the production of defective DNA and abortive reproduction of cells. Although alkylating agents are most effective on rapidly proliferating cells, they are not *phase specific* and may act on cells at any stage of the cell cycle. The drugs are used concurrently or sequentially with other antineoplastics and are indicated, in general, in the palliative* treatment of malignancies susceptible to the drugs. The conditions include malignant lymphomas, leukemias, germ cell and progressive testicular, ovarian, and prostate cancers, myelomas, and brain tumors. Other conditions amenable to alkylating agents are metastatic carcinomas of the stomach, colon, and bladder, neuroblastomas, and nonmalignant nephritic syndrome in children (cyclophosphamide, Cytoxan®).

19.4.2 Acute Toxicity

As with the antimetabolites, the most common and serious toxic effects of the alkylating agents are related to their alkylating properties of rapidly dividing cells (Table 19.2). Adverse reactions are seen at any dose and include GI, dermatologic, hematologic (myelosuppression, especially with busulfan), metabolic, and CNS reactions. Although their cytotoxicities have become more manageable recently, experience dictates an adequately established diagnosis, recognition of signs of ADRs, and supportive care.

TABLE 19.2
Classification of Selected Alkylating Agents and Predominant Adverse Drug Reactions (ADRs)

Category	Nonproprietary Name	Predominant Target of Inhibition	Predominant ADRs
Nitrogen mustards (NM)	Cyclophosphamide Melphalan Chlorambucil	Interfere with DNA integrity by formation of DNA adducts; also inhibit several key enzymes by carbamoylation of amino acids in proteins	GI, GU, renal, hematologic, hepatic, CNS, dermatologic toxicity; secondary carcinogenesis
Nitrosoureas	Carmustine (BCNU) Lomustine (CCNU) Streptozotocin		
Triazenes	Dacarbazine (DTIC)		otoxicity (Pt),
Platinum (Pt) coordination complexes	Cisplatin Carboplatin	Form interstrand DNA cross-links	anaphylactic reactions (Pt)
Alkyl sulfonates	Busulfan	Granulocytes	

Note: CNS = central nervous system, GI = gastrointestinal, GU = genitourinary.

---

* Palliative therapy is designed to relieve or reduce intensity of signs and symptoms, rather than to produce a cure.

19.4.3 CLINICAL MANAGEMENT OF ADRs

Management of patients treated with alkylating agents involves monitoring for signs and symptoms of toxicity, including clinical measurements of hematological, renal, and metabolic functions, as well as general supportive treatment. Adjustment of dosage, discontinuation of the regimen, or replacement with another chemotherapeutic agent, are some of the recourse actions taken to alleviate drug toxicity.

19.5 MISCELLANEOUS CHEMOTHERAPEUTIC DRUGS

19.5.1 NATURAL PRODUCTS

These antineoplastic agents include a diverse group of naturally derived compounds of plant or prokaryotic origin with unique mechanisms of action and toxicity (Table 19.3).

The vinca alkaloids, named after the beneficial effects derived from the parent periwinkle plant,* are cell cycle-specific agents *(M phase)*. Vinca alkaloids, like

---

TABLE 19.3
Classification of Selected Natural Product Antineoplastic Agents and Predominant Adverse Drug Reactions (ADRs)

Category	Nonproprietary Name	Predominant Target of Inhibition	Predominant ADRs
Vinca alkaloids	Vinblastine Vincristine (V)	Inhibits microtubular assembly (V); enhances	CNS, CV, GI, dermatologic, hematologic, metabolic,
Taxoids	Paclitaxel (P)	tubulin polymerization (P); mitotic inhibitors	i.v. extravasation and hypersensitivity reactions
Epidophyllotoxins	Etoposide (E) Teniposide (T)	Inhibits DNA synthesis at G_2 (E); inhibits type II topoisomerase (T)	
Antibiotics	Actinomycin D Daunorubicin Doxorubicin	DNA intercalation; inhibits DNA/RNA synthesis; antimitotics	Extremely corrosive to soft tissue; myocardial toxicity
	Bleomycin	DNA lesions at G_2, inhibits DNA repair	Pulmonary fibrosis
	Mitomycin C	Formation of DNA adducts	Myelosuppression, hemolytic uremic syndrome (see text)
	Pentostatin	Adenosine deaminase	CNS, liver, renal, pulmonary toxicity

Note: CV = cardiovascular, CNS = central nervous system, GI = gastrointestinal, GU = genitourinary.

---

* The anticancer potential of the family of *Catharanthus roseus*, formerly *Vinca rosea*, was recognized early in 1958. The plant's ability of producing peripheral granulocytopenia and bone marrow depression in rodents then prompted the subsequent isolation of a large number of alkaloids.

vinblastine (Velban®) and vincristine (Vincasar PFS®), specifically bind to tubulin, the protein subunits of the microtubules that polymerize to form the mitotic spindle. Thus, vinca alkaloids interrupt microtubular assembly and produce metaphase arrest. Normal and malignant cells exposed to the plant alkaloids express apoptotic changes. The characteristic neurotoxicity displayed by patients receiving the drugs may be explained, in part, by disruption of microtubules normally involved in intracellular movement, axonal transport, and phagocytosis. Considerable irritation results from improper positioning of the i.v. needle or catheter. These compounds are used by injection only.

Paclitaxel (Taxol®) is a naturally derived *M phase-specific* antimitotic product.* Paclitaxel promotes the assembly of microtubules by stimulating tubulin polymerization, rendering stable, nonfunctioning microtubules. The resulting network "bundles" of microtubules are incapable of dynamic reorganization, thus inhibiting cellular mitosis and proliferation. ADRs associated with paclitaxel are similar to those of the vinca alkaloids.

Etoposide (VePesid®) is a semisynthetic derivative of podophyllotoxin** with selective activity at the G_2 *phase* of the cell cycle. At high concentrations, the compound causes cytolysis of cells entering mitosis, while at low concentrations, it prevents the cells from entering prophase. Teniposide (Vumon®) causes single and double-stranded DNA breaks by inhibiting type II topoisomerase activity, but does not intercalate DNA. Severe myelosuppression and hypersensitivity reactions are noted with both drugs.

Unlike the antibacterial, antifungal, and antiviral antibiotic drugs, antibiotic antineoplastics are capable of disrupting DNA-dependent RNA synthesis and inhibiting mitosis. This class of natural products is derived from a variety of eubacterial and actinomycetes genuses.*** The drugs act on rapidly proliferating normal and neoplastic cells and, with one exception (bleomycin), are *phase nonspecific*. In addition to the GI, hematologic, dermatologic, and metabolic toxicities, some of the more peculiar ADRs associated with these antibiotics are listed in Table 19.3. For example, hemolytic uremic syndrome, mostly observed with mitomycin C, is characterized by microangiopathic hemolytic anemia (anemia within small blood vessels), thrombocytopenia (decrease in platelet count), and irreversible renal failure.

Pentostatin is often classified as an antimetabolite, although it is derived from microorganisms. It acts as a transition state analog and interferes with adenosine deaminase. The enzyme specific inhibition results in accumulation of ATP and deoxyadenosine nucleotides, blockage of ribonucleotide reductase, and suspension

---

* Paclitaxel was first isolated in 1971 from the bark of the Western yew tree.

** Podophyllotoxin is derived from the rhizomes and root of the mandrake plant, *Podophyllum peltatum* (mayapple), which should not be confused with mandragora. The latter is referred to as mandrake in ancient Greek and Asian literature. The mandrake (mayapple) plant was used by the American Indians, and introduced to colonial settlers for its emetic and cathartic properties. It was later developed as a caustic agent in a 25% dispersion in compound benzoin tincture and used topically for the treatment of papillomas.

*** Compounds and their species of derivation include: actinomycin D (dactinomycin, Cosmegen®) from *Streptomyces parvullus*; pentostatin (Nipent®) from *S. antibioticus*; anthracycline antibiotics (daunorubicin, Cerubidine®, and doxorubicin, Adriamycin®) from *S. peucetius*; bleomycin (Blenoxane®) from *S. verticillus*; and, mitomycin C (Mutamycin®) from *S. caespitosus*.

of DNA synthesis. Interestingly, although most of the antineoplastic antibiotics have antibacterial and antifungal properties, their toxicities preclude their routine use in the treatment of infectious diseases.

19.5.2 HORMONES AND ANTAGONISTS

The basis of hormonal anticancer therapy is the interaction of synthetic nonsteroidal chemicals with nuclear and cell membrane growth stimulatory receptor proteins. The drugs have the advantage of greater specificity for tissues responsive to their counterbalancing effects, such as breast, endometrium, testes, and prostate. Consequently, they are capable of occupying nuclear or membrane steroid receptors, redirecting the feedback mechanism, and inhibiting the normal or abnormal function of the tissue. The therapeutic advantage lies in their proclivity to inhibit uncontrolled cell proliferation without significant direct cytotoxic effects. The major ADRs are listed in Table 19.4. Antineoplastic hormones are used initially or as adjunctive therapy in the palliative treatment of malignancies susceptible to the drugs, as noted in Table 19.5.

19.5.3 PLATINUM COORDINATION COMPLEXES

Carboplatin (Paraplatin®) and cisplatin (Platinol AQ®) are platinum coordination compounds whose action is similar to that of the alkylating agents. Platinum coordination complexes are *phase-nonspecific* drugs that produce interstrand DNA cross-links rather than DNA-protein intercalation. Their toxicities (Table 19.2) and net effect (interference with DNA synthesis and integrity) are similar to the alkylating agents. The compounds are used in the initial and secondary treatment of ovarian carcinoma, testicular tumors, and advanced bladder cancer.

TABLE 19.4
Classification of Selected Hormonal Antineoplastic Agents and Predominant Adverse Drug Reactions (ADRs)

Category	Nonproprietary Name	Predominant Target of Inhibition	Predominant ADRs
Progestins	Medroxyprogesterone, megestrol acetate	Interact with cell membrane and	Weight gain, thromboembolism
Estrogens	DES, ethinyl estradiol	nuclear growth	Thromboembolism
Androgens	Testolactone	stimulatory receptor	CNS, GI
Antiestrogens	Tamoxifen	proteins in tissues responsive to their	Thromboembolism, hot flashes
Antiandrogens	Flutamide, bicalutamide	counterbalancing effects	Liver, GI, blood, gynecomastia
GRH analog	Leuprolide (LHRH agonist)		CV, CNS, GI, GU, gynecomastia

Note: CV = cardiovascular, CNS = central nervous system, GI = gastrointestinal, GRH = gonadotropin-releasing hormone, GU = genitourinary.

TABLE 19.5
Antineoplastic Hormones Used in the Palliative Treatment of Malignancies

Hormone	Malignancy Susceptible to the Drug
Medroxyprogesterone (Depo-Provera®)	Endometrial or renal carcinoma
Megestrol acetate (Megace®)	Breast or endometrial carcinoma, appetite enhancement for AIDS patients
DES, estradiol (various)	Progressing prostatic cancer
Testolactone (Teslac®)	Advanced breast carcinoma
Tamoxifen (Nolvadex®)	Breast cancer, treatment and preventive
Flutamide (Eulexin®)	Prostate carcinoma
Bicalutamide (Casodex®)	
Leuprolide (LHRH agonist, Lupron®)	Advanced prostatic carcinoma

19.5.4 SUBSTITUTED UREA

Hydroxyurea (Hydrea®) is a substituted urea with antimetabolite actions (Table 19.1). It is *S phase-specific* and interferes with the conversion of ribonucleotides to deoxyribonucleotides by selectively blocking the enzyme ribonucleotide reductase. In addition, it inhibits the incorporation of thymidine into DNA. The drug is indicated in the treatment of melanomas and leukemias. It is also used concomitantly with irradiation therapy in the management of squamous cell carcinoma of the head and neck.

REFERENCES

SUGGESTED READINGS

Drug Facts and Comparisons, 56th ed., Kluwer, St. Louis, 2002, chap. 13.
Eckhardt, S., Recent progress in the development of anticancer agents, *Curr. Med. Chem. Anti-Canc. Agents.*, 2, 419, 2002.

REVIEW ARTICLES

Blankenship, J.R. et al., Teaching old drugs new tricks: reincarnating immunosuppressants as antifungal drugs, *Curr. Opin. Investig. Drugs*, 4, 192, 2003.
Bodo, A. et al., The role of multidrug transporters in drug availability, metabolism and toxicity, *Toxicol. Lett.*, 140, 133, 2003.
Chabner, B.A., Cytotoxic agents in the era of molecular targets and genomics, *Oncologist*, 7, 34, 2002.
Dy, G.K., Haluska, P., and Adjei, A.A., Novel pharmacological agents in clinical development for solid tumours, *Expert Opin. Investig. Drugs*, 10, 2059, 2001.
Elsayed, Y.A. and Sausville, E.A., Selected novel anticancer treatments targeting cell signaling proteins, *Oncologist*, 6, 517, 2001.
Furst, A., Can nutrition affect chemical toxicity? *Int. J. Toxicol.*, 21, 419, 2002.

Gilligan, T. and Kantoff, P.W., Chemotherapy for prostate cancer, *Urology,* 60, 94, 2002.

Hogberg, T., Glimelius, B., and Nygren, P., A systematic overview of chemotherapy effects in ovarian cancer, *Acta Oncol.,* 40, 340, 2001.

Iqbal, S. and Lenz, H.J., Targeted therapy and pharmacogenomic programs, *Cancer,* 97, 2076, 2003.

Langebrake, C., Reinhardt, D., and Ritter, J., Minimising the long-term adverse effects of childhood leukaemia therapy, *Drug Saf.,* 25, 1057, 2002.

Medina, P.J., Sipols, J.M., and George, J.N., Drug-associated thrombotic thrombocytopenic purpura-hemolytic uremic syndrome, *Curr. Opin. Hematol.,* 8, 286, 2001.

Nabholtz, J.M. and Riva, A., Taxane/anthracycline combinations: setting a new standard in breast cancer? *Oncologist,* 6, 5, 2001.

Prinz, H., Recent advances in the field of tubulin polymerization inhibitors, *Expert Rev. Anticancer Ther.,* 2, 695, 2002.

Royce, M.E., Hoff, P.M., and Pazdur, R., Novel oral chemotherapy agents, *Curr. Oncol. Rep.* 2, 31, 2000.

Zucchi, R. and Danesi, R., Cardiac toxicity of antineoplastic anthracyclines, *Curr. Med. Chem. Anti-Canc. Agents,* 3, 151, 2003.

20 Vitamins

20.1 INTRODUCTION

Vitamins, as the Latin derivation of the name implies,[*] are essential for maintenance of adequate health and life. They are diverse organic substances provided in small quantities in the diet, and are found in a variety of chemical forms and structures. Vitamins have assorted essential biochemical roles in contributing toward maintenance of health, and have unique therapeutic places in the treatment of related disorders. Originally, most vitamins were used for the prevention of deficiency syndromes associated with inadequate nutritional intake. For instance, in the presence of a deficiency of a particular nutrient and the subsequent induction of the corresponding condition, adequate replacement of the deficient substance resulted in a cure. And, until recently, it was reasonable to conclude that by following a balanced diet, no additional vitamin supplementation was necessary. This assumption was valid for normal healthy children, adolescents, and adults, in the absence of deficiency (with the exception of pregnancy and lactation). This message has not been heeded in recent years, however, as evidenced by the growing consumption (*megadoses*) and infatuation with vitamin supplementation in the U.S. This was encouraged by the misinformation that, if vitamins are important for maintenance of health, then greater ingestion must necessarily provide better health. The belief has been defended by the equivocal results of clinical and scientific studies interpreted out-of-context. In particular, such studies have concluded that clinical benefits, such as prevention of aging, can be obtained from the beneficial effects of antioxidants against factors that contribute to oxidative stress.

The Food and Nutrition Board[**] publishes the recommended dietary allowances (RDA) as standards for essential nutrients. The standards are based on periodic review of the scientific evidence for most healthy persons under normal daily stresses. Almost all of these nutrients are provided with a well-balanced dietary intake plan that includes the four basic food groups. In addition, RDA information is included in individual vitamin monographs. Table 20.1 outlines an abbreviated listing of RDA ranges of vitamins and minerals for children (ages 1 to 10 years) and adult males and females (ages 11 to 51+ years). The values are based on normal healthy, height-and-weight-adjusted individuals.

In general, vitamin supplementation is warranted in situations where a suspected vitamin deficiency contributes to the condition. In the U.S., the *relative risk* for the development of vitamin deficiencies may be higher in the following individuals:

---

[*] *Vita (L.)*, vital, for life.
[**] U.S. National Research Council, Institute of Medicine of the National Academy of Sciences.

TABLE 20.1
Recommended Dietary Allowances of Vitamins and Minerals

Nutrient	Infants	Children	Males	Females	Pregnant/ Lactating
Protein (g)	13–14	16–28	45–63	46–50	60–65
Fat-Soluble Vitamins					
Vitamin A (µg RE)	375	400–700	1000	800	800–1300
Vitamin D (IU)	300–400	400	400–200	400–200	400
Vitamin E (IU)	4–6	9–10	15	12	15–18
Vitamin K (µg)	5–10	15–30	45–80	45–65	65
Water-Soluble Vitamins					
Vitamin C (mg)	30–35	40–45	50–60	50–60	70–95
Thiamine (B_1, mg)	0.3–0.4	0.7–1.0	1.3–1.5	1.0–1.1	1.5–1.6
Riboflavine (B_2, mg)	0.4–0.5	0.8–1.2	1.4–1.8	1.2–1.3	1.6–1.8
Niacin (B_3, mg)	5–6	9–13	15–20	13–15	17–20
Pyridoxine (B_6, mg)	0.3–0.6	1.0–1.4	1.7–2.0	1.4–1.6	2.1–2.2
Folic Acid (µg)	25–35	50–100	150–200	150–180	260–400
Vitamin B_{12}[a] (µg)	0.3–0.5	0.7–1.4	2	2	2.2–2.6
Minerals					
Calcium (mg)	400–600	800	1200–800	1200–800	1200
Phosphorus (mg)	300–500	800	1200–800	1200–800	1200
Magnesium (mg)	40–60	80–170	270–400	280–300	320–355
Iron (mg)	6–10	10	10–12	15–10	30–15
Zinc (mg)	5	10	15	12	15–19
Iodine (µg)	40–50	70–120	150	150	175–200
Selenium (µg)	10–15	20–30	40–70	45–55	65–75

Note: Age ranges, in years: infants, 0–1; children, 1–10; males and females, 11–51+. Ranges of daily allowances are determined by age, height and weight (not shown) within group; in general, requirements increase with age, except with some vitamins (e.g., vitamins D, B_1, B_2, B_3, calcium, and phosphorus) where requirement drops for adult males and females over 25 years old. Requirements are usually higher during the 1st 6 months of lactation than during the 2nd 6 months.

Note: RE = retinol equivalents where 1 RE = 1 µg all-trans-retinol, or = 6 µg β-carotene, or 12 µg carotenoid provitamins; IU: 10 µg cholecalciferol = 400 IU vitamin D; 1 mg d-α-tocopherol (α-TE) = 1.49 IU vitamin E.

[a] Cyanocobalamin.

Adapted and condensed from *Recommended Dietary Allowances*, 10th ed., National Academy of Sciences, National Academy Press, Washington D.C., 1989.

1. Those living below the poverty level
2. Patients with malabsorption syndromes
3. Patients undergoing treatment with antibiotics that alter normal vitamin-synthesizing bacterial flora
4. Individuals with behavioral problems that encourage poor dietary intake (e.g., anorexia nervosa)
5. Inadequate intake of nutritionally rich foods that leads to decreased ingestion or poor absorption of vitamins (poorly-planned vegetarian diets, weight-reducing diets, among alcoholics and the elderly)

Vitamin toxicity due to overdose is documented in clinical situations, but relies on experimental scientific evidence for an adequate description of such conditions. More recently, the adverse drug reactions (ADRs) of retinoic acid derivatives of vitamin A have been well documented, the toxicology and pharmacology of which are discussed below.

Vitamins are classified according to their biological inclination for distribution and elimination from the body. The *water-soluble* vitamins are readily eliminated in the urine and consequently have a low incidence of toxic effects. Biochemically, they act as cofactors in most physiologically important reactions. In contrast, the *fat-soluble* vitamins are readily distributed throughout the body, with a propensity for storage in lipid-rich tissue. As a result, they tend to accumulate in physiologic compartments, risking potential cumulative toxicity. Biochemically, they elicit hormone-like activity at physiologic targets.

This chapter emphasizes the toxicity and deficiencies associated with vitamins and vitamin supplementation whose adverse reactions have been historically and therapeutically documented. It is important to note that natural diets are rarely deficient in single nutrients, and it is rare for clinical manifestations to develop from single causes. Consequently, detection and diagnosis of vitamin deficiency, or chronic toxicity, is not without ambiguity.

20.2 FAT-SOLUBLE VITAMINS

20.2.1 VITAMIN A AND RETINOIC ACID DERIVATIVES

Vitamin A, along with its derivatives, is essential for proper maintenance of vision acuity, for dental development, skeletal muscle and bone growth, corticosteroid synthesis, embryonic development, and reproduction. Vitamin A also influences differentiation of epithelial membranes, particularly corneal, gastrointestinal (GI), and genitourinary epithelia. Derivatives of vitamin A include retinol, retinal, retinoic acid, and β-carotene (a precursor). These physiologically important factors support proper functioning of the reproductive cycle, visual acuity, somatic growth and differentiation, and visual adaptation to darkness, respectively. β-carotene is a naturally occurring vitamin A precursor. β-carotene is found primarily in dark-green and yellow-orange vegetables and possesses antioxidant and immuno-stimulating (anticancer) activity. A balanced diet consisting of fish, liver, meat, carrots, and dairy products, provides the RDA for vitamin A.

Oral or parenteral administration of vitamin A (Aquasol A® injection, various tablet and capsule formulations) is indicated for the treatment of conditions associated with, but not exclusive to, vitamin A deficiency states. Deficiency syndromes have been associated with kwashiorkor,[*] xerophthalmia,[**] keratomalacia,[***] and malabsorption syndromes.

Hypervitaminosis A syndrome develops with chronic ingestion of *megadoses* of the vitamin, or in the presence of hepatic disease.[****] Table 20.2 lists the toxic manifestations of hypervitaminosis syndromes, as well as the deficiency states. In general, acute doses of 25,000 IU/kg results in toxicity. Prolonged excessive consumption of vitamin A for 6 to 15 months (4000 IU/kg) also produces a toxic syndrome, although chronic adverse reactions are more insidious and protracted. Most symptoms resolve with prompt withdrawal of vitamin supplementation, although increased intracranial pressure requires further palliative measures.

As noted above, the retinoids are derivatives of retinoic acid that promote epithelial cell differentiation, keratinization, and local inflammation. These properties are advantageous in topical or oral treatment of acne vulgaris or psoriasis, attributable to the compounds' ability to normalize follicular epithelial cell differentiation. Therapeutically, the desired effect results in the reduction of the severity and formation of microcomedones[*****] characteristic of acne. Adverse effects of most of the topical products are related to transient or temporary local inflammatory responses (Table 20.2). Oral retinoids, such as isotretinoin, are reserved for severe recalcitrant nodular acne. The retinoids, however, are contraindicated in women of childbearing potential because of teratogenic risk. Major human fetal abnormalities have been reported with oral isotretinoin ingestion, including skeletal, neurological, and cardiovascular anomalies. In addition, a variety of adverse effects appear with routine therapeutic use of oral isotretinoin.

20.2.2 Vitamin D

Vitamin D is a fat-soluble vitamin with hormone-like activity. Calcitriol is the most active form of vitamin D_3.[******] In conjunction with parathyroid hormone (PTH) calcitriol maintains blood calcium levels by promoting GI absorption of calcium, phosphorus, and magnesium. Calcitriol stimulates renal tubular reabsorption of calcium and mobilizes calcium from bone. Negative feedback of blood calcium controls secretion of calcitonin from the thyroid gland and PTH from the parathyroid

---

[*] A disease of very young African natives as a result of severe protein deficiency. It is characterized by anemia, edema, swollen abdomen, skin and hair depigmentation, and hypoalbuminemia.

[**] Excessive conjunctival and corneal dryness.

[***] Cornea becomes softened and vulnerable to ulceration and infection, and may lead to blindness.

[****] Although mostly innocuous, consumption of megadoses greater than 180 mg/day of β-carotene is manifested by yellow-orange skin discoloration.

[*****] Dilated hair follicles filled with keratin and sebum (pustules).

[******] Calcitriol, also known as 1,25-dihydroxy vitamin D_3, is converted from 7-dehydrocholesterol to cholecalciferol (vitamin D_3), by initial action of UV light on skin. Intermediate metabolic reactions in liver and kidney follow. Similarly, the major transport form of vitamin D, 1,25-dihydroxyergocalciferol (vitamin D_2) is similarly converted from provitamin D_2 by exposure of skin to UV light, followed by liver and kidney metabolism.

TABLE 20.2
Fat-Soluble Vitamins and Toxic Manifestations of Excessive Consumption or Administration

Vitamins	Derivatives	Proprietary Name	Deficiency State	Common ADRs Associated with Excessive Consumption
Vitamin A	Retinol, retinal, retinoic acid	Palmitate A 5000 tablets, Aquasol A injection, various tablets and capsules	Kwashiorkor, xerophthalmia, keratomalacia	Acute: anorexia, nervousness, increased intracranial pressure, blurred vision; chronic: hepatomegaly, allopecia, dry scaly skin, bone pain & demineralization, cheilitis[a]
	β-carotene	Various capsules		Yellow-orange skin discoloration
Retinoids	Adapalene Tretinoin Tazarotene	Differen gel Retin-A gels, creams Tazorac gel, cream	None	Erythema, scaling, dryness, pruritis, burning, photosensitivity, skin discoloration
	Isotretinoin[b]	Accutane capsules	None	Major human fetal malformations involving neurological, skeletal, muscular, hormonal, and CV systems; ADRs include pancreatitis, psychiatric disorders, visual impairment, dermatologic, CNS, GI, GU, IBS
Vitamin D	Calcitriol (D₃) Cholecalciferol (D₃) Ergocalciferol (D₂)	Rocaltrol Delta-D Drisdol, Calciferol	Rickets (children) Osteomalacia (adults)	Acute: weakness, headache, NV, constipation, bone pain; Chronic: anorexia, polydipsia, polyuria, nephrocalcinosis, vascular calcification; chronic OD: hypercalcemia, hypercalciuria, hyperphosphatemia
Vitamin E	dl-α-tocopherols	Aquavit-E, various products and dosage forms	Anemia, thrombocytosis, increased platelet aggregation (uncommon)	Hypervitaminosis E: NVD, weakness, thrombophlebitis, increased lipids and hormone levels, breast tumors, gynecomastia, altered immunity
Vitamin K	Phytonadione (K₁)	Mephyton, AquaMEPHYTON	Hemorrhagic disorders (uncommon)	Severe allergic reactions, especially upon injection; transient flushing, pain at site; hemolytic anemia in infants; scleroderma-like lesions, hyper-bilirubinemia

Note: CNS = central nervous system, CV = cardiovascular, GI = gastrointestinal, GU = genitourinary, IBS = inflammatory bowel syndrome, NVD = nausea, vomiting, diarrhea, OD = overdose.

[a] Inflammation of the lips.
[b] Category X = should not be used during pregnancy or in women with the potential for becoming pregnant.

TABLE 20.3
Causes and Effects of Rickets in Children, and Osteomalacia in Adults, Resulting from Vitamin D Deficiency

Metabolic, Physiologic, or Behavioral Cause	Pathologic or Net Effect on Vitamin D
Inadequate exposure to sunlight; races or descendants of African or other dark-skinned nations	Reduced endogenous synthesis
Poor or inadequate nutrition (poor diet)	Poor GI absorption
Cytochrome P-450 inducing drugs[a]	Enhanced degradation
Liver, renal disease	Impaired synthesis
Chronic antacid ingestion; renal disease	Phosphate depletion

[a] Isoniazid, phenobarbital.

gland. Vitamin D_2 is a plant vitamin used to fortify milk and cereal products. The role of the parathyroid glands and their interaction with calcium, vitamin D, and PTH secretion are discussed in some recent reviews.

Oral or parenteral administration of the active forms of vitamin D are indicated in the management of hypocalcemia. The condition is prevalent in renal dialysis patients and individuals with hypoparathyroidism (treated with calcitriol), refractory *rickets*, and hypophosphatemia (treated with vitamin D_2). In addition, the compounds are used as dietary supplements or in the management of vitamin D deficiency (vitamin D_3).

Deficiency states of vitamin D result in *rickets* in growing children and *osteomalacia* in adults, the causes and effects of which are summarized in Table 20.3. In both cases, limited exposure to sunlight is probably the most important reason for development of a deficiency state leading to hypocalcemia. Hypocalcemia, in turn, stimulates PTH secretion, which promotes renal α1-hydroxylase activity (responsible for conversion of precursors to D_2 and D_3 in kidney). The net effect is the enhancement of GI calcium absorption, increased calcium mobilization from bone, and stimulation of renal excretion of phosphate. Thus, although calcium blood levels may return to normal, loss of renal phosphate and hypophosphatemia further imperil bone mineralization. Persistent failure of bone formation in adults risks eventual loss of skeletal mass (*osteopenia*),[*] producing weak, fracture-sensitive long bones and vertebrae. In children, gross skeletal changes depend on age and severity of the deficiency. In neonates, abnormalities are manifested as softened, flattened, buckled bones resulting from pressure stress. Deformation of cranial bones, pelvic bones, and the chest cavity (*pigeon breast deformity*) complete the presentation. In older children, deformities are more likely to affect the spine, pelvis, and long bones (*lumbar lordosis* and *bowing of the legs*).

Administration of vitamin D in excess of daily requirements may cause clinical signs of acute or chronic overdosage (*hypervitaminosis D syndrome*) most

---

[*] Although *osteopenia* is an osteomalacia that is histologically similar to other forms of osteoporosis, the hallmark characteristic is an excess of persistent unmineralized osteoid, the protein matrix of the bone.

of which are related to elevated calcium levels (Table 20.2).* Concomitant high intake of calcium and phosphate may cause the development of similar abnormalities. Treatment of accidental overdose requires general supportive measures, whereas treatment of hypervitaminosis D with hypercalcemia consists of prompt withdrawal of vitamin D supplements, low calcium diet, laxatives, and attention to serum electrolyte imbalances and cardiac function. Major blood vessels, myocardium, and kidneys are at risk of developing ectopic calcification. Hypercalcemic crisis with dehydration, stupor, and coma requires more immediate attention, such as prompt hydration, diuretics, short-term hemodialysis, corticosteroids, and urine acidification.

20.2.3 VITAMIN E

The most biologically active form of vitamin E, a fat-soluble vitamin, is *dl*-α-tocopherol. The antioxidant properties of vitamin E help to protect cells from oxidative processes. For example, it preserves the integrity of the red blood cell membrane, stimulates production of cofactors in steroid metabolism, and suppresses prostaglandin synthesis and platelet aggregation. Vitamin E has numerous unlabelled uses, including the prevention of cancer, preservation of ageless skin, and stimulation of sex drive. However, it is only indicated for the treatment of nutritional states related to vitamin E deficiency. It is widely distributed in nature, predominantly found along with polyunsaturated fatty acids in vegetables and their oils, meat, dairy, wheat, soy, and nuts. Its ubiquitous presence, coupled with a low RDA, makes clinical deficiency of vitamin E a rare phenomenon. Premature infants and patients with malabsorption syndromes, however, are more likely to develop deficiency, defined as having tocopherol levels less than 0.5 mg/dl. Signs and symptoms of deficiency, particularly in premature infants, include hemolytic anemia, thrombocytosis, and increased platelet aggregation.

Symptoms associated with hypervitaminosis E are summarized in Table 20.2 and are usually experienced at doses greater than 3000 IU.

20.2.4 VITAMIN K

Vitamin K and its equally active synthetic analog, K_1 (phytonadione), are fat-soluble vitamins. Vitamin K promotes the hepatic synthesis of coagulation factors II (prothrombin), VII (proconvertin), IX (plasma thromboplastin), and X (Stuart factor). The vitamin acts as a cofactor for hepatic post-translation carboxylation of glutamic acid residues to the active γ-carboxyl glutamate moieties of the clotting proteins, as well as anticoagulant proteins C, S, and osteocalcin (bone matrix).

Phytonadione is indicated in the treatment of coagulation disorders related to vitamin K-associated decreased synthesis of coagulation factors. It is also valuable in the treatment of prothrombin deficiency (hypoprothrombinemia) induced by oral or parenteral anticoagulants, salicylates, or antibiotics. Sources of the vitamin are provided in various foods, particularly green vegetables, dairy products, meats, grains, and fruits. In addition, it is synthesized by normal intestinal bacterial flora.

---

* Interestingly, prolonged exposure to sunlight does not produce excess vitamin D.

As with vitamin E, vitamin K deficiency is uncommon, except in premature and breast-fed newborns, patients with malabsorption syndromes, and patients receiving chronic anticoagulant, or broad spectrum antibiotic therapy.

Hypervitaminosis K is rare principally because the drug is not available over-the-counter (OTC) as a dietary supplement.

20.3 WATER-SOLUBLE VITAMINS

20.3.1 THIAMINE

Thiamine (vitamin B_1) is essential for normal aerobic metabolism and tissue development, proper transmission of nerve impulses, and synthesis of acetylcholine. It combines with adenosine triphosphate (ATP) to form thiamine pyrophosphate, the active form of thiamine. As such, it serves as a coenzyme in many α-ketoacid decarboxylation reactions (such as with pyruvate) and transketolation (pentose-phosphate pathway) reactions.

Thiamine is indicated in the oral or parenteral treatment of B_1 deficiency syndromes (*beriberi*) and in neuritis of pregnancy. Sources of the vitamin include brewer's yeast, meats, nuts, grains, and dairy products.

Beriberi is the classic deficiency syndrome frequently associated with chronic alcoholism, renal dialysis patients, individuals with liver and biliary dysfunction, or poor diets (polished rice). The syndrome is characterized by peripheral neuritis, muscle wasting (*dry beriberi*), and cardiac failure and edema (*wet beriberi*). Other conditions due to thiamine deficiency include lactic acidosis and *Wernicke-Korsakoff* syndrome.[*]

Hypersensitivity reactions, anaphylactic shock, and hypervitaminosis syndrome are rare with oral or i.v. doses. Toxic manifestations, proprietary names, and deficiency states of water-soluble vitamins are summarized in Table 20.4

20.3.2 RIBOFLAVIN

Vitamin B_2 is a component of flavin mononucleotide (FMN) and flavin adenine dinucleotide (FAD). These two coenzymes catalyze a variety of oxidation-reduction reactions, including glucose oxidation and amino acid deamination. The vitamin is found in fish, poultry, dairy products, and leafy vegetables. Poor intestinal absorption of riboflavin limits its toxicity. Deficiency state (ariboflavinosis) is rare and often masked by other nutritional insufficiency. Early symptoms include cheilosis (fissures in the mouth), glossitis (inflammation of the tongue), interstitial ophthalmic keratosis, and dermatitis.

20.3.3 NIACIN

Vitamin B_3[**] (nicotinic acid) is a component of nicotinamide adenine dinucleotide (NAD, coenzyme I) and nicotinamide adenine dinucleotide phosphate (NADP, coen-

---

[*] The syndrome is characterized by encephalopathy and psychosis manifested primarily by ophthalmic nerve and muscle paralysis.

[**] The active forms, niacinamide and nicotinamide, are used synonymously.

TABLE 20.4
Water-Soluble Vitamins, Deficiency States, and Toxic Manifestations of Excessive Consumption or Administration

Vitamin	Compound	Proprietary Name	Deficiency State	ADRs Associated with Excessive Ingestion
Vitamin B_1	Thiamine	Thiamilate, various	Beriberi, lactic acidosis, *Wernicke-Korsakoff*	Pruritis, weakness, nausea, urticaria, hypersensitivity, anaphylactic shock
Vitamin B_2	Riboflavine	Various	Ariboflavinosis (rare)	No toxicity noted, limited absorption
Vitamin B_3	Niacin	Various	Pellagra	Dermatologic: cutaneous flushing, rash, dry skin; GI: ulcer, NVD, abdominal pain; hepatoxicity, hyperglycemia
Vitamin B_6	Pyridoxine HCl	Various	Dermatologic, hematologic, CNS	Sensory neuropathy, ataxia, digital and perioral numbness, paraesthesias
Folic Acid	Pteroylglutamic acid (folate)	Folvite, various	Megaloblastic anemia	CNS: altered sleep patterns, irritability, confusion; GI: N, anorexia, abdominal distention
Vitamin B_{12}	Cyanocobalamin	Various (oral) Nascobal (I.N.) LA-12 (injection)	Pernicious anemia	Nontoxic Paresthesia, headache, glossitis, nausea Pulmonary edema, CHF, itching, anaphylactic shock
Vitamin C	Ascorbic acid	Various	Scurvy	GI disturbances, poor wound healing, urinary calculi

Note: CNS = central nervous system, CHF = congestive heart failure, GI = gastrointestinal, GU = genitourinary, I.N. = intranasal, NVD = nausea, vomiting, diarrhea.

zyme II). The two coenzymes catalyze oxidation-reduction reactions that act as electron acceptors and hydrogenases. Niacin is derived from niacinamide or tryptophan and occurs naturally in most red meats, fish, poultry, dairy products, nuts, and vegetables. Niacin deficiency (*pellagra*, Ital. *rough skin*) is characterized by dermatitis, dementia, and diarrhea (*3Ds*). It is often seen in chronic alcoholism, malabsorption syndrome, and in patients receiving isoniazid (an antituberculosis antibiotic). Pharmacologically, nicotinic acid, but not nicotinamide, is effective in reducing serum lipids. In addition, it triggers peripheral vasodilation and increases blood flow by stimulating histamine release. These properties are distinct from its nutrient role. Consequently, nicotinic acid is useful in the treatment of hypercholesterolemia, hyperlipidemia, and in the management of niacin deficiency and *pellagra*.

20.3.4 FOLIC ACID

Pteroylglutamic acid (folate) is found in leafy vegetables, organ meats, and yeast. Physiologically, folic acid is required for nucleoprotein synthesis and maintenance of hematopoiesis. It is converted intracellularly to tetrahydrofolic acid, which acts as a cofactor in the biosynthesis of purines and thymidylates of nucleic acids. Consequently, deficiency of folic acid (along with vitamin B_{12}), is often seen during pregnancy and in malabsorption conditions, and is responsible for defective DNA synthesis. The condition is manifested by the production of enlarged immature red cells characteristic of megaloblastic anemia. Although folic acid is relatively nontoxic, some allergic, CNS, and GI reactions have been noted with large doses (Table 20.4).

20.3.5 CYANOCOBALAMIN (VITAMIN B_{12})

Dietary deficiency of vitamin B_{12} is rare, since the nutrient is found in all meats and dairy products but is absent from plant foods. Strict vegetarians and individuals with malabsorption syndrome, especially those experiencing atrophic gastritis who cannot absorb B_{12}, are prone to developing pernicious anemia. Presence of intestinal parasitic infections has been noted to induce B_{12} deficiency.[*] Signs and symptoms of the syndrome, however, may not be evident for 3 to 5 years. Pernicious anemia develops principally because of the lack of secretion of intrinsic factor in the stomach, which is necessary for absorption of cyanocobalamin in the ileum.

Vitamin B_{12} is essential for cell growth, hematopoiesis, and nucleic acid and neuronal myelin synthesis. Several preparations of cyanocobalamin are available and are indicated for the management of B_{12} deficiency (all dosage forms) and pernicious anemia (intranasal gel and injection only).

20.3.6 ASCORBIC ACID (VITAMIN C)

Vitamin C is abundant in citrus fruits, strawberries, tomatoes, and leafy vegetables. It is involved in numerous oxidation-reduction reactions, including the synthesis of

---

[*] *Diphyllobothrium latum*, the broad or fish tapeworm, extracts vitamin B_{12} from the intestinal lumen, preventing its normal absorption.

connective tissue components such as chondroitin sulfate and collagen. Ascorbic acid supports the hydroxylation of proline to hydroxyproline in collagen. In addition, it improves the absorption of iron from the GI tract, promotes the synthesis of catecholamine neurotransmitters, and is an important cofactor in the wound healing process. Because of the latter role of vitamin C and its antioxidant properties, it was one of the first nutritional supplements sensationalized for these properties. It has been proclaimed to thwart many conditions, from the common cold to cancer, none of which have been substantiated.

Deficiency of ascorbic acid (*scurvy*) is well documented and occurs in individuals with inadequate dietary intake, including chronic alcoholism and the elderly. Some suppression of ascorbate blood levels appears in situations such as extreme cold, heat, fever, physical trauma, tuberculosis, cigarette smoking, and in women taking oral contraceptives. Scurvy is characterized by impaired wound healing, petechial hemorrhage (pinpoint, minute spots in the skin), and perifollicular hemorrhage (surrounding the hair follicles). It is also demonstrated by inflammatory bleeding gums, loss of teeth, arrested skeletal development (in children), dry skin, joint pain, and increased susceptibility to infections and fatigue.

Although the incidence is low, long-term effects of doses greater than the RDA are associated with cataracts and coronary artery disease, increased iron absorption, and development of renal oxalate stones. Interestingly, sudden curtailing of vitamin C ingestion after chronic megadose administration may precipitate signs of scurvy.

20.3.7 Pyridoxine (Vitamin B₆)

Found primarily in vegetables, peanuts, eggs, soy, and cereals, vitamin B_6 (pyridoxal, pyridoxamine) appears to enact a significant role in neuronal development. It is particularly important in the formation of pyridoxal-dependent decarboxylase necessary for the synthesis of the neurotransmitter γ-aminobutyric acid (GABA). In fact, pyridoxine deficiencies, although rare, are characterized by unremarkable features of dermatologic, hematologic, and nervous system anomalies. Vitamin B_6 deficiencies occur in individuals who are also susceptible to deficiencies of other B-vitamins, including chronic alcoholism and malabsorption syndrome. Patients receiving isoniazid, cycloserine (antituberculosis antibiotics), hydralazine (antihypertensive), and oral contraceptives are also prone to B_6 deficiency. Pyridoxine is indicated solely for the management of pyridoxine deficiency states. Sensory neuropathies, ataxia, and numbness are possible in subjects receiving megadoses for several months.

20.3.8 Pantothenic Acid (Vitamin B₅)

Vitamin B_5 is important as a cofactor in enzyme-catalyzed reactions involving carbohydrates, gluconeogenesis, fatty acids, and steroids. It is distributed in many food products, is nontoxic, and deficiencies are seen only in association with severe multiple B-complex malnutrition.

Toxicity associated with minerals and trace metals is discussed in detail in Chapter 24, "Metals."

REFERENCES

SUGGESTED READINGS

Drug Facts and Comparisons, 56th ed., Kluwer, St. Louis, 2002, chap. 1.

Hardman, J., Limbird, L., and Gilman, A., *Goodman & Gilman's The Pharmacological Basis of Therapeutics*, 10th ed., McGraw-Hill, New York, 2001, chap. 63 and 64.

Rubin, E., and Farber, J., *Pathology*, 2nd ed., Lippincott-Raven, Philadelphia, 1999, chap. 8.

REVIEW ARTICLES

Backstrand, J.R., The history and future of food fortification in the United States: a public health perspective, *Nutr. Rev.*, 60, 15, 2002.

Bast, A. et al., Antioxidant effects of carotenoids, *Int. J. Vitam. Nutr. Res.*, 68, 399, 1998.

Bates, C.J., Diagnosis and detection of vitamin deficiencies, *Br. Med. Bull.*, 55, 643, 1999.

Blot, W.J., Vitamin/mineral supplementation and cancer risk: international chemoprevention trials, *Proc. Soc. Exp. Biol. Med.*, 216, 291, 1997.

Fairfield, K.M. and Fletcher, R.H., Vitamins for chronic disease prevention in adults: scientific review, *JAMA*, 287, 3116, 2002.

Fletcher, R.H. and Fairfield, K.M. Vitamins for chronic disease prevention in adults: clinical applications, *JAMA*, 287, 3127, 2002.

Fukugawa, M. and Kurokawa, K., Calcium homeostasis and imbalance, *Nephron*, 92, 41, 2002.

Garewal, H.S. and Diplock, A.T., How 'safe' are antioxidant vitamins?, *Drug Saf.*, 13, 8, 1995.

Haenen, G.R. and Bast, A., The use of vitamin supplements in self-medication, *Therapie.*, 57, 119, 2002.

Hathcock, J.N., Vitamins and minerals: efficacy and safety, *Am. J. Clin. Nutr.*, 66, 427, 1997.

Marks, J., The safety of the vitamins: an overview, *Int. J. Vitam. Nutr. Res. Suppl.*, 30, 12, 1989.

Mawer, E.B. and Davies, M. Vitamin D nutrition and bone disease in adults, *Rev. Endocr. Metab. Disord.* 2, 153, 2001.

Meyers, D.G., Maloley, P.A., and Weeks, D., Safety of antioxidant vitamins, *Arch. Intern. Med.*, 156, 925, 1996.

Nagai, K., et al., Vitamin A toxicity secondary to excessive intake of yellow-green vegetables, liver and laver, *J. Hepatology*, 31, 142, 1999.

Omaye, S.T., Safety of megavitamin therapy, *Adv. Exp. Med. Biol.*, 177, 203, 1984.

Rolig, E.C., Vitamins: physiology and deficiency states, *Nurse Pract.*, 11, 38, 1986.

Swain, R. and Kaplan, B., Vitamins as therapy in the 1990s, *J. Am. Board Fam. Pract.*, 8, 206. 1995.

Truswell, A.S., ABC of nutrition. Vitamins II., *Br. Med. J. (Clin. Res. Ed.)*, 291,1103, 1985.

21 Herbal Remedies

21.1 INTRODUCTION

The popularity of self-medication or prescribed therapeutic intervention with herbal products has burgeoned. These "natural" supplements* have been traditionally promoted and used for centuries in Asian and Indian medicine, and later in American folk medicine. The belief that carefully measured amounts of the leaves, flowers, bark, stems, or seeds of botanicals can treat or prevent diseases has encouraged generations to trust the beneficial effects of ingredients contained within nature's packages. As society questions the limitations, abilities, efficacy, and safety of Western medicine, it creates an opportunity for alternative therapies to demonstrate their potential. The platform for the introduction of alternative medicines into the Western medical establishment is based particularly on the prevention of diseases and the avoidance of adverse reactions associated with Western therapeutic modalities.

It is interesting how the practice of pharmacy has come full circle, particularly since the days of the medieval European apothecaries. Pharmacy's first specific and peculiar contribution to the art of healing was the recognition that botanicals contained substances which could prevent or treat disease. American folk medicine and the early colonists relied on the Native American botanicals to help the ailing. One of the earliest American folk medicine publications was Peter Smith's *Indian Doctor's Dispensatory, Being Father Smith's Advice Respecting Diseases and Their Cure* (1812). It documented a series of diseases commonly accepted as therapeutic categories of the times and recommended herbs for their remedy. In time, detailed descriptions of plants, flowers, and shrubs were systematically categorized and incorporated as part of the discipline of *pharmacognosy.*** As the practice of medicine and pharmacy matured from the era of empiricism, the emphasis shifted from handling of the bulk plant to procedures for isolating the crude drug. Eventually, identification and isolation of the active constituents, and structure-activity relationships, defined the modern age of pharmaceutical development. Another driving force for modernization was the recognition that plants and their derivatives were as likely to be poisonous as they were beneficial. Thus, systematic scientific studies of the unseen chemicals contained within the powdered compounds forged the path toward

---

* The terms natural/dietary supplements, botanicals, and herbal remedies/medicines are used interchangeably. The use of herbal products, particularly in Chinese medicine, is considered to be part of the total approach to maintaining the body in a state of well being, and thus is incorporated into the practice of "alternative" medicine. The latter also includes the Asian practices and procedures of acupuncture, meditation, *tai chi chuan*, massage and aromatherapies.

** The art of pharmacognosy, which means knowledge of pharmaceuticals, developed from the ancient civilizations. These societies used parts of plants and animals to concoct healing potions to prevent or eliminate disease.

modern pharmacology, toxicology, and therapeutics. Today, botanical remedies are desirable as a way of returning to the holistic art of healing. Thus, it has taken over 500 years for Western medicine to complete the "circle" and reacquaint itself with the power that nature always possessed. Ultimately the goal is, perhaps, to complement the tremendous advances achieved in Western medicine.

The use of herbal remedies incorporates numerous botanical products, each espoused to contain curative or preventative compounds for a variety of disease states. The effectiveness of the herbs, however, is mostly based on empirical experience gathered over time. Documentation of the history of the medicines as recorded in Chinese and Indian pharmaceutical compendia has also contributed to the empirical database. An important Chinese herbal manuscript, for instance, dates back to the third millennium BC and the emperor Shen Nung. He was deified by the people as the "God of Agriculture" and is credited with authorship of the first Chinese pharmacopoeia, Pen Ts'ao ("Great Herbal"). The manuscript is a vast Chinese medical volume containing descriptions of vegetable, animal, and mineral medicines. Huang Ti (Yellow Emperor, circa 2800 BC), the father of Chinese internal medicine, systematically classified diseases into therapeutic categories, thus advancing the practice of treatment with herbal medicines. Today, Chinese compendia list over 5800 natural products and their ingredients. However, rigorous scrutiny, as defined by Western scientific investigations, has shown that herbal product claims are not firm or final. This understanding of the limitations of herbal claims has impeded the smooth acceptance of alternative medicine into Western society. In addition, as their use increases and information accumulates, it is apparent that the products carry significant adverse reactions, hazards, contraindications, precautions, drug interactions, and consequences of overdose. Several documented instances of adulterated or mislabeled natural products have surfaced, resulting in serious poisoning from unsuspected reactions to mislabeled botanicals. Also, hypersensitivity reactions have been attributed to ingestion of plant components resulting in anaphylactic responses.

Much of the information relied upon in the U.S. is based on current summaries categorized by the German Regulatory Authority's herbal watchdog agency, "Commission E." The Commission's assessment of the peer-reviewed literature encompasses over 300 herbs and botanicals. The Commission compares the quality of the clinical evidence regarding their indications, effectiveness, and toxicity. This chapter, therefore, summarizes the currently accepted knowledge, attributes, and therapeutic usefulness associated with some frequently encountered herbal products and the reported toxicities observed with their use.

21.2 NOMENCLATURE AND CLASSIFICATION

21.2.1 NOMENCLATURE

Herbal products are listed according to their common, scientific (biological), and brand names. Common names are readily recognizable and generally accepted. The scientific name refers to the taxonomic botanical designation of the plant. Commercial preparations of the product are assigned trade names.

21.2.2 THERAPEUTIC CATEGORY

Many of the botanical products were originally categorized in ancient compendia and folk medicine publications according to the ailments for which they were prescribed. Similarly today, herbal products are listed according to standard accepted treatment categories — i.e., organs that are affected by a disease and amenable to treatment with an herbal product. It should be noted, however, that in the U.S., herbal products are marketed under the provision of the Dietary Supplement and Health Education Act of 1994. This legislation defines herbs, vitamins, minerals, amino acids, and biochemical components of tissues and organs as food supplements, rather than drugs, thus relieving them from many of the efficacy and safety requirements necessary for FDA drug approval. In addition, therapeutic claims of herbal products are restricted to the enhancement of general health that affects normal physiologic processes. The compounds, however, are not permitted to claim or warrant efficacy for the diagnosis, treatment, cure, or prevention of any disease.

21.3 INDICATIONS

Indications for which an herbal product is deemed useful are listed under several major categories. Primary indications are those approved by Commission E. Homeopathic indications refer to some disease symptoms that could be treated by very small doses of medicine. Asian indications are based on traditional Chinese and Indian compendia and may or may not be recognized as primary indications by Western medicine. Finally, there are many unproven uses for which a botanical has empirically been used, but lacks sufficient data to determine otherwise.

21.4 OTHER THERAPEUTIC AND TOXICOLOGIC INFORMATION OF HERBAL PRODUCTS

Other information that is available for most common herbal products includes actions and pharmacology of the known active ingredients, their dosages, adverse drug reactions, side effects, drug/herb interactions, precautions, and where available, treatment of acute intoxication.

Table 21.1 lists accepted and well-documented herbal preparations according to their common, scientific, and proprietary names. Botanicals that are used primarily as culinary spices, flavoring agents, fruits, or vegetables or that lack documented Chinese, Indian, or Western therapeutic uses or toxicity are not included. The principal components or parts of the botanical used in the preparation of the medicinal are listed. The major active ingredients contained within the herb are outlined, most of which are structurally classified as aromatic or polycyclic glycosides.

Table 21.2 summarizes the therapeutic effects, indications, and adverse reactions of the botanicals listed in Table 21.1. The most common indications are: (1) those approved by Commission E and (2) those documented in traditional Chinese or Indian medicine compendia or in American folklore. Many other historical applications for which the compounds have claimed usefulness are not included. Among the most common adverse reactions noted with ingestion or application of herbal

TABLE 21.1
Names and Major Active Ingredients of Various Herbal Products

Common Name	Scientific Name[a]	Other Common Names	Herbal Component	Major Active Ingredients
Acacia	Acacia arabica	Babul bark	Bark	Tannins
Agrimony	Agrimonia eupatoria	Stickwort, sticklewort	Leaves	Catechin tannins
Aloe	Aloe vera	Various oral and topical preparations	Topical products	Anthracene & flavanoid derivatives
Amaranth	Amaranthus hypochondriacus	Velvet flower, Lady bleeding	Plant	Saponins, β-cyans
American bittersweet	Celastrus scandens	Waxwork	Root, bark	Tannins, celastrol
Anise	Pimpinella anisum	Aniseed oil	Oil of fruit	Anetholes, flavanoids
Arnica	Arnica montana	Wolfsbane	Oil of flowers	Sesquiterpine lactones
Belladonna	Atropa belladonna	Deadly nightshade, poison black cherry	Leaves, root	(-)-Hyoscyamine, atropine, scopolamine
Benzoin	Styrax benzoin	Benjamin tree	Resin	Benzoate esters
Betel nut	Piper betle	Betel	Dried leaves	Betel phenol, eugenol
Brewer's yeast	Saccharomyces cerevisiae	Various preparations	Dried yeast cells	B-complex vitamins, polysaccharides, protein
Calamus	Acorus calamus	Sweet flag, myrtle flag	Rhizome, oil	Asarone
Camphor tree	Cinnamomum camphora	Gum camphor	Oil	D(+)-camphor
Cardamom	Elettaria cardamomum	Various preparations	Oil, fruit, seeds	Cineol
Cascara sagrada	Rhamnus purshiana	Sacred bark, dogwood bark	Dried bark	Anthracene
Castor oil plant	Ricinus communis	Castor bean, Palma Christi	Oil, seeds	Ricin D, ricinoleic acid
Cat's claw	Unicaria tomentosa	Una de gato	Root bark	Strictosidine alkaloids, triterpines
Cayenne	Capsicum annuum	Capsicum, Chili pepper, Paprika	Dried fruit	Capsaicinoids
Clove	Syzygium aromaticum	Various preparations	Oil, leaves	Eugenol
Coca	Erythroxylon coca	Cocaine	Leaves	Cocaine
Colchicum	Colchicum autumnale	Meadow saffron, upstart	Flowers, seeds	Colchicine
Devil's claw	Harpagophytum procumbens	Grapple plant, wood spider	Roots, tubers	Harpagoside

Digitalis[b]	*Digitalis lanata, D. purpurea*	Foxglove, Dog's finger	Leaves	Digitoxigenin glycosides
Dong Quai	*Angelica sinensis*	Chinese angelica, dang gui, tang kuei	Root	Vitamins: B-complex, E, folic acid
Echinacea	*Echinacea angustifolia, E. purpurea*	Black Sampson, Purple coneflower	Root, leaves	Arabinoxylan polysaccharides
Ergot[b]	*Claviceps purpurea*	Cockspur rye, Hornseed	Fungal sclerotium	Indole (ergot) alkaloids
Eucalyptus	*Eucalyptus globulus*	Blue gum, fever tree	Oil, dried leaves	1,8-cineol, limonene, camphene
Flax	*Linum usitatissimum*	Flaxseed, linseed	Stem, oil, seeds, flowers	Arabinoxylans (mucilages), fatty acids
Garlic	*Allium sativum*	Stinking rose, Poor man's treacle	Oil, fresh bulb	Alliins (sulfoxides)
Ginger	*Zingiber officinale*	Various preparations	Root	Zingiberene, farnesene, camphor, gingerols
Ginkgo	*Ginkgo biloba*	Maidenhair tree	Leaves, seeds	Quercetin, myristicins
Ginseng	*Panax ginseng*	American, Chinese and Korean ginseng	Root	Ginsenoside (aglycone)
Goldenseal	*Hydrastic canadensis*	Orange root, yellow root	Rhizome	Hydrastine, berberine
Gotu kola	*Centella asiatica*	Indian pennywort	Leaves, stems	Asiatocides, asiatic acid
Green tea	*Camellia sinensis*	Black tea, Chinese tea	Leaves	Methyl xanthines, theaflavins
Guaiac	*Guaiacum officinale*	Pockwood	Resin	Oleanolic acid, guaiaretic acids
Hemlock[b]	*Conium maculatum*	Cicuta, poison parsley	Dried leaves	Piperidin alkaloids (conine)
Henbane	*Hyoscyamus niger*	Devil's eye, stinking nightshade	Dried leaves	Tropane alkaloids (hyoscyamine)
Hibiscus	*Hibiscus sabdariffa*	Guinea sorrel, red sorrel	Flowers	Fruit acids, anthocyans
Ipecac	*Cephaelis ipecacuanha*	Ipecacuanha, matto grosso	Dried root	Emetine, cephalin
Jimson weed	*Datura stramonium*	Jamestown weed, devil's apple	Dried leaves	Tropane alkaloids (hyoscyamine)
Juniper	*Juniperus communis*	Juniper berry, enebro	Oil, berry cones	α-pinene, β-myrcene, limonene
Kava kava	*Piper methysticum*	Ava pepper, tonga	Dried rhizome	Kavain, methysticin
Khat[b]	*Catha edulis*	None	Leaves	Khatamine (alkyl amine)
Licorice	*Glycyrrhiza glabra*	Sweet root, sweet wort	Dried root	Glycyrrhetic acid, glycocoumarin, glabridin

(continued)

TABLE 21.1 (CONTINUED)
Names and Major Active Ingredients of Various Herbal Products

Common Name	Scientific Name[a]	Other Common Names	Herbal Component	Major Active Ingredients
Ma-huang	Ephedra sinica	Ephedrine, desert herb	Cane, root	Ephedrine, pseudoephedrine
Mandrake	Mandragora officinarum	Mandragora, Satan's apple	Dried root, fresh herb	Tropane alkaloids (hyoscyamine)
Marijuana	Cannabis sativa	Cannabis, pot, bhang, grass, weed	Flowering twigs	Δ^9-tetrahydrocannabinol (THC)
Morning glory	Ipomoea hederacea	None	Seeds, root	Ergoline alkaloids (lysergol, chanoclavine)
Nutmeg	Myristica fragrans	Mace	Seeds, oil	Sabinene, α-pinene, myristicin, fatty acids
Nux vomica	Strychnos nux vomica	Poison nut, Quaker buttons	Dried seeds, bark	Strychnine, brucine
Periwinkle	Vinca minor	None	Dried leaves	Vincamine
Peyote[b]	Lophophora williamsii	Mescal buttons, sacred mushroom	Dried shoot, fresh plant	Mescaline
Poison ivy	Rhus toxicodendron	Poison oak, poison vine	Dried leaves, shoots	Urushiol (alkyl phenol)
Poke	Phytolacca americana	Pokeweed, American nightshade	Dried root, berries	Phytolaccoside, lectins, histamine
Poppy seed	Papaver somniferum	Garden poppy, opium poppy	Seed capsule extract	Morphine, codeine, papaverine, narcotine, thebaine
Psyllium	Plantago ovata, P. afra	Plantain, fleaseed	Husk, seed	Arabinoxylans
Pyrethrum	Chrysanthemum cinerariifolium	Dalmation insect flowers	Flower	Pyrethrines I, II; cinerines I, II
Quinine	Cinchona pubescens	Peruvian bark, cinchona	Dried bark	Quinine, quinidine, cinchonine
Rauwolfia	Rauwolfia serpentina	Various proprietary names	Dried root	Reserpine, serpentine
Sarsaparilla	Smilax sp.	Various proprietary names	Dried root	Sarsapilloside
Saw palmetto	Serenoa repens	Various proprietary names	Dried ripe fruit	β-sitosterol
Senna	Cassia senna	India senna, Alexandria senna	Leaves, fruit, flowers	Sennosides A,B,C, D (anthracenes)
Soybean	Glycine soja, G. max	Soya, tofu, miso	Bean, seed, legume, oil	Phospholipids (PC, PE, PI)
Squill	Urginea maritime	Scilla	Bulbs	Cardiac glycosides (scillarene A)

St. John's wort	*Hypericum perforatum*	Amber, goatweed	Buds, flowers	Xanthones, hypericin, napthodianthrone, procyanidines
Thyme	*Thymus vulgaris*	Various proprietary names	Oil, dried leaves	Thymol, *p*-cymene, carvacrol
Tobacco	*Nicotiana tabacum*	Various formulations	Dried leaves	Nicotine
Tragacanth	*Astragalus gummifer*	Gum dragon	Exudate from branch	Tragacanthine
Uva-ursi	*Arctostaphylos uva-ursi*	Arberry, mountain cranberry	Dried leaves	Arbutin (hydroqinone glycoside), tannins
Valerian	*Valeriana officinalis*	Amantilla, Vandal root	Dried root	Valepotriates, isovaltrate, valerenate
White mustard	*Sinapis alba*	Mustard	Dried seeds	Sinalbin (*p*-hydroxy-benzylglucosinolates)
Witch hazel	*Hamamelis virginiana*	Hazel nut, tobacco wood	Plant distillates	Hamamelitannin
Yerba santa	*Eriodyctyon californicum*	Bear's weed, sacred herb	Dried leaves	Eriodictyonin
Yohimbe bark	*Pausinystalia yohimbe*	Various proprietary names	Bark	Yohimbine

Note: PC = phosphatidylcholine, PE = phosphatidylethanolamine, PI = phosphatidylinositol.

[a] Botanicals may incur several scientific names for different species of the genus. The most popular designations are noted.

[b] Because of toxicity and unreliable control of dose/effect, this herb is no longer recommended for use as an herbal preparation (see Effects, Table 21.2).

TABLE 21.2
Therapeutic Effects, Indications, and Adverse Reactions of Common Botanicals

Common Name[a]	Desirable Therapeutic Effects	Indications	Adverse Reactions
Acacia	Astringent	Diarrhea, inflammation	Gastric disturbances
Agrimony	Astringent	Diarrhea, inflammation	Gastric disturbances
Aloe	Laxative, antibacterial, antineoplastic, anti-inflammatory, analgesic	Constipation, antibacterial, inflammation	Gastric and electrolyte disturbances, hypersensitivity, possible malignancy
Amaranth	Astringent	Diarrhea, inflammation	No significant ADRs
American bittersweet	Diuretic	Inflammation, menstrual disorders	No significant ADRs, botanical is obsolete
Anise	Expectorant, antispasmodic, antibacterial	Cough, colds, fever, inflammation, rheumatism	Allergic reactions
Arnica	Analgesic, antiseptic, ↓ respiratory secretions	Cough, colds, fever, inflammation, rheumatism	Allergic reactions, ↑ skin sensitivity
Belladonna	Anticholinergic, GI antispasmodic, positive chronotropy	Liver & gall bladder disorders	Mydriasis, dryness of mouth, perspiration, arrhythmias
Benzoin	Expectorant	Respiratory cold, stroke, syncope	No significant ADRs
Betel nut	Antibacterial, anti-inflammatory	Cough, asthma, bronchitis	None, compound is obsolete
Brewer's yeast	Antibacterial, immuno-stimulant	Dyspepsia, eczema	Gastric bloating, allergic reactions
Calamus	Aromatic, cholinergic, antispasmodic, sedative	Dyspepsia, gastritis, rheumatism	Possible carcinogen with chronic use
Camphor tree	Hyperemic, antispasmodic, ↑ bronchial secretions	Bronchitis, rheumatism, arrhythmias	Dermal irritation, delirium, spasms, dyspnea
Cardamom	Antimicrobial, cholinergic	Cough, colds, fever, inflammation	Gastric colic
Cascara sagrada	Laxative, cholinergic	Constipation	Gastric spasms, edema, electrolyte disturbances, nephropathy
Castor oil plant	Laxative, cholinergic	Constipation, dyspepsia, dermal inflammation	NVD, electrolyte disturbances, gastroenteritis, shock, fatal with OD

	Actions	Indications	Adverse Effects
Cat's claw	Anti-inflammatory, immuno-stimulant, ↓ platelet aggregation, anti-HT, contraceptive	Inflammation, antiviral	Interference with gonadotropin levels
Cayenne	Hyperemic, antibacterial, thrombolytic anti-neoplastic	Rheumatism, muscular tension	Diarrhea, dermal ulcers, anaphylaxis, hypocoagulation
Clove	Antiseptic, antispasmodic, local anesthetic	Oral inflammation, dental analgesia	Allergic reactions, local irritation
Coca	Local anesthetic, CNS stimulant	Local anesthesia	Hallucinations, depression, addictive, embryo-toxic
Colchicum	Anti-inflammatory, inhibits phagocytizing lymphocytes	Gout, Mediterranean fever	NVD, hemorrhage, kidney, liver, CNS, BM pathology
Devil's claw	Cholinergic, anti-inflammatory	Dyspepsia, anorexia, rheumatism	Allergic reactions
Digitalis	Cardioactive, positive inotropy, negative chronotropy	Cardiac insufficiency[b]	NVD, HA, anorexia, arrhythmias, visual disorders, confusion[b]
Dong Quai	Relaxes uterine smooth muscle, coronary vasodilator	Menopause, irregular menstruation, Raynaud's syndrome	Photosensitization, abortifacient, anticoagulant
Echinacea	Anti-inflammatory, promotes wound healing, antibacterial, immuno-stimulant	Cough, colds, fever, inflammation, UTI, rheumatism	NV, fever, hypersensitivity, dyspnea, hypotension
Ergot	Smooth muscle contraction	Hemorrhage, migraine, uterine and muscle spasm[b]	NVD, muscle pain, multiple systemic pathology[b]
Eucalyptus	Expectorant, diuretic, aromatic	Chronic bronchitis, rheumatism	NVD, asthmatic attacks with facial application
Flax	Bulk laxative, hypolipidemic	Constipation, dermal inflammation	Delayed GI absorption
Garlic	Antibacterial, hypolipidemic, antioxidant, antiplatelet	Hypertension, hypercholesterolemia	Gastric irritation, allergic reactions, bleeding disorders
Ginger	Antiemetic, anti-inflammatory	Dyspepsia, anorexia, motion sickness	Gastric irritation, allergic reactions
Ginkgo	Antiplatelet, antioxidant, improves cognitive function, thrombolytic	Inflammation, tinnitus, intermittent claudication, vertigo	Gastric irritation, allergic reactions
Ginseng	Improves cognitive function, antineoplastic, antioxidant, antiplatelet, hypolipidemic	Malaise	HT, insomnia, edema

(continued)

TABLE 21.2 (CONTINUED)
Therapeutic Effects, Indications, and Adverse Reactions of Common Botanicals

Common Name[a]	Desirable Therapeutic Effects	Indications	Adverse Reactions
Goldenseal	Antiparasitic, antiseptic, antibacterial	Infection (antiseptic, cold sores), acute diarrhea	Gastric disorders, constipation, hallucinations
Gotu kola	Anti-inflammatory, antineoplastic, promotes wound healing, anti-HT	Inflammation, neoplasms, gastric ulcers	Allergic contact dermatitis
Green tea	CNS stimulation, diuresis, positive inotropic, anticancer	Cancer prevention	Gastric irritation, reduction of appetite
Guaiac	Antifungal	Rheumatism	Diarrhea, gastroenteritis
Hemlock	Autonomic stimulant	Rheumatism, cramps, bronchial spasms[b]	Tonic contractions, hypotension, cramps, paralysis[b]
Henbane	Anticholinergic, smooth muscle relaxation	Dyspepsia	Mydriasis, dryness of mouth, perspiration, arrhythmias
Hibiscus	Hypotensive, uterine relaxation	Anorexia, colds, constipation, dermal inflammation	No significant ADRs
Ipecac	Emetic, gastric irritation	Asthma, bronchitis, cough, colds, poisoning	Allergic reactions, myopathy
Jimson weed	Anticholinergic, parasympatholytic	Stomach complaints, colic, dyspnea	Restlessness, irritability, hallucinations, delirium
Juniper	Antihypertensive, diuretic, antidiabetic	Anorexia, dyspepsia	Kidney irritation
Kava kava	Anticonvulsant, antispasmodic, sedative/hypnotic	Nervousness, spasms, insomnia	GI upset, allergic reactions
Khat	CNS stimulant, sympathomimetic	Depression, headache, asthma, fever, obesity[b]	Irritability, hypertonia nervousness, insomnia[b]
Licorice	Anti-inflammatory, antiplatelet, antifungal, mineralocorticoid	Cough, bronchitis, gastritis	Hypokalemia, hypernatremia, edema, HT
Ma-huang	Sympathomimetic	Cough, bronchitis, asthma, edema, fever	Irritability, HT, arrhythmias, restlessness, HA
Mandrake	Anticholinergic	Stomach complaints, colic, whooping cough	Drowsiness, delirium, excitation, tachycardia, hallucinations

Marijuana	Psychotropic, antiemetic, analgesic, anticonvulsive, CV stimulant, ↓IOP	Anorexia, depression, insomnia, vomiting	Alterations of perception, sensory disturbances
Morning glory	Laxative	Constipation, intestinal parasitic infections	Abdominal cramps
Nutmeg	Antidiarrheal, anti-inflammatory	Diarrhea, vomiting, stomach cramps	Allergic contact dermatitis
Nux vomica	↑CNS and muscular excitability	Anorexia, depression, CV stimulant, pain, respiratory disorders	Anxiety, tonic-clonic spasms & convulsions, nervousness
Periwinkle	Hypotension, hypoglycemia, sympatholytic	Circulatory disorders, memory loss	GI upset, skin flushing, hypotension
Peyote	Hallucinogenic	Used as a hallucinogen	Visual, auditory, sensory disturbances[b]
Poison ivy	Dermal immuneo-stimulant	Rheumatism, muscle strain, inflammation	Skin irritation, swelling, blisters
Poke	Immuneo-stimulant, antiedemic, emetic	Rheumatism, dermal ulcers, inflammation	NV, diarrhea, hypotension, tachycardia
Poppyseed	Analgesic, sedative, euphoric antitussive	Pain, nervousness, muscle spasms, cough, diarrhea	Constipation, weakness, dizziness, clonic twitching
Psyllium	Laxative, antidiarrheal (swelling)	Constipation, diarrhea, hyper-cholesterolemia, hemorrhoids	Allergic reactions, GI obstruction
Pyrethrum	Neurotoxic, contact insecticide	Mite and lice infestation (scabies, pediculosis)	NV, paresthesia, tinnitus, HA
Quinine	Anti-inflammatory, appetite stimulant	Anorexia, dyspepsia, malaria, fever	Eczema, itching, arrhythmias, tinnitus, NV
Rauwolfia	Sympatholytic, hypotensive effect	Hypertension, nervousness, insomnia	Nasal congestion, depression, erectile dysfunction
Sarsaparilla	Diuretic, diaphoretic	Dermal inflammation, rheumatism, edema	GI upset
Saw palmetto	Antiandrogenic, antiestrogenic	Prostate and urinary complaints, irritable bladder	GI upset
Senna	Stimulant laxative	Constipation	Spastic GI upset, electrolyte & CV abnormalities
Soybean	Lipid-lowering effects	Hypercholesterolemia	GI upset
Squill	Positive inotropy, negative chronotropy	Cardiac insufficiency, arrhythmias, venous conditions	Arrhythmias, depression, confusion
St. John's wort	Antidepressant, sedative, anxiolytics	Anxiety, depression, dermal inflammation, wounds, burns	Photosensitization, drug interactions (see text)
Thyme	Relaxes bronchial smooth muscle	Cough, bronchitis	No significant ADRs

(continued)

TABLE 21.2 (CONTINUED)
Therapeutic Effects, Indications, and Adverse Reactions of Common Botanicals

Common Name[a]	Desirable Therapeutic Effects	Indications	Adverse Reactions
Tobacco	CV, respiratory & CNS stimulant	Dental pain, angina pectoris, diarrhea, skin parasites	Habituation, nicotine poisoning
Tragacanth	Laxative	Constipation	No significant ADRs
Uva-ursi	Diuretic, antibacterial	UTI, biliary tract disorders	GI irritation, NV
Valerian	Sedative, anxiolytics, muscle relaxant, spasmolytic	Nervousness, insomnia	Headache, restlessness, mydriasis
White mustard	Dermal hyperemia, decongestant, swelling	Cough, bronchitis, cold, rheumatism	Skin necrosis, nerve damage
Witch hazel	Astringent, hemostatic, anti-inflammatory	Inflammation, wounds, burns, hemorrhoids	No significant ADRs
Yerba santa	Diuretic	Asthma, masks bitter taste	No significant ADRs
Yohimbe bark	Aphrodisiac, analgesic, sympatholytic (α-2 antagonist)	Impotence, sexual dysfunction	Anxiety, HT, mydriasis

Note: BM = bone marrow; CV = cardiovascular; HT = hypertension; GI = gastrointestinal; NVD = nausea, vomiting, diarrhea; HA = headache; IOP = intraocular pressure; OD = overdose.

[a] Botanicals may incur several scientific names for different species of the genus. The most popular designations are noted in Table 21.1.

[b] Because of toxicity and unreliable control of dose/effect, this botanical is not recommended for use as an herbal preparation.

TABLE 21.3
Some Significant Drug-Drug Interactions Associated with Therapeutic Use of Common Botanicals

Botanical	Generic Therapeutic Drug	Drug-Drug Interaction: Potential Influence of Botanical on Drug
Belladonna	Anticholinergic agents (eg. tricyclic antidepressants, atropine)	↑ anticholinergic effects
Castor oil plant	Cholinergic agents, oral medications, diuretics	↑ cholinergic effects, ↑ GI motility (produces diarrhea); delays absorption of oral medications, ↑ potential for electrolyte disturbances (diuretics)
Digitalis	Cardioactive agents	Counteracts effectiveness of cardioactive agents; potentiates effect of cardiac stimulants
Dong Quai	Oral anticoagulants	Enhances anticoagulant effects
Echinacea	Immunosuppressant agents	Reduces immunosuppression activity
Flax	Oral medications	Delays absorption and oral bioavailability
Garlic	Oral anticoagulants	Enhances anticoagulant effects, ↑ risk of bleeding episodes
Ginkgo	Oral anticoagulants	Enhances anticoagulant effects, ↑ risk of bleeding episodes
Ginseng	Oral anticoagulants; oral hypoglycemics	Enhances anticoagulant effects, ↑ risk of bleeding episodes; enhances hypoglycemic effect, raises risk of diabetic shock
Jimson weed	Anticholinergic agents (eg. tricyclic drugs, atropine)	↑ anticholinergic effects
Kava kava	Anesthetics, opioids, sedative/hypnotics	Enhances sedative effects
Ma-huang	CNS stimulants, sympathomimetics, MAOI	Enhances CNS stimulation, potential for HT, vascular complications, arrhythmias, hemodynamic instability
Rauwolfia	Anti-HT agents, antidepressants	Enhances anti-HT effect (syncope, dizziness, shock); may counteract effect of antidepressants
Saw palmetto	Oral anticoagulants	Enhances anticoagulant effects, increases risk of bleeding episodes
St. John's wort	Drugs requiring cytochrome P_{450} inactivation	Cytochrome P_{450} enzyme inducer, ↓ bioavailability of many therapeutic drugs
Valerian	Anesthetic, opioids, sedative/hypnotics	Enhances sedative effects
Yohimbe bark	CNS stimulants, sympathomimetics, MAOI	Enhances CNS stimulation, potential for HT, vascular complications, arrhythmias, hemodynamic instability

Note: MAOI = monoamine oxidase inhibitor.

products is the propensity for development of allergic reactions. In particular, the lectin, glycosidic, or peptide components of the herbs behave as haptens. Haptens, by definition, are incapable of inducing inflammatory reactions alone, but can stimulate an antigenic response by binding to circulating proteins. Toxicity of some herbs has also resulted from contamination of the product with metals and pharmaceutical agents. Because of the lenient federal oversight for these products, some poisonings have resulted from misidentification, mislabeling, and inadequate purification of herbal components. In addition, toxic effects of herbal compounds generally result from ingestion of higher doses than recommended or of recommended doses for extended periods.

As more information is gathered with the increasing popularity of these agents, notable drug interactions are surfacing, some of which are summarized in Table 21.3. In general, several classes of drugs have the potential for undesirable interactions with botanical preparations. These include anticoagulants and other medications requiring therapeutic drug monitoring, drugs that require P450 biotransformation, drugs that sensitize the myocardium, or compounds that increase risk of systemic allergic reactions.

REFERENCES

SUGGESTED READINGS

Blumenthal, M., Ed., *The Complete German Commission E Monographs: Therapeutic Guide to Herbal Medicines*, American Botanical Council, Austin, TX, 1999, p. 218.

Dietary Supplement Health and Education Act of 1994, Public Law 103-417, U.S. Food and Drug Administration.

Haller, C., Herbal preparations, in *Toxicology Secrets*, Ling, L.J. et al., Eds., Hanley and Belfus, Inc., Philadelphia, 2001, chap. 58.

Keys, J.D., *Chinese Herbs: Their Botany, Chemistry, and Pharmacodynamics*, Charles E. Tuttle Co., Boston, MA, 1993.

Meyer, C., *American Folk Medicine*, Plume Books, 1973.

PDR for Herbal Medicines, 2nd ed., Medical Economics, 2000.

PDR Physicians' Desk Reference for Nonprescription Drugs and Dietary Supplements, 23rd ed., Medical Economics, 2002.

REVIEW ARTICLES

Durante, K.M. et al., Use of vitamins, minerals and herbs: a survey of patients attending family practice clinics, *Clin. Invest. Med.*, 24, 242, 2001.

Ernst, E., Heavy metals in traditional Indian remedies, *Eur. J. Clin. Pharmacol.*, 57, 891, 2002.

Ervin, R.B., Wright, J.D., and Kennedy-Stephenson, J., Use of dietary supplements in the United States, 1988–94, *Vital Health Stat.* 11, 1, 1999.

Haller, C.A. et al., An evaluation of selected herbal reference texts and comparison to published reports of adverse herbal events, *Adverse Drug React. Toxicol. Rev.*, 21, 143, 2002.

Huxtable, R.J., The harmful potential of herbal and other plant products, *Drug Saf.*, 5, 126, 1990.

Lee, K.H., Research and future trends in the pharmaceutical development of medicinal herbs from Chinese medicine, *Public Health Nutr.*, 3, 515, 2000.

Nelson, L. and Perrone, J., Herbal and alternative medicine, *Emerg. Med. Clin. North Am.*, 18, 709, 2000.

Palmer, M.E. et al., Adverse events associated with dietary supplements: an observational study, *Lancet,* 361, 101, 2003.

Perharic, L. et al., Toxicological problems resulting from exposure to traditional remedies and food supplements, *Drug Saf.*, 11, 284, 1994.

Perharic, L., Shaw, D. and Murray, V., Toxic effects of herbal medicines and food supplements, *Lancet,* 342, 180, 1993.

Shaw, D. et al., Traditional remedies and food supplements. A 5-year toxicological study (1991–1995), *Drug Saf.*, 17, 342, 1997.

Part III

Toxicity of Nontherapeutic Agents

22 Alcohols and Aldehydes

Zhuoxiao Cao, Yunbo Li, and Michael A. Trush

Alcohols are carbon compounds containing hydroxyl groups (–OH). Alcohols are common types of chemicals, and exposure to alcohols can cause diverse biological effects, either indirectly through metabolic products or directly through the parent molecules. Ethanol, methanol, and isopropanol are the important alcohols due to their wide availability. These alcohols are able to induce toxicity both in animals and humans. Chemically, carbon chains with carbonyl groups (H–C=O) are classified as aldehydes. Among the aldehydes, formaldehyde is ubiquitously distributed in the environment. Human exposure to this chemical has received considerable attention due to its established carcinogenicity and developmental toxicity in laboratory animals. Accordingly, this chapter will focus on the clinical toxicology of ethanol, methanol, isopropanol, and formaldehyde.

22.1 ETHANOL

Ethanol (ethyl alcohol) has been produced from fermented grain, fruit juice, and honey for thousands of years. The presence of ethanol in wine, beer, and liquor and the use of it as a common solvent make it widely available to adults. The consumption and abuse of ethanol is not only a serious public health problem but also one of the major social problems, especially in Western countries.

22.1.1 CHEMICAL CHARACTERISTICS

Ethanol is a colorless aliphatic hydrocarbon molecule. This weakly polar molecule is both water and lipid soluble. The average apparent volume of distribution (V_d) of ethanol is about 0.6 l/kg, which is nearly equivalent to that of water. Ethanol diffuses across cell membranes easily and is absorbed from the gastrointestinal (GI) tract rapidly. As such, ethanol is able to distribute throughout the body. It penetrates the blood brain barrier and placenta and exerts its effects on most organ systems. Because oxidation of ethanol yields 7.1 kcal/g, sufficient calories can be obtained from ethanol alone for chronic drinkers if the daily intake of ethanol exceeds 5 g/kg of body weight. However, malnourishment can occur in chronic drinkers due to the absence of other important nutrients, which are present in a normal, complete diet.

22.1.2 TOXICOKINETICS

The absorption of ethanol from the GI tract is within 30 to 60 min after its ingestion. The stomach extracts about 20%, with the remainder of absorption occurring in the

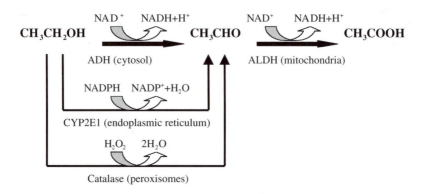

FIGURE 22.1 Metabolic pathways of ethanol.

small intestine. The absorption of ethanol from the GI tract may be delayed by various factors, including coingested food, drugs, and medical conditions that inhibit gastric emptying. After it enters the portal vein, ethanol first passes through the liver before it distributes to the rest of the body. More than 90% of the ingested ethanol is oxidized to acetaldehyde by liver and gastric mucosal cells; 5 to 10% is excreted unchanged by kidneys, lungs, and sweat. Oxidation of ethanol to acetaldehyde occurs predominantly in the liver by alcohol dehydrogenase (ADH). In addition, hepatic cytochrome P450, principally the isoform 2E1 (CYP2E1) in endoplasmic reticulum, and catalase in peroxisomes, are also able to catalyze the oxidation of ethanol to acetaldehyde. The acetaldehyde formed is further converted to acetate via the action of aldehyde dehydrogenase (ALDH) present in liver mitochondria (Figure 22.1).

Generally, women have a higher peak ethanol concentration than men if exposed to the same amount of ethanol, due to their lower body water content and the lower level of ADH in gastric mucosal cells. ADH, ALDH, and CYP2E1 exhibit genetic polymorphisms. Polymorphisms of these alcohol-metabolizing enzymes may lead to alterations in the ethanol elimination rate. For example, some Asian people have a facial flushing reaction when they drink alcohol, which is caused by the lower efficiency of their ALDH, leading to accumulated acetaldehyde in blood. In addition, polymorphisms of ethanol-metabolizing enzymes may influence the susceptibility to ethanol-induced diseases such as pancreatitis, liver cirrhosis and esophageal cancer. The average rate of ethanol metabolism in adults is 100 to 125 mg/kg/h in occasional drinkers, and can be up to 175 mg/kg/h in chronic drinkers. For medium-sized adults, the blood ethanol level drops at an average rate of 15 to 20 mg/dl/h.

22.1.3 CALCULATION OF BLOOD ALCOHOL CONCENTRATIONS (BAC)

Estimation of the blood concentrations of ethanol provides useful information regarding the severity of its intoxication. BAC can be calculated according to the following equation, where V_d is the apparent volume of distribution.

$$BAC \text{ (mg/dl)} = [\text{amount of ethanol ingested (mg)}/V_d \text{ (l/kg)}] \times \text{body weight (kg)} \times 10$$

22.1.4 Mechanisms of Toxicity

22.1.4.1 General Mechanisms of Toxicity

A multifactorial setting is responsible for the mechanisms of ethanol's toxic effects on individuals. The liver, nervous, gastrointestinal (GI), and cardiovascular (CV) systems are the principal targets of ethanol toxicity. Several cellular processes have been proposed to be crucially involved in ethanol-induced toxicity:

1. Ethanol directly affects cell membrane fluidity and modifies membrane proteins, which may result in alterations in the liquid-crystal state of membranes, membrane ion transport (i.e., Na^+ channel), transmembrane signal transduction (i.e., N-methyl-D-aspartate receptor), and activities of intrinsic membrane enzymes (i.e., Na^+-K^+-ATPase).

2. Recently, substantial evidence suggests that free radicals and reactive oxygen species (ROS) may contribute significantly to ethanol-induced toxicity. Metabolism of ethanol by microsomal enzymes, especially CYP2E1, has been shown to result in the formation of 1-hydroxyethyl radicals. Alternatively, induction of CYP2E1 by ethanol has been repeatedly demonstrated to lead to the increased production of ROS, including superoxide, hydrogen peroxide, and hydroxyl radicals. In this context, among various microsomal enzymes, CYP2E1 is an effective producer of ROS, possibly due to the high rate of electron leakage of the enzyme. The above reactive species, generated either from the metabolism of ethanol or the ethanol-induced CYP2E1, are able to attack important biomolecules, including lipids, proteins and nucleic acids, leading to oxidative cell injury.

3. Ethanol toxicity is also attributable to the formation of phosphatidylethanol (PE), a unique phospholipid formed in cell membranes in the presence of ethanol. The reaction is catalyzed by phospholipase D, an enzyme that normally catalyzes the hydrolysis of phospholipids, leading to the formation of phosphatidic acid. However, phospholipase D can also utilize ethanol as a substrate, resulting in the formation of the phosphatidylethanol. In view of the critical roles played by phospholipase D and phosphatidic acid in a number of cell signal transduction pathways, formation of phosphatidylethanol may be an important mechanism by which ethanol interferes with cell signaling, leading to cell dysfunction. In addition, the PE accumulated in membranes may also cause direct effects on the functions of cell membranes. Thus, both the inhibition of phospholipase D-mediated signal transduction and the accumulation of PE in membranes represent possible pathways through which ethanol may disturb cell function.

4. Fatty acid ethyl esters (FAEEs) produced from conjugations of ethanol and fatty acids are also implicated in ethanol-mediated toxicity in various organs, including heart, brain, pancreas, and liver. The synthesis of FAEEs from ethanol is catalyzed by FAEE synthase, a widely distributed enzyme. FAEEs have been shown to be cytotoxic species. Due to their lipophilicity,

FAEEs accumulate in cell membranes and are able to alter the properties of cell membranes and membrane-associated proteins. FAEEs may also accumulate in mitochondria, resulting in impaired mitochondrial oxidative phosphorylation.

5. Mitochondrial dysfunction is an important mechanism of ethanol-induced toxicity. Ethanol can change the permeability of inner mitochondrial membrane and may inhibit the expression of some components of the mitochondrial electron transport chain (METC), such as NADH dehydrogenase and cytochrome c oxidase, promoting ROS formation and resulting in decreased ATP synthesis. Moreover, ethanol may decrease mitochondrial glutathione levels and, as such, make them more vulnerable to the oxidative stress. ROS can cause damage to mitochondrial DNA and alteration of the METC, which further increases ROS production from the defective METC in the cells, leading to a vicious cycle of accumulating cell damage.

22.1.4.2 Mechanisms of Organ-Specific Toxicity

The liver is the most important target organ of ethanol-induced toxicity, especially chronic ethanol intoxication. The increased NADH level resulting from ethanol oxidation not only reduces gluconeogenesis but also accelerates triglyceride synthesis from free fatty acids, which leads to an accumulation of fat in the liver parenchyma. Ethanol stimulates release of endotoxin by Gram-negative bacteria in the gut, which has also been implicated in the ethanol-induced liver toxicity. Endotoxin is absorbed from the gut and enters the liver through the hepatic portal vein. Inside the liver, endotoxin activates Kupffer cells, resulting in release of the cytotoxic ROS and a number of cytokines, including tumor necrosis factor-α, interleukins, and prostaglandins. These cytokines can elicit inflammatory responses that may further lead to hepatic injury. Another mechanism of ethanol hepatotoxicity is through the formation of acetaldehyde. Acetaldehyde interacts with diverse cellular macromolecules, leading to the formation of protein adducts and enzyme inactivation. Moreover, acetaldehyde promotes GSH depletion, free-radical-mediated toxicity, and lipid peroxidation. Acetaldehyde has also been shown to stimulate collagen synthesis by liver stellate cells, which might be involved in the pathogenesis of ethanol-induced liver cirrhosis.

Central Nervous System (CNS) — Ethanol is a CNS depressant. Numerous different types of ion channels in CNS are important targets of ethanol, including ligand-gated, G-protein-regulated, and voltage-sensitive channels. The effects of ethanol on CNS are primarily attributed to the alteration of neurotransmission, including glutamate and GABA. Glutamate and GABA are major excitatory and inhibitory neurotransmitters in CNS. Acute ethanol exposure was shown to augment the GABA action at ligand-gated GABA$_A$ receptors. Excitatory glutamate receptors are classified into the NMDA and nonNMDA receptors. In addition to the activation of GABA receptors, ethanol inhibits the activation of NMDA glutamate receptors that are involved in cognition such as learning and memory.

Cardiovascular System — Ethanol-induced cardiotoxicity may involve several factors. Ethanol or its metabolite, acetaldehyde, may alter the myocardial stores of catecholamines and decrease the synthesis of cardiac contractile protein, leading to a depression of myocardial contractility. Ethanol may also have adverse effects on cardiac conduction (i.e., prolonged QT interval and ventricular repolarization) and cause cardiac arrhythmias.

GI Tract — Ingestion of ethanol impairs the mucosal barrier directly and increases gastric and pancreatic secretion. In addition, FAEEs may play a major role in the disposition of ethanol in the pancreas and the development of pancreatitis. In this regard, the enzyme that catalyzes the formation of FAEEs (i.e., FAEE synthase), was found to have the highest activity in the pancreas.

22.1.5 Clinical Manifestations of Acute Toxicity

In the U.S., the level for ethanol intoxication is defined as 80 to 100 mg/dl in most of the states, and 400 mg/dl is the average lethal blood concentration. For chronic drinkers who become tolerant to the effects of ethanol, the corresponding concentrations to elicit the same degree of toxicity might be much higher than those for casual drinkers. The clinical manifestations of acute intoxication include sedation and relief of anxiety, reduced tension and coordination, impaired concentration and reaction time, tachycardia, and more severely, slurred speech, ataxia, and altered emotions. At high concentrations, it can cause breathing difficulties. Consumption of very large amounts of ethanol (>300 mg/dl) can produce metabolic and toxic coma that presents clinically as muscular hypotonia, respiratory depression, hypotension, and hypothermia. Clinical laboratory testing reveals hypoglycemia, ketosis, and electrolyte derangements in patients with severe ethanol intoxication.

22.1.6 Management of Acute Intoxication

The severity of acute alcohol intoxication is the basis for treatment, which is dependent on the blood ethanol concentration, the rising rapidity of ethanol level, and the duration of its high blood level. In the management of acute ethanol intoxication, the crucial goal is to prevent the severe respiratory depression and the pulmonary aspiration of vomitus that occurs. Respiratory and cardiovascular systems must be supported by protecting airway and establishing ventilatory and circulatory assistance. Glucose is administered to treat the hypoglycemia and ketosis. An electrolyte solution should be given to alcoholic patients who are vomiting and dehydrated. Severe vomiting causes the loss of potassium; thus supplementation of potassium is required if renal function is to remain normal. Moreover, for chronic drinkers, nutrients such as thiamine, folate, and magnesium should be given. Other strategies, including hemodialysis and gastric decontamination, have limited efficacy in the management of ethanol intoxication. Usually BAC falls at an average rate of 15 to 20 mg/dl/h. Most patients can recover with clinically supportive care.

22.1.7 Clinical Manifestations of Chronic Toxicity

Long-term consumption of ethanol impairs almost all of the organ systems (Table 22.1). It should be noted that alcoholics have a nearly two times higher risk of death than that of nondrinkers, due to alcoholic liver cirrhosis, infections, accidents, cancers, and cardiovascular diseases.

TABLE 22.1
Major Systemic Effects of Chronic Ethanol Consumption

Liver	Steatosis
	Alcoholic hepatitis
	Cirrhosis
	Liver cancer
Cardiovascular System	Alcoholic cardiomyopathy
	Cardiac arrhythmias
	Hypertension
Central Nervous System	Wernicke-Korsakoff syndrome
	Dementia
	Tolerance, dependence and withdrawal
Gastrointestinal System	Esophagitis
	Gastritis
	Malabsorption
	Pancreatitis
	Cancer of mouth, pharynx, and esophagus
Endocrine and Metabolic Systems	Hypoglycemia
	Alcoholic Ketoacidosis
	Hypomagnesemia
	Hypokalemia
	Malnutrition
	Gynecomastia
	Menstrual cycle abnormalities
Reproductive System	Hypogonadism
	Impotence
	Infertility
Hematologic System	Iron, folate, B_{12} deficiency anemias
	Leukopenia

Nervous System — Chronic use of ethanol profoundly affects the central and peripheral nervous system. Chronic alcoholic patients may be detected with damage to the frontal lobes of the brain, brain shrinkage, and an increase in the size of ventricles. Wernicke-Korsakoff syndrome resulting from alcohol abuse is classically characterized by a triad of paralysis of external eye muscles, cerebellar ataxia, and mental confusion, but the full clinical presentation is rarely encountered. It is thought to be associated with thiamine deficiency due to reduced thiamine (vitamin B1) absorption in alcoholics. Wernicke's encephalopathy is the acute phase of this disease, with longer duration of the confusional state in comparison to acute ethanol intoxication. Administration of thiamine alleviates the ataxia, ocular signs, and confusion; however, a memory deficit, known as Korsakoff psychosis, may be still present. Moreover, ethanol may cause bilateral and symmetrical visual impairment because of optic nerve degeneration.

Peripheral nerve damage is also an important characteristic of chronic ethanol intoxication. Ethanol-related neuropathy, especially when subclinical, seems to be frequent and mostly characterized by axonal degeneration of peripheral nerve fibers, with earlier and more frequent involvement of sensory fibers and lower limbs. It usually begins with symmetrical paresthesias of hands and feet.

Liver — Liver disease is the most frequent clinical complication of chronic ethanol abuse. About 90% of chronic drinkers have fatty liver that is characterized by the abnormal accumulation of triglycerides in hepatocytes. While fatty liver is reversible, it may develop into alcoholic hepatitis, cirrhosis, or liver cancer. Alcoholic hepatitis refers to hepatocyte degeneration and necrosis. Clinically, patients may present with nausea, vomiting, jaundice, abdominal pain, and hepatosplenomegaly. Alcoholic cirrhosis, characterized by fibroblastic proliferation and the production of connective tissue in the periportal and centrilobular regions, is the most common type of cirrhosis in North America. The amount and the duration of ethanol consumption are highly correlated with the development of liver diseases. Moreover, concurrent infection with hepatitis B or C viruses aggravates the progress of liver diseases in alcoholics.

GI Tract — Long-term ingestion of ethanol increases the occurrence of gastritis and pancreatitis and causes intestine injury, leading to vitamin deficiencies, diarrhea, and loss of weight. In addition to liver cancer, alcoholism may also be associated with the development of cancer of the tongue, oral cavity, pharynx, larynx, or esophagus.

Cardiovascular System — Chronic heavy alcohol intake can result in dilated cardiomyopathy with ventricular hypertrophy and fibrosis. It may also induce atrial and ventricular arrhythmias. In addition, chronic consumption of ethanol, especially in large amounts, is associated with an increased incidence of hypertension.

Other Systems — Chronic alcoholics may also develop reproductive disorders, fluid disorders and electrolyte derangements, and hematologic disorders (Table 22.1). Alcoholics have a higher rate of infection, particularly respiratory infections (i.e., pneumonia and tuberculosis).

22.1.8 MANAGEMENT OF CHRONIC INTOXICATION

The most common approach to prevent and treat ethanol-related diseases is to maintain abstinence by the administration of drugs that interfere with ethanol metabolism.

Disulfiram — Disulfiram (tetraethylthiuram) is the most commonly used drug to deter drinking. Disulfiram is an inhibitor of aldehyde dehydrogenase. It causes the accumulation of acetaldehyde, which elicits extreme discomfort soon after the intake of ethanol, including flushing, throbbing, headache, nausea, vomiting, sweating, hypotension, and confusion. Although disulfiram is rapidly absorbed, it has little effect in nondrinkers. It takes about 12 h to exert its full effect. This drug is long-lasting (a few days) due to its slow elimination. Administration of disulfiram should begin at least 24 h after patients have been free of ethanol. Disulfiram inhibits the metabolism of other therapeutic agents such as phenytoin, isoniazid, and oral anticoagulants. Compliance is often a problem with disulfiram treatment. Additionally, the drug may influence liver function and cause mild alterations in liver function tests. Due to poor compliance and side effects, disulfiram is becoming less favored in alcoholism therapy.

Naltrexone — Naltexone works as an opioid receptor antagonist with high oral availability and a long duration of action. It was approved by the FDA for alcoholism treatment in 1994. Animal research and clinical experience indicate that there is a link between alcohol consumption and opioids. Opioids may increase the craving for ethanol, while opioid receptor antagonists can reduce the urge to drink and decrease ethanol intake. Typically, naltrexone should be administrated in conjunction with psychosocial therapy. The major side effects of naltrexone are nausea, dizziness, and headache. These appear more commonly in women than in men. Considering that an overdose of naltrexone can cause severe liver damage, acute hepatitis and liver failure are contraindications of naltrexone administration. In contrast to disulfiram, naltrexone has good compliance in alcoholism therapy. Due to the potential hepatotoxicity for both drugs, the combination of naltrexone and disulfiram should be avoided.

Nalmefene — Nalmefene is a promising opioid antagonist in preliminary clinical tests. It has some advantages over naltrexone, including greater oral availability, longer duration of action, and lack of dose-dependent liver toxicity.

Other Drugs — In addition to the opioid system, the glutamate, serotonergic, and dopaminergic neurotransmitter systems might be also involved in the regulation of ethanol consumption. For example, acamprosate, a competitive inhibitor of the NMDA receptor, can decrease the rate of relapse and enhance the duration of abstinence. Buspirone, a serotonin receptor antagonist, fluoxetine, a serotonin reuptake inhibitor, and antagonists of D1 and D2 dopamine receptors are being studied as new agents for treating alcoholism. In addition to pharmacotherapy, magnesium, potassium phosphate, multivitamins, and folate should be administrated to alcoholics to correct the hypomagnesemia, hypophosphatemia, hypokalemia, and vitamin deficiency associated with chronic alcohol abuse.

22.1.9 FETAL ALCOHOL SYNDROME (FAS)

FAS is the most common preventable cause of mental retardation and congenital malformation in humans. It is estimated that FAS affects 4000 infants per year in the U.S., and an additional 7000 cases show fetal alcohol effects. The typical features of FAS include retarded body growth, craniofacial abnormalities, and CNS dysfunction. The mechanism underlying the teratogenic effects caused by chronic ethanol abuse remains uncertain.

22.1.10 TOLERANCE, DEPENDENCE, AND WITHDRAWAL

Tolerance refers to the situation where a higher dose of ethanol is required to elicit the same behavioral or physiological response. **Dependence** is defined as a compulsive desire to avoid the appearance of withdrawal syndrome when ethanol ingestion is ceased. **Withdrawal syndrome** consists of sleep disruption, anxiety, sweating, tremors, even seizures and hallucinations. It is thought that the development of tolerance to ethanol involves complex mechanisms and occurs in part via the induction of alcohol-metabolizing enzymes. Downregulation of the GABA-mediated response and upregulation of NMDA receptor function appear to account for the CNS hyperexcitability in ethanol withdrawal.

22.1.11 Methods of Detection

To detect and quantify ethanol, many methods have been established. Blood alcohol levels can be determined accurately by immunoassay or gas chromatography in most hospitals, but it takes longer to obtain these results than from other methods. An electrochemical meter has been applied to test alcohol concentration in venous blood, and this method has high sensitivity but poor specificity. Breath alcohol analyzers are widely used as alcohol screening tools, especially by law-enforcement agencies. This test is performed by microprocessors and infrared spectral analysis with good accuracy and precision. To sample the breath of unconscious patients, breath-alcohol devices with mouth cups and nasal tubes should be used. Another method to determine ethanol exposure is the fatty acid ethyl esters (FAEEs) test. This test is highly sensitive and works as a hallmark of recent ethanol use since FAEEs can be detected even after ethanol is completely metabolized.

22.2 METHANOL

Methanol (methyl alcohol) is readily available at variable concentrations in numerous industrial and household products, including windshield washer fluid. It is also used in the manufacture of formaldehyde and methyl tert-butyl ether. Exposure to methanol commonly occurs in the workplace and household. In addition, methanol may be intentionally ingested by alcoholics.

22.2.1 Toxicokinetics

Methanol is absorbed via the skin, GI, and respiratory routes. When ingested, peak levels of methanol in blood occur within 30 to 60 min. Methanol is oxidized to formaldehyde by ADH in liver, which in turn is converted to formate via the action of formaldehyde dehydrogenase. Formation of formate is largely responsible for the toxicity of methanol. Formate can be eliminated by formyl-tetrahydrofolate-synthetase (formyl-THF-synthetase) by combining with tetrahydrofolate (THF) to form 10-formyl-THF. This is then converted to carbon dioxide by the catalytic action of formyl-THF-dehydrogenase (F-THF-DH). The elimination half-life of formate is about 3.5 h. Ethanol and the ADH inhibitor, fomepizole can competitively inhibit the metabolism of methanol by ADH, thus delaying its elimination. The metabolic pathway of methanol is illustrated in Figure 22.2.

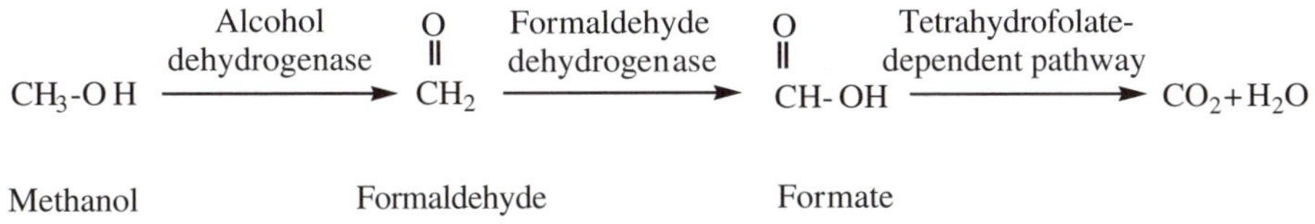

FIGURE 22.2 Metabolism of methanol.

22.2.2 MECHANISMS OF TOXICITY

Most of the toxic effects of methanol are attributed to the formation of formate. Formate inhibits the mitochondrial cytochrome c oxidase complex and concomitantly decreases ATP production, resulting in increased anaerobic glycolysis and production of lactate. The accumulation of formate and lactate causes systemic acidosis, which facilitates the formation of nonionized formate, leading to its increased cellular accumulation and cytotoxic effects. In addition, production of hydroxyl radicals and induction of lipid peroxidation may also be implicated in the cellular damage induced by methanol intoxication. Ocular tissues such as optic nerve and retina are more susceptible to the toxicity of formate, probably because the retina is able to metabolize methanol to formate. Histologically, the optic nerve and retina edema occurs in methanol intoxication.

22.2.3 CLINICAL MANIFESTATIONS OF ACUTE INTOXICATION

Methanol primarily affects the nervous, ocular, and GI systems. While intoxication symptoms appear within a few hours after methanol intake, they can be delayed more than 30 h due to varied individual response and/or coingestion of ethanol.

Ocular — Among the symptoms induced by methanol, the most typical clinical presentation is visual disturbance, including blurred vision, visual hallucination, and even visual loss. Upon eye examinations, retinal edema, visual field constriction, and nonreactive pupils might be found in patients.

Nervous System — Methanol may elicit various and nonspecific neurological manifestations, such as headache, dizziness, bradycardia, impaired consciousness, seizures, and even coma.

Others — Methanol-mediated effects on the GI system may include abdominal pain, diarrhea, GI hemorrhage, and pancreatitis. Systemic acidosis induced by methanol intoxication may also increase the respiratory rate and cause Kussmaul respiration in severe cases.

22.2.4 MANAGEMENT OF ACUTE INTOXICATION

General Supportive Care — Respiratory support, cardiac monitoring and circulatory assistance should be established. Sedative agents such as phenobarbital should be administrated to patients with seizures.

Antidote Therapy — Ethanol and the ADH inhibitor, fomepizole, are used as antidotes in methanol intoxication. They effectively block the metabolism of methanol and reduce its toxic effects. As such, the antidote should be given i.v. to all patients with methanol intoxication. The use of ethanol may cause CNS depression and hypoglycemia, and its dose is not easily manipulated. However, fomepizole has great efficacy and fewer side effects than ethanol; hence it is the favored antidote in the treatment of methanol intoxication.

Correction of Acidosis — Sodium bicarbonate may be administrated i.v. to ameliorate metabolic acidosis, especially in severe cases.

Others — If the blood concentration of methanol is higher than 50 mg/dl, hemodialysis should be carried out to enhance its elimination. Moreover, folinic acid (leucovorin) can be given i.v. to facilitate the elimination of formate.

22.3 ISOPROPANOL

Isopropanol (isopropyl alcohol) is a colorless and volatile alcohol with fruity odor and a slight bitter taste. It is present in rubbing alcohol, industrial solvents, paints, disinfectants, and drugs. It may be ingested accidentally by nonalcoholics and intentionally by alcoholics.

22.3.1 TOXICOKINETICS

Isopropanol can enter the body by ingestion, inhalation of the vapors, or through the skin. GI absorption is a major route of exposure leading to toxicity, while inhalational or dermal absorption may also elicit toxic effects. Blood isopropanol reaches peak levels 30 min after ingestion. It is metabolized by hepatic ADH, and 80% is converted to acetone (Figure 22.3). Acetone is excreted primarily through the renal route (20% being excreted unchanged), and a small amount through lungs, saliva, and gastric juices. The range of elimination half-life for isopropanol is 2.5 to 6.6 h and 10 to 31 h for acetone. Because acetone cannot be further converted to an acid, isopropanol intoxication is not considered to cause metabolic acidosis.

22.3.2 MECHANISMS OF TOXICITY

Studies on mechanisms of isopropanol-induced toxicity are lacking in the literature. The principal toxic effect of isopropanol is CNS depression that is twice as potent as ethanol. In this context, acetone, the by-product of isopropanol, is a potent central nervous system depressant.

22.3.3 CLINICAL MANIFESTATIONS OF ACUTE TOXICITY

The presentation of CNS depression with isopropanol intoxication includes inebriation with drowsiness, poor balance, staggering gait, slurred speech, and poor coordination, as well as sweating, stupor, coma, and even death due to respiratory depression. GI responses such as nausea, vomiting, and abdominal pain and hemorrhage into the bronchi and the chest cavity may occur. In addition, the patient may have a distinct odor of acetone. In severe intoxication, CV compromise may occur, including myocardial depression and severe hypotension. Less common presentations include renal tubular necrosis, hemolytic anemia, acute myopathy, and hypothermia. For young children with isopropanol ingestion, irritability, hypotonia, and seizures may be indicators of intoxication.

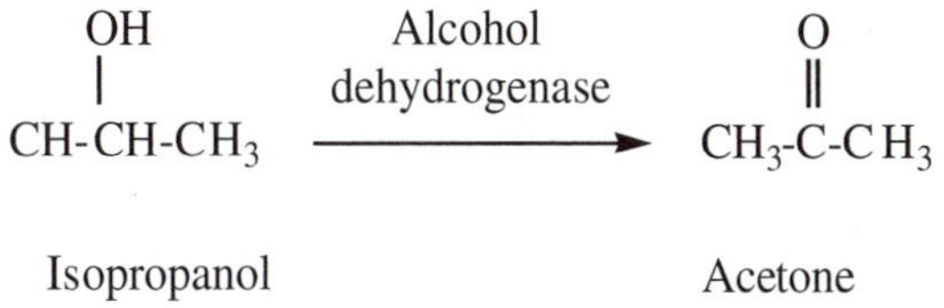

FIGURE 22.3 Metabolism of isopropanol.

22.3.4 MANAGEMENT OF ACUTE INTOXICATION

Respiratory support and cardiac monitoring are required in the treatment of isopropanol toxicity. For respiratory depressed patients, endotracheal intubation and ventilatory support should be applied. For severe intoxication, gastric lavage and hemodialysis may be useful to remove the isopropanol.

22.4 FORMALDEHYDE

Formaldehyde is a nearly colorless gas with a pungent odor. It dissolves easily in water and is found in formalin (a formaldehyde solution containing water) and methanol (wood alcohol). Formaldehyde is used as a preservative, a hardening and reducing agent, a corrosion inhibitor, and a sterilizing agent. It is also found in glues, pressed wood products, foam insulation, and a wide variety of molded or extruded plastic items. Indoor sources include permanent press fabrics, carpets, pesticide formulations, and cardboard and paper products. Outdoor sources include emissions from fuel combustion, oil refining processes, and environmental tobacco smoke.

22.4.1 TOXICOKINETICS

Formaldehyde can enter the body by inhalation, ingestion, or skin contact. Formaldehyde is readily absorbed via the respiratory and GI routes. Dermal absorption of formaldehyde appears to be very slight. Absorbed formaldehyde is metabolized quickly to formate by a glutathione-dependent formaldehyde dehydrogenase. Formate can either be further converted to carbon dioxide as described in Section 22.2.1 or can enter the one-carbon cycle, incorporated as a methyl group into nucleic acids and proteins. Metabolites of formaldehyde are mainly excreted through respiratory and renal routes.

22.4.2 MECHANISMS OF TOXICITY

Formaldehyde can cause multiorgan toxicity upon either acute or chronic exposure. Acute toxicity is largely attributable to its irritating and corrosive properties. The mechanisms underlying formaldehyde-induced chronic toxicity remain to be elucidated. The binding of formaldehyde to endogenous proteins may result in the formation of neoantigens. Such neoantigens may elicit an immune response that might account for the occurrence of asthma and other health complaints associated with formaldehyde exposure. In this regard, long-term exposure to formaldehyde is associated with the formation of formaldehyde-albumin adducts, autoantibodies, and immune activation in patients occupationally exposed, or residents of mobile homes or homes containing particleboard sub-flooring. In addition, formaldehyde has been shown to cause cancer, especially nasal cancer in laboratory animals. The carcinogenicity of formaldehyde may be due to its high reactivity with DNA. However, its carcinogenicity in humans remains to be established. Formaldehyde may also cause genotoxicity in humans. For example, a higher frequency of the DNA-protein crosslinks (DPCs) and sister chromatid exchanges (SCEs) was observed in peripheral-blood lymphocytes of workers occupationally exposed to formaldehyde, as compared to unexposed workers. It appears unlikely that formaldehyde reaches concentrations sufficient to cause reproductive and developmental damages in humans, due to its rapid metabolism.

22.4.3 CLINICAL MANIFESTATIONS OF ACUTE INTOXICATION

Formaldehyde primarily affects the mucous membranes of the upper airways and eyes. The manifestations include watery eyes, burning sensations in the eyes and throat, nausea, wheezing, coughing, chest tightness, and difficulty in breathing at elevated levels (above 0.1 ppm). Drinking formalin can cause severe burns to the throat and stomach, and as little as 30 ml of formalin can cause death.

22.4.4 MANAGEMENT OF ACUTE INTOXICATION

There is no antidote for formaldehyde poisoning. Supportive care constitutes the primary management of patients with acute formaldehyde intoxication. With supportive care, most patients fully recover.

REFERENCES

SUGGESTED READINGS

Ford, M.D. et al., *Clinical Toxicology,* W.B. Saunders Company, Philadelphia, 2001, chap. 74, 93, and 94.

Goldfrank, L.R. et al., *Goldfrank's Toxicologic Emergencies,* 6th ed., Appleton & Lange, Stamford, CT, 1998, chap. 62.

Harsman, J.G. and Limbird, L.E., *Goodman & Gilman's The Pharmacological Basis of Therapeutics,* 10th ed., McGraw-Hill, New York, 2001, chap. 18.

Katzung, B.G., *Basic & Clinical Pharmacology,* 8th ed., McGraw-Hill, New York, 2001, chap. 23.

Williams, P.L., James, R.C., and Roberts, S.M., *Principles of Toxicology,* 2nd ed., John Wiley & Sons, Inc., New York, 2000, chap. 16.

REVIEW ARTICLES

Agarwal, D.P., Genetic polymorphisms of alcohol metabolizing enzymes, *Pathol. Biol.,* 49, 703, 2001.

Ansari, G.A., Kaphalia, B.S., and Khan, M.F., Fatty acid conjugates of xenobiotics, *Toxicol. Lett.,* 75, 1, 1995.

Baker, R.C. and Kramer, R.E., Cytotoxicity of short-chain alcohols, *Annu. Rev. Pharmacol. Toxicol.,* 39, 127, 1999.

Barceloux, D.G. et al., American Academy of Clinical Toxicology practice guidelines on the treatment of methanol poisoning, *J. Toxicol. Clin. Toxicol.,* 40, 415, 2002.

Beckemeier, M.E. and Bora, P.S., Fatty acid ethyl esters: potentially toxic products of myocardial ethanol metabolism, *J. Mol. Cell Cardiol.,* 30, 2487, 1998.

Collins, J.J. et al., A review of adverse pregnancy outcomes and formaldehyde exposure in human and animal studies, *Regul. Toxicol. Pharmacol.,* 34, 17, 2001.

Cowan, J.M., Jr. et al., Determination of volume of distribution for ethanol in male and female subjects, *J. Anal. Toxicol.,* 20, 287, 1996.

Daniel, D.R., McAnalley, B.H., and Garriott, J.C., Isopropyl alcohol metabolism after acute intoxication in humans, *J Anal Toxicol.,* 5, 110, 1981.

Garner, C.D. et al., Role of retinal metabolism in methanol-induced retinal toxicity, *J. Toxicol. Environ. Health,* 44, 43, 1995.

Henderson, G.I., Chen, J.J., and Schenker, S., Ethanol, oxidative stress, reactive aldehydes, and the fetus, *Front. Biosci.,* 4, D541, 1999.

Hoek, J.B., Cahill, A., and Pastorino, J.G., Alcohol and mitochondria: a dysfunctional relationship, *Gastroenterology,* 122, 2049, 2002.

Hoek, J.B. and Pastorino, J.G., Ethanol, oxidative stress, and cytokine-induced liver cell injury, *Alcohol,* 27, 63, 2002.

Johnson, B.A. and Ait-Daoud, N., Neuropharmacological treatments for alcoholism: scientific basis and clinical findings, *Psychopharmacology,* 149, 327, 2000.

Kaphalia, B.S. and Ansari, G.A., Fatty acid ethyl esters and ethanol-induced pancreatitis, *Cell Mol. Biol.,* 47, 173, 2001.

Kril, J.J. and Halliday, G.M., Brain shrinkage in alcoholics: a decade on and what have we learned? *Prog. Neurobiol.,* 58, 381, 1999.

Lang, C.H. et al., Alcohol myopathy: impairment of protein synthesis and translation initiation, *Int. J. Biochem. Cell Biol.,* 33, 457, 2001.

Liesivuori, J. and Savolainen, H., Methanol and formic acid toxicity: biochemical mechanisms, *Pharmacol. Toxicol.,* 69, 157, 1991.

Patel, V.B. et al., The effects of alcohol on the heart, *Adverse Drug React. Toxicol. Rev.,* 16, 15, 1997.

Ramchandani, V.A., Bosron, W.F., and Li, T.K., Research advances in ethanol metabolism, *Pathol. Biol.,* 49, 676, 2001.

Sanghani, P.C. et al., Kinetic mechanism of human glutathione-dependent formaldehyde dehydrogenase, *Biochemistry,* 39, 10720, 2000.

Sherman, D.I. and Williams, R., Liver damage: mechanisms and management, *Br. Med. Bull.,* 50, 124, 1994.

Song, B.J., Ethanol-inducible cytochrome P450 (CYP2E1): biochemistry, molecular biology and clinical relevance: 1996 update, *Alcohol Clin. Exp. Res.,* 20, 138A, 1996.

Szabo, G., Consequences of alcohol consumption on host defense, *Alcohol,* 34, 830, 1999.

Thrasher, J.D., Broughton, A., and Madison, R., Immune activation and autoantibodies in humans with long-term inhalation exposure to formaldehyde, *Arch. Environ. Health,* 45, 217, 1990.

Wax, P.M., Hoffman, R.S., and Goldfrank, L.R., Rapid quantitative determination of blood alcohol concentration in the emergency department using an electrochemical method, *Ann. Emerg. Med.,* 21, 254, 1992.

Zachman, R.D. and Grummer, M.A., The interaction of ethanol and vitamin A as a potential mechanism for the pathogenesis of Fetal Alcohol syndrome, *Alcohol Clin Exp Res.,* 22, 1544, 1998.

23 Gases

23.1 INTRODUCTION

Pulmonary irritants, simple asphyxiants, toxic products of combustion, lacrimating agents, and chemical asphyxiants constitute a diverse group of toxic gases capable of causing a variety of local and pulmonary reactions. The sources of these compounds are as varied, encompassing both naturally occurring and synthetic chemicals developed over the last 50 years. In addition, exposures to the gases are encountered *accidentally*, at home or in the workplace with industrial products, as environmental hazards, or *intentionally*, as commercial sprays for individual protection, for law enforcement, or as potential bioterrorist weapons. The most common routes of exposure to these agents occurs through oral ingestion, local dermal or mucous membrane contact, or deep inhalation. Because of their seemingly unrelated chemical structures and properties, the gases are classified principally according to the clinical effects and metabolic consequences of exposure.

Physiologically, the respiratory system is composed of (1) the upper respiratory tract (URT), consisting of the nasal and oral cavities, pharynx, and larynx and (2) the lower respiratory tract (LRT), namely the trachea, bronchi, bronchioles, and lungs. Two main functions of the respiratory system are ventilation (inspiration and expiration of air down to the level of the alveoli) and gas exchange.* In support of these functions, the mucociliary system produces mucus. This tenacious fluid captures inhaled particles and transports them to the nasal and oral mucosa by ciliary action of epithelial cells of the URT and LRT. The cough reflex then acts to expectorate the sequestered mucus. Together, these innate reflex responses cooperate in the *clearance mechanism* of pulmonary function. For effective gas exchange, therefore, ventilation and perfusion must match closely (calculated as the *V/Q ratio*). Consequently, any alteration of the V/Q ratio, or interference with the *clearance mechanism* due to the presence of toxic gases, results in altered lung mechanics. This explains the ensuing clinical effects.

23.2 PULMONARY IRRITANTS

As the label implies, pulmonary irritants are chemicals that, when in contact with mucous membranes, produce an inflammatory response and cytotoxicity. The extent of trauma ranges from mild to severe irritation and depends on the nature of the chemical (solubility, concentration, pH). Table 23.1 lists commonly encountered

---

* Gas exchange involves the passage of gas molecules through the respiratory membranes. Oxygen diffuses from air in the alveoli, across the alveolar membranes, and into the capillary circulation. Carbon dioxide diffuses from the capillaries to the alveolar space. Gas exchange is driven by partial pressures of the gases in inspired air.

TABLE 23.1
Pulmonary Irritants: Sources, Chemical and Clinical Properties

Agent	Source	Industrial[a] or Household Uses	Chemical Properties	Acute Effects
Acrolein	Petroleum by-product, synthetic	Plastics, metals, aquatic herbicide	WS, F liquid	Local irritation, delayed pulmonary edema
Acrylonitrile	Synthetic	Acrylics, fumigant, chemical intermediate	WS, LS, F, explosive	Cyanide toxicity, skin vesiculation, dermatitis
Ammonia	Synthetic	Plastics, refrigerants, household cleaners, petroleum products	Alkaline, WS gas	Liquifaction necrosis, hemoptysis, ARDS, RADS[a]
Arsine (AsH$_3$)	Petroleum by-product	Glass, enamels, herbicides, textiles, preservative	Neutral gas, slightly WS (*garlic odor*)	Local irritation, hemolysis, renal failure, peripheral neuropathy
Carbon disulfide	Petroleum by-product, natural gas	Electroplating, degreaser, production of rayon	F liquid	Peripheral neuropathy, euphoria, restlessness, NV
Chlorine	Synthetic chemical intermediate	Bleach, chlorination of water, rubber, plastics, disinfectant	Greenish-yellow gas, oxidizing agent	Local, URT, LRT irritation
Formaldehyde	Environmental, synthetic, wood/coal smoke	Disinfectant, histological preservative (fixative)	Reducing agent, 37% gas in water	Local, URT, LRT irritation, convulsions, coma, respiratory failure
Hydrogen fluoride	Photographic film, solvents, plastics	Insecticide, bleach, metal and glass industry	Colorless gas, WS, LS	Local, URT, LRT irritation; cardiac arrhythmias

Agent	Source	Use	Properties	Clinical effects
Hydrogen sulfide	Naturally occurring, organic decomposition	Petroleum, paper industries, metallurgy	F gas (*rotten egg odor*)	Irritant and asphyxiant, respiratory paralysis; mechanism similar to CN
Metal fumes (zinc chloride)	Welding	Undesirable product of welding and metal industries	Lustrous metal, WS	Local, URT, LRT irritation (*metal fume fever*)
Nitrogen dioxide	Synthetic, photochemical smog	Chemical intermediate, nitration	Reddish-brown gas, oxidizing agent	Local, URT, LRT irritation; pulmonary edema and arrest
Nitrogen oxide	Welding, farming, explosives	Undesirable product of welding and farming industries	Oxidizing agent	Pulmonary edema, methemoglobinemia
Ozone (O_3)	Welding, sewage treatment plants, air pollution	Disinfectant, bleaching, oxidizing agent	Bluish explosive gas or liquid, oxidizing agent	Irritation, pulmonary edema, chronic respiratory disease
Phosgene	Welding	Production of solvents, plastics, pesticides	Colorless gas, poor WS	Pulmonary edema, URT irritation
Sulfur dioxide	Synthetic	Preservative, disinfectant, bleaching	Colorless gas	Local, URT irritation
Sulfur oxide	Industrial, air pollution	Bleaching, paper industry	Oxidizing agent	Bronchoconstriction, cough, chest tightness

Note: F = flammable, WS = water soluble, N = nausea, V = vomiting, LS = lipid soluble, URT = upper respiratory tract, LRT = lower respiratory tract; ARDS = adult respiratory distress syndrome.

[a] Used in manufacturing, synthesis, or as part of industrial processes; RADS, reactive airway dysfunction, develops secondary to massive, acute, accidental, high-level irritant exposure. It is manifested by persistent, nonspecific hyperreactivity.

TABLE 23.2
Presentation of Signs and Symptoms of Pulmonary Irritants Depending on Site of Exposure

Pulmonary Target	Pathological Effects
Nasal, oral, ocular mucous membranes	Local irritation: rhinitis, conjunctivitis, sneezing, coughing, lacrimation
URT: nasal and oral cavities, pharynx, larynx	Burning throat, sinusitis, laryngitis, swelling, laryngoedema, dyspnea, epistaxis
LRT: trachea, bronchi, bronchioles, lungs	Nausea, vomiting, dyspnea, bronchospasm, chest pain, bronchitis, chemical pneumonitis, epithelial denudation, intravascular thrombosis, pulmonary edema, development of secondary infections

Note: LRT = lower respiratory tract, URT = upper respiratory tract.

pulmonary irritants, sources, and major pathophysiologic effects. Presentation of signs and symptoms of exposure to pulmonary irritants, summarized in Table 23.2, appears progressively. Toxicity depends on several factors: the extent of exposure (local contact or deep inhalation), duration of exposure, degree of remedial measures (physiologic clearance, availability of treatment), and development of secondary complications (such as infections).

23.3 SIMPLE ASPHYXIANTS

23.3.1 INTRODUCTION

Unlike the pulmonary irritants or the chemical asphyxiants (described below), simple asphyxiants are nonirritating, chemically inert gases. Simple asphyxiants interfere with pulmonary function by overwhelming the oxygen concentration in inspired air. The net result is a lowered oxygen content of inspired air and decreased oxygen availability for gas exchange. The toxicity of these agents depends on the available oxygen concentration remaining.

23.3.2 GASEOUS AGENTS

The characteristics and properties of the simple asphyxiants are summarized in Table 23.3. The agents are naturally occurring atmospheric components, or are produced as products of industrial combustion. Toxic concentrations, however, are encountered in areas where the gases tend to accumulate. The acute effects and corresponding signs and symptoms of simple asphyxiants, therefore, result from replacing oxygen in inspired air with the gas, causing a decrease in oxygen concentration (Table 23.4).

Administration of therapeutic oxygen (O_2) is associated with toxicity, depending on the concentration, duration of inhalation, and the forced pressure. Respiratory asphyxiation or irritation occurs with prolonged inhalation (>24 h) of 100% O_2 at 1 atm of pressure. This concentration is capable of raising the partial pressure of

TABLE 23.3
Simple Asphyxiants, Sources, Chemical and Clinical Properties

Agent	Source	Industrial[a] or Household Uses	Chemical Properties
Carbon dioxide	Atmospheric, fermentation, mammalian metabolism, coal mines (*afterdamp*)	Carbonation, propellant, fumigation, aerosols, fire prevention	Colorless, odorless noncombustible gas heavier than air
Ethane	Petroleum by-product, constituent of natural gas	Fuel gas, refrigerant	Colorless, odorless flammable gas
Helium	Constituent of natural gas	Cryogen, lasers, welding, metal processing, carrier in GC, fill balloons and airships	Colorless, odorless nonflammable gas
Hydrogen	Electrolysis of water, action of HCl on Fe or Zn, hydrolysis of metal hydrides	Welding, chemical production, fill balloons and airships, coolant, thermonuclear reactors	Colorless, odorless flammable, explosive gas
Methane	Constituent of natural gas, action of aluminum carbide and water, coal mines (*firedamp*)	Illuminating and cooking gas, organic synthesis	Colorless, odorless flammable gas, lighter than air
Nitrogen	Atmospheric, mine gases, heating of Na azides	Inorganic synthesis, explosives, incandescent bulbs, cryogen, pharmaceutic aid	Odorless gas
Oxygen	Atmospheric, liquefaction of air	Welding, propellant, lighting, liquid fuels, therapeutic administration	Colorless, odorless gas, supports combustion
Radon (^{220}Rn)	Naturally occurring, decay product of ^{235}U	Study of chemical reactions, source of neutrons, study of radium	Radioactive isotope, α-emitter, colorless, odorless, tasteless gas
Xenon	Naturally occurring distillation/liquefaction of air	Gas lamps, leak detection systems for nuclear reactors	Colorless, odorless noncombustible tasteless gas

Note: GC = gas chromatography.

[a] Used in manufacturing, synthesis, or as part of industrial processes.

TABLE 23.4

Oxygen Concentration and Corresponding Signs and Symptoms Associated with Simple Asphyxiants

Oxygen Concentration in Inspired Air (%)	Acute Pathologic Effects
16–21 (normal)	No signs and symptoms
12–16	Tachypnea, tachycardia, muscular incoordination
10–12	Hypoxia; confusion, fatigue, dizziness
6–10	Hypoxia and decreased oxygen saturation; nausea, vomiting, lethargy, unconciousness
<6	Convulsions, apnea, cardiac arrest

oxygen (PO_2) in arterial blood to 600 mmHg.[*] Oxygen toxicity also occurs with administration of hyperbaric 100% O_2 (about 8 h at 2 atm of pressure or 1 h at 3 atm of pressure). With hyperbaric oxygen, arterial and venous plasma are at risk of complete saturation. For instance, at 2 to 3 atm of hyperbaric oxygen for 1 h, the volume percent O_2 dissolved in plasma is 6.1%; normal breathing at sea level is 0.3 to 0.5%. For these high pressures, the PO_2 increases to 1500 to 2000. At this saturation level, patients experience signs and symptoms related to O_2 apnea, i.e., sore throat, coughing, retraction of eardrums, and obstruction of paranasal sinuses. Tracheobronchitis, pulmonary edema, and atalectasis (complete alveolar collapse) follow progressively. Other adverse reactions resulting from inhalation of high concentrations or hyperbaric oxygen include retrolental fibroplasia,[**] paresthesias, vertigo, loss of consciousness, nausea, and vomiting. The conditions are reversible upon discontinuation before onset of permanent damage.

Distinct among the simple asphyxiants is radon, a naturally occurring radioactive gas. Radon is a liquid below 211K but is found in the atmosphere at a concentration of 6×10^{-14} parts per million (ppm) in air. Although the isotopes (^{220}Rn and ^{222}Rn) are short-lived ($t_{1/2} = 3.825$ days for ^{222}Rn), these α-emitters release ionizing radiation and are strongly adsorbed onto various surfaces. These properties account for radon's ubiquitous and resilient presence in the earth's crust and atmosphere. Radon is a known carcinogen suspected to produce lung cancer in occupational exposures to hard rock mine workers. The EPA has established an action level of 4 pCi/l (0.02 working level) for home indoor radon, with a maximum permissible concentration of ^{222}Rn in air of 10^{-8} μCi/cc.

Normal atmospheric concentrations of carbon dioxide (CO_2) range between 0.027 and 0.036% v/v. Inhaling 2 to 5% carbon dioxide stimulates the medullary respiratory center in the brain stem, resulting in an increase in the respiratory minute volume (RMV). Initial local peripheral and skeletal muscle vasodilation and

---

[*] Normal PO_2 for arterial and venous blood, breathing air at sea level, is 100 and 40 mmHg, respectively.
[**] Characterized by retinal detachment in premature infants administered high oxygen at birth; a cause of blindness.

hypotension soon develop. In addition, since CO_2 freely diffuses between plasma and tissue, an increase in blood PCO_2 (hypercapnia) risks the development of respiratory acidosis. This development promotes medullary and peripheral chemoreceptors and sympathetic innervation. The net result is an increased tachycardia, arrythmias, and seizure activity[*] (5 to 10% CO_2 further stimulates RMV and produces a characteristic acidic oral taste).

Inhalation of 10% CO_2 for one minute causes *carbon dioxide narcosis*, a condition characterized by dizziness, dyspnea, sweating, malaise, restlessness, paresthesias, coma, convulsions, and death. Because it is heavier than air, CO_2 accumulates in low-lying, enclosed compartments, such as in mines, wells, and caverns.

23.4 TOXIC PRODUCTS OF COMBUSTION (TCP)

23.4.1 INTRODUCTION

TCPs are by-products of combustion, generated from a variety of mostly synthetic materials,[**] that are released with the smoke. TCPs include ammonia, acids, aldehydes, cyanide and isocyanates, carbon monoxide, halogenated hydrocarbons, oxides of nitrogen and sulfur, and styrene. Smoke inhalation of these substances produces toxicity from the heat in the gases, vapors, and fumes (thermal damage), or may act as simple asphyxiants or pulmonary irritants. As with the pulmonary irritants, URT and LRT injury depends on duration of exposure, respiratory minute volume (RMV[***]), and solubility.

23.4.2 CLINICAL TOXICITY

URT and LRT toxicity are distinguished based on signs and symptoms. Upper airway injury is characterized primarily by local inflammation and irritation of ocular, oral, and nasal mucous membranes. Symptoms include conjunctivitis, lacrimation, rhinitis, pharyngitis, and stridor (an abnormal, high pitched musical sound caused by an obstruction in the larynx or trachea). Lower respiratory tract symptoms entail wheezing, deep chest pain, and carbonaceous sputum (material coughed up by the lungs, expectorated, and accompanied by the presence of particulate residues of combustion).

Treatment of smoke inhalation victims is primarily supportive, including decontamination (removal of clothes, washing or showering of patient) and removal of the individual from the source. This is followed by endotracheal intubation and administration of humidified oxygen, β-agonists and/or steroids for bronchospasm, and epinephrine for stridor. Carbon monoxide or cyanide poisoning, which often accompany smoke inhalation, may complicate the case (see below).

---

[*] Interestingly, about 50% of patients receiving general anesthetics hypoventilate (decrease in normal respirations per minute, rpm), a state accompanied by depressed alveolar ventilation and retention of CO_2. Thus, hypoventilation increases blood PCO_2. Hyperventilation (increase in rpm) enhances elimination of blood CO_2 and causes respiratory alkalosis. The response here is peripheral vasodilation and a fall in blood pressure. Kidney, CNS, and intestinal arteries, however, constrict.

[**] Burning of cellulose acetate film, resins, paper, polystyrene, nylon, petroleum products, rubber, wool, polyurethane, acrylics, wood, and organic material generates TCPs.

[***] RMV is a product of number of respirations per minute (rpm) by volume of air inspired per respiration (V_T, tidal volume).

23.5 LACRIMATING AGENTS (TEAR GAS)

23.5.1 INTRODUCTION

Before World War I, the mechanisms of biological and chemical alkylating agents were surfacing. The search for less toxic, yet severely irritating compounds was already progressing. Law enforcement and governing bodies were convinced that such chemicals could be used in domestic (personal protection, crowd control) or in military situations (war). This understanding prompted the effort to develop agents that could be effective tools for law enforcement while avoiding life-threatening force. Thus spawned the introduction of lacrimating agents, popularly referred to as tear gas or pepper spray. Unlike the pulmonary irritants or asphyxiants that have practical industrial and commercial applications, lacrimating agents were developed specifically to cause irritation.

23.5.2 CHEMICAL AGENTS

The compounds consist mostly of chemically invariable groups of brominated or chlorinated, simple or aromatic hydrocarbons that cause severe local, upper respiratory, and lower respiratory illness. Most of the agents are highly lipid-soluble powders. They are dissolved in organic solvents to effect aerosol delivery, or burned and exploded for military use. Table 23.5 summarizes the properties, chemistry, and clinical effects of popular lacrimating agents currently used for domestic and military use. Today, the compounds are all organically synthesized and have otherwise limited commercial or industrial utility.

23.6 CHEMICAL ASPHYXIANTS

As noted above, chemical asphyxiants produce toxicity through induction of cellular hypoxia or anoxia. The agents alter the oxygen-carrying capacity of hemoglobin (such as with carbon monoxide) or inhibit cellular metabolic enzymes (cyanide, hydrogen sulfide), ultimately interfering with normal physiologic respiration. Among the chemical asphyxiants, carbon monoxide, cyanide, and hydrogen sulfide are the most frequently encountered chemical asphyxiants and are discussed below.

23.7 CARBON MONOXIDE (CO)

23.7.1 INCIDENCE

Each year, nearly 500 unintentional deaths, and more than 1,700 suicides are related to carbon monoxide poisoning in the U.S. An estimated 3,000 to 5,000 people are treated annually for CO poisoning in emergency departments (EDs). Thousands more are either misdiagnosed or do not seek medical care. The statistics support the conclusion that CO poisoning is a serious public health issue.

TABLE 23.5
Lacrimating Agents: Chemical and Clinical Properties

Agent	Chemical (or *Common Name*)	Chemical Properties[a]	Uses	Acute Clinical Effects
Benzyl bromide	bromomethyl-benzene	Liquid, decomposed by water	Chemical war gas	Intense local irritation; large doses cause CNS depression
Bromoacetone	1-bromo-2-propanone	Liquid, turns violet in air	Chemical war gas	Intense local irritation
α-Bromobenzyl cyanide	α-bromobenzene acetonitrile; *camite*	Crystalline powder, odor of soured fruit	Chemical war gas	Intense local irritation
Chloroacetone	1-chloro-2-propanone	Liquid, pungent odor, turns dark with light	Tear gas component for police and military use; insecticide; lead, perfume and drug manufacturing	Intense local irritation
ω-Chloroaceto-phenone	2-chloro-1-phenylethanone; *chemical mace*	Crystalline powder	Riot control agent	Intense local irritation; URT and LRT irritation, pulmonary edema
o-Chlorobenzyl-idenemalononitrile	[(2-chloro-phenyl)methylene] propanedinitrile	Crystalline solid	Riot control agent, chemical warfare agent	Intense local irritation; URT and LRT irritation plus erythema, chest constriction, vesiculation
Chloropicrin	trichloronitro-methane; *acquinite*	Oily liquid	War gas, insecticide, disinfectant, fumigant	URT irritation and lacrimation, potent skin irritant, NVD (orally)

Note: NVD = nausea, vomiting, diarrhea, URT = upper respiratory tract, LRT = lower respiratory tract.

[a] At standard temperature and pressure (STP); All of the compounds are miscible or soluble in acetone, alcohol, chloroform or ether, and are poorly or slightly soluble in water; URT and LRT symptoms are as described in Table 23.2.

23.7.2 CHEMICAL CHARACTERISTICS AND SOURCES OF EXPOSURE

CO is odorless, colorless, and nonirritating, and an abundant product of industrial combustion,[*] thus appropriately labeled as the *silent killer.*

Principal sources of the gas include commercial and passenger motor vehicle exhaust fumes (1% from new automobiles, above 10% in older models) as well as other gasoline, diesel, and propane-powered engines. Smoke from charcoal fires and organic materials, tobacco smoke (3 to 6% CO), and methylene chloride, account for the majority of sources. Methylene chloride is a useful industrial solvent in paint, cleaning, and food processing industries, as well as an aerosol propellant and insecticide. In fact, upon ingestion, methylene chloride is metabolized by hepatic mixed function oxidases (MFO) to carbon monoxide and carbon dioxide. Because of the wide distribution of the pollutant, it is not surprising to detect normal adult blood CO levels between 0.40% and 0.55%.

23.7.3 TOXICOKINETICS

Although CO has low aqueous (plasma) solubility, its binding affinity, particularly for hemoglobin (Hb), is high. Like other toxic gases, absorption and binding of CO to hemoglobin depends on the same factors that increase exposure to the substance — i.e., percent CO in ambient air, duration of exposure, and RMV. The degree of binding is estimated according to the following formula:

$$\% \text{ COHb} = \text{RMV} \times [\text{CO}] \times \text{time}$$

where % COHb is the percent carboxyhemoglobin formed, RMV is the respiratory minute volume (described above and equals about 6 l/min in average adults), [CO] is the CO concentration in ambient air, and time of exposure is in minutes. According to this formula, inhaling 500 ppm CO from exhaust fumes (0.05% in a typical open garage with a running motor vehicle engine) for 30 min yields a percent COHb concentration in blood equal to 15%. The compound is not metabolized, and its half-life is approximately 4 to 5 h.

23.7.4 MECHANISM OF TOXICITY

The net effect of CO toxicity is tissue hypoxia. This is mediated through its reversible but high affinity for ferrous ion (Fe^{+2}) in hemoglobin in the red blood cell. The binding is estimated to range from 200 to 250 times that of molecular oxygen for Hb. The strength of the binding results in the formation of a stable carboxyhemoglobin (COHb) moiety. COHb then displaces the oxygen-carrying capacity of Hb, and shifts the *oxygen-Hb dissociation curve* leftward (Figure 23.1). The diagram illustrates the normal sigmoidal relationship between Hb saturation and the partial pressure of oxygen (PO_2, mmHg) dissolved in blood at normal body temperature.[**] At normal atmospheric pressure, the higher the PO_2, the more oxygen combines

---

[*] It is the most abundant pollutant, accounting for 0.001% atmospheric gases.
[**] The percent saturation expresses the average saturation of Hb with oxygen.

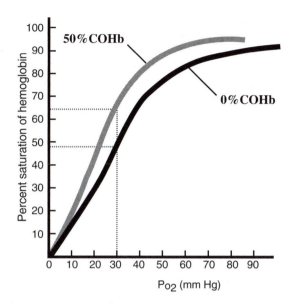

FIGURE 23.1 Oxygen-hemoglobin and carboxyhemoglobin dissociation curves.

with Hb. The curve reaches a plateau at 100 mmHg PO_2, where Hb is almost completely saturated (98%). In the presence of CO, oxygen is displaced from Hb binding sites, rendering less oxygen available for delivery to tissues. The oxygen remaining within the Hb molecule combines more tightly with Hb. At any given PO_2, in the presence of CO, Hb is more saturated with oxygen. This phenomenon is known as the *Bohr effect* (the *Bohr effect* also occurs in metabolic alkalosis, and is stimulated by high blood pH or low blood PCO_2). In addition, CO also binds myoglobin and cytochrome oxidase enzymes with high intensity.

23.7.5 SIGNS AND SYMPTOMS OF ACUTE TOXICITY

Clinical presentation of CO poisoning depends on the time of exposure and the concentration of CO in the area, as noted above. Acute, high-concentration exposure, such as might occur in an enclosed space (automobile exhaust in a closed garage) will produce more severe signs and symptoms than chronic, low-concentration exposure (as with faulty heating systems). The latter scenario may be misdiagnosed as mimicking a bacterial or viral infection. Symptoms from acute, mild exposure range from asymptomatic to headache, dizziness, malaise, and fatigue. Moderate exposure may present with confusion, lethargy, ataxia, syncope, and nystagmus.[*] Severe intoxication manifests as seizures, pulmonary edema, myocardial infarction, and coma. The classic cherry-red discoloration of the face and extremities, due to uncompensated peripheral vasodilation, is evident only in severe poisoning. Blood samples for gas analysis must be obtained immediately after exposure (using blood gas CO-oximetry). Calculation of percentage of arterial

---

[*] Pendular or jerky rhythmical oscillation of the eyeballs.

blood oxyhemoglobin (SaO_2), based on blood gas analysis, is often falsely elevated because of COHb high affinity binding. Other routine clinical laboratory values may also lead to inaccurate conclusions.

Although recovery following nonfatal acute exposure is often complete within several days, subacute complications develop, depending on the severity of exposure. The complications include persistent neurologic and myocardial dysfunction, peripheral neuropathy, aspiration pneumonitis, and ischemic skin. Approximately 10 to 30% of victims of severe acute poisoning will display delayed-onset neurobehavioral dysfunction, also known as *CO-induced delayed neuropsychiatric syndrome* (CO-DNS). The condition is characterized by impaired cognitive function, personality changes, dementia, and symptoms resembling Parkinson's disease. Individuals at greater risk for development of complications are patients with a history of heart disease, anemia, and chronic obstructive pulmonary disease (COPD), and patients exposed in the presence of alcohol or respiratory depressants. Infants are also at greater risk for CO-DNS.

23.7.6 TREATMENT OF ACUTE POISONING

As with any agent suspected of causing CNS depression or disrupting cardiovascular function, clinical history and evaluation should determine other etiologies, such as intoxication with alcohol or other CNS depressants. Presence of concurrent cyanide poisoning (particularly in burn victims) may aggravate the complications. The goal of treatment of CO inhalation victims, then, is to reduce the development of cerebral and cardiovascular ischemia and to increase the dissociation of COHb. Initial management includes removal of the individual from the source (while minimizing muscle and spinal movement, if possible), followed by administration of supplemental humidified oxygen soon after. Maintenance of respiration, fluid and electrolyte replacement, and clinical chemistry determination are largely supportive. Administration of 100% normobaric* oxygen reduces the half-life of 50% COHb level from about 4 h in room air to approximately 50 to 60 min,** although longer periods may be required in high-risk patients. Treatment continues until COHb levels drop to within normal range.

23.8 CYANIDE

23.8.1 CHEMICAL CHARACTERISTICS, OCCURRENCE, AND USES

Cyanic acid (hydrogen cyanate, HCNO) is the starting chemical principle for the various salt forms of cyanide, including the sodium (cyanogran, NaCN), potassium (KCN), and calcium (CaCN) salts. Hydrogen cyanide (HCN, hydrocyanic acid, prussic acid) is a gas and a catalyst and is prepared from the cyanate salts. In addition, the compounds occur naturally as cyanogenic glycosides. The compounds are found

---

* At 1 atm of pressure.

** Although some studies have demonstrated a further reduction of the half-life to less than 40 min with hyperbaric oxygen (i.e., 100% oxygen at 3 atm of pressure), the results from this mode of therapy are equivocal. As noted above, hyperbaric oxygen is associated with signs and symptoms of oxygen toxicity.

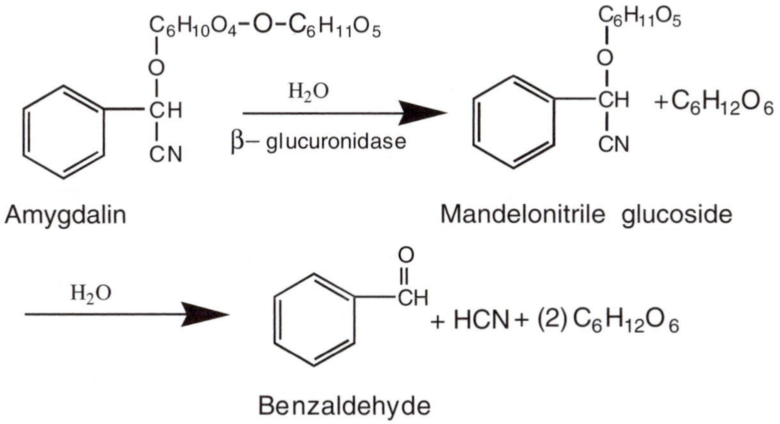

FIGURE 23.2 Cyanogenic glycosides and hydrolysis of amygdalin.

from 0.01 to 14% in the seeds of various nuts, including almonds (highest concentration, 2 to 14%), cherries, plums, apples, peaches, apricots, pears, plums, and rosaceous plants, as well as in bamboo sprouts and cassava. Figure 23.2 illustrates the hydrolysis of amygdalin, the most widely distributed cyanogenic glycoside. Most hydrolyzing agents, in the presence of the enzyme β-glucuronidase, are capable of producing the hydrolysis products of amygdalin, i.e., mandelonitrile glucoside (an intermediate) plus glucose, benzaldehyde, and hydrocyanic acid.

Cyanide compounds are also valuable industrial chemicals used in electroplating and electropolishing, manufacturing of plastics, extraction of gold and silver from ores, as fumigants, in fertilizer, and in artificial nail glue removers. Therapeutically, sodium nitroprusside, a direct arterial vasodilator used in the treatment of emergency hypertension, releases five molecules of CN when metabolized, which also accumulates with fast infusion rates (see Chapter 18, "Cardiovascular Drugs"). As with CO poisoning, fire victims are also prone to CN intoxication.

23.8.2 MECHANISM OF TOXICITY

Cyanide produces histotoxic anoxia by inhibiting oxidative phosphorylation, resulting in arrest of cellular respiration (see Figure 16.3, Chapter 16). By binding to cytochrome a/a3, CN forms a CN–cytochrome oxidase–Fe^{+3} complex. The complex interferes with the transfer of electrons to O_2, the final electron acceptor. Ultimately, CN blocks the electron transport chain and inhibits metabolic respiration. It provokes a decrease in cellular oxygen utilization, prevents oxidative phosphorylation of ADP to ATP, and prompts an increase in venous PO_2 (arterialization of venous blood).[*] The decrease in aerobic respiration forces the cell to revert to anaerobic metabolism, which generates excess lactic acid, triggering metabolic acidosis.

---

[*] Interestingly, the patient is not **cyanotic**, and availability and binding of oxygen are not compromised. In fact, arterial PO_2 appears normal (100 mmHg).

23.8.3 TOXICOKINETICS

Acute lethal toxicity results within 1 h from an oral dose of 100 to 200 mg, while inhalation of 150 to 200 ppm of HCN gas is fatal (approximately only 60% of the population can smell 0.2 to 5.0 ppm). Trace amounts of CN are generally detoxified slowly by binding to circulating methemoglobin (methHb). The resulting cyanomethemoglobin complex prevents access to the cytochrome enzymes. Normally circulating rhodanese enzyme (thiosulfate cyanide sulfur transferase) transfers a sulfur group to the cyanomethemoglobin complex, forming a relatively nontoxic thiocyanate ion that is eventually eliminated by renal excretion. Chronic, low dose intoxication is more insidious.

23.8.4 SIGNS AND SYMPTOMS OF ACUTE TOXICITY

Signs and symptoms precipitate rapidly with exposure to HCN vapors. Initially symptoms of neurological toxicity appear, including headache, nausea, vomiting, weakness, and dizziness. The chemical stimulates chemoreceptors in the carotid artery, triggering reflex hyperpnea (increase in respirations), tachypnea (gasping for air), and pulmonary edema. Hypotension with reflex tachycardia completes the cardiovascular presentation. With high doses, the victim is stuporous yet responsive, where the condition may deteriorate to hypoxic convulsions, hypotension, coma, and death.

23.8.5 TREATMENT OF ACUTE POISONING

As with CO poisoning, initial management of patients with CN intoxication includes removal of the individual from the source, decontamination (removal of clothes, flushing with water, if necessary), and administration of activated charcoal or gastric lavage if the victim is encountered soon after ingestion. The goal of treatment is to immediately decrease CN binding to cytochrome enzymes with the specific antidote available. The Cyanide Antidote Package (various manufacturers) consists of three major components:

1. Amyl nitrite inhalant, 0.3 ml (12 aspirols)
2. Sodium nitrite, 300 mg in 10 ml (2 ampoules)
3. Sodium thiosulfate, 12.5 g in 50 ml (25% solution, 2 ampoules)

plus disposable syringes, stomach tube, tourniquet, and instructions. The primary mechanism of detoxification involves conversion of CN to the nontoxic thiocyanate ion, in preparation for renal elimination. Initially, either i.v. sodium nitrite (300 mg over 3 to 5 min)* or amyl nitrite inhalant (1 or 2 crushed aspirols every 2 to 3 min, if i.v. route is not accessible) are administered. Thus, the nitrites induce formation of cyanomethemoglobin-Fe^{+3} (CN–Hb–Fe^{+3}) complex in preference to CN–cytochrome oxidase–Fe^{+3}. Nitrites convert reduced Hb–Fe^{+2} ([H]) to oxidized methHb

---

*In children, initial dose of sodium nitrite (mg/kg) is calculated according to the patient's Hb level (g/dl).

([O]), freeing cytochrome oxidase enzyme to resume oxidative phosphorylation. The sequence is outlined in Reaction 1:

$$Hb\text{-}Fe^{+2} + NO_2 \rightarrow Hb\text{-}Fe^{+3} + NO \qquad (23.1)$$

Since methHb has a greater affinity for CN than cytochrome oxidase, it induces the transfer of CN from the cytochrome enzyme complex to methHb, forming cyanomethemoglobin ($CN\text{-}Hb\text{-}Fe^{+3}$) according to Reaction 2:

$$Hb\text{-}Fe^{+3} + CN\text{-}cytochrome\text{-}Fe^{+3} \rightarrow CN\text{-}Hb\text{-}Fe^{+3} + cytochrome\text{-}Fe^{+3} \quad (23.2)$$

Peak methHb levels are reached within 30 min of i.v. administration in adults. Since cyanomethemoglobin is relatively unstable and reversible, the subsequent step is to force renal excretion of the CN moiety by administration of sodium thiosulfate. As mentioned above, this requires the rhodanase enzyme reaction that naturally detoxifies trace amounts of circulating CN ions. This reaction (3, below) is accelerated by supplying exogenous sulfur from the administration of sodium thiosulfate ($Na_2S_2O_3$). $Na_2S_2O_3$ (12.5 g i.v. over 10 min) is administered immediately after sodium nitrite (400 mg/kg, up to 12.5 g total in children). The treatment results in the formation of thiocyanate, sodium sulfite, and regenerated methemoglobin, respectively.

$$CN\text{-}Hb\text{-}Fe^{+3} + Na_2S_2O_3 \rightarrow CN\text{-}S + Na_2SO_3 + Hb\text{-}Fe^{+3} \qquad (23.3)$$

Adverse reactions associated with nitrites involve hypotension and the risk of production of excess, life-threatening amounts of methemoglobin. In excess, methemoglobin decreases availability of oxyhemoglobin (reduced form) necessary for oxygen transport. Other antidotes for CN poisoning, such as 4-methylaminophenol (4-DMAP), hydroxycobalamin, dicobalt-EDTA, and hyperbaric oxygen, are not FDA approved or recommended.

Permanent neurological damage (Parkinson-like syndrome) is a complication of severe CN toxicity. Higher levels of thiocyanate are also implicated in the development of tobacco amblyopia (in chronic smokers) and tropical ataxic neuropathy (in diets rich in cassava).

23.9 METHODS OF DETECTION

Clinical chemistry analysis, hematology assays (including hemoglobin and hematocrit tests) and arterial blood gas determinations are not clinically useful indicators for CO poisoning. Routine blood gas analysis (pulse oximetry), used to measure changes in oxyhemoglobin content, may not be sensitive enough, due to the high affinity COHb complex. Carboxyhemoglobin blood levels are useful if performed soon after acute exposure. Automated spectrophotometric devices (CO-oximeters) provide valuable measures of carboxyhemoglobin, oxyhemoglobin, and methemoglobin, the levels of which are correlated with severity of CO exposure. The technique estimates simultaneously total hemoglobin, percent oxyhemoglobin, and percent carboxyhemoglobin. The procedures are recommended for most clinical purposes. For the investigation of low-level exposure and the detection of increased hemolysis in neonates, more sensitive methods involving the release of CO and its measurement by gas chromatography are required.

As with CO, pulse oximetry may not be suitable for therapeutic management of CN poisoning. In fact, the onset and rate of CN toxicity is often too rapid to allow CN blood levels to be of any utility. Consequently, determination of hemoglobin levels is a better indicator of the progress of CN poisoning, and can be used to manage initial treatment with sodium nitrite. Elevated plasma lactate, associated with cardiovascular collapse, should also suggest cyanide intoxication. Other clinical chemistry and hematology tests can be of value as indicators of supportive measures.

REFERENCES

SUGGESTED READINGS

Bui, L., Cyanide and hydrogen sulfide, in *Toxicology Secrets*, Ling, L.J. et al., Eds., Hanley & Belfus, Inc., Philadelphia, 2001, chap. 53.

Budavari, S., Ed., *The Merck Index*, 12th ed., Merck & Co., Inc., Whitehouse Station, NJ, 1996.

Fung, F., Simple asphyxiants and pulmonary irritants, in *Toxicology Secrets*, Ling, L.J. et al., Eds., Hanley & Belfus, Inc., Philadelphia, 2001, chap. 50.

Holmes, H.N., Ed., Respiratory System, in *Handbook of Pathophysiology*, Corwin, E.I., Ed., Springhouse Corp., PA, 2001, chap. 7.

Wallace, K.L., Carbon monoxide, in *Toxicology Secrets*, Ling, L.J. et al., Eds., Hanley & Belfus, Inc., Philadelphia, 2001, chap. 52.

REVIEW ARTICLES

Beasley, D.M. and Glass, W.I., Cyanide poisoning: pathophysiology and treatment recommendations, *Occup. Med. (Lond).* 48, 427, 1998.

Borron, S.W. and Baud, F.J., Acute cyanide poisoning: clinical spectrum, diagnosis, and treatment, *Arh. Hig. Rada. Toksikol.,* 47, 307, 1996.

Choi, A.M. and Otterbein, L.E., Emerging role of carbon monoxide in physiologic and pathophysiologic states, *Antioxid. Redox. Signa,* 4, 227, 2002.

Friederich, J.A. and Butterworth, J.F., IV, Sodium nitroprusside: twenty years and counting, *Anesth. Analg.,* 81, 152, 1995.

Gonzales, J. and Sabatini, S., Cyanide poisoning: pathophysiology and current approaches to therapy, *Int. J. Artif Organs,* 12, 347, 1989.

Hartzell, G.E., Overview of combustion toxicology, *Toxicology,* 115, 7, 1996.

Holland, M.A. and Kozlowski, L.M., Clinical features and management of cyanide poisoning, *Clin. Pharm.,* 5, 737, 1986.

Jones, J., McMullen, M.J., and Dougherty, J., Toxic smoke inhalation: cyanide poisoning in fire victims, *Am. J. Emerg. Med.,* 5, 317, 1987.

Medinsky, M.A. and Bond, J.A., Sites and mechanisms for uptake of gases and vapors in the respiratory tract, *Toxicology,* 160, 165, 2001.

Olajos, E.J. and Salem, H., Riot control agents: pharmacology, toxicology, biochemistry and chemistry, *J. Appl. Toxicol.,* 21, 355, 2001.

Omaye, S.T., Metabolic modulation of carbon monoxide toxicity, *Toxicology,* 180, 139, 2002.

Opresko, D.M., et al., Chemical warfare agents: estimating oral reference doses, *Rev. Environ. Contam. Toxicol.,* 156, 1, 1998.

Prien, T. and Traber, D.L., Toxic smoke compounds and inhalation injury — a review, *Burns Incl. Therm. Inj.,* 14, 451, 1988.

Shifrin, N.S., et al., Chemistry, toxicology, and human health risk of cyanide compounds in soils at former manufactured gas plant sites, *Regul. Toxicol. Pharmacol.,* 23, 106, 1996.

Shusterman, D., Toxicology of nasal irritants, *Curr. Allergy Asthma Rep.,* 3, 258, 2003.

Strickland, J.A. and Foureman, G.L., US EPA's acute reference exposure methodology for acute inhalation exposures, *Sci. Total Environ.,* 288, 51, 2002.

Widdop, B., Analysis of carbon monoxide, *Ann. Clin. Biochem.,* 39, 378, 2002.

24 Metals

Diane Hardej and Louis D. Trombetta

24.1 INTRODUCTION

Metals are the most numerous of all elements. Even though some are necessary in biological systems, they are usually required only in trace amounts. Even essential metals in excess can be toxic if not fatal. They are involved in enzymatic reactions or, as in the case of iron, are involved with oxygen transport. Some metals such as Na^+, K^+ and Ca^{2+} act as ions in neurotransmission and muscle contraction. Most metals function as metal complexes and are involved in electron transfer reactions. It is the misplacement of these electrons or competition between metals that results in toxicity. Metals are known to generate free radicals, which may result in membrane and organelle degradation. They are also known to combine with normally occurring molecules, such as proteins, and inhibit or alter their activity. The metals discussed in this chapter represent the toxicologically important ones (Table 24.1) of those present in the Periodic Table.

24.2 CHELATION THERAPY

24.2.1 DESCRIPTION

Exposure to metals and metallic elements can be a source of serious toxicological effects. These effects will largely depend on the type of exposure (inhalation, dermal absorption, or ingestion), the species (salt, element, vapor), dose, and time of exposure. Whenever possible, removal of the individual from the source of exposure is the first course of action. For some cases of metal exposure, gastric lavage and induction of vomiting are recommended. This can only be safely and effectively accomplished if the toxicant is not corrosive and the exposure is recent.

Once absorption occurs, chelation therapies are often suggested to lessen body burdens of metals that have been absorbed and distributed to body tissues.* The chelator may have one or more attachment points for the metal, and its affinity for a particular metal will vary with its structure and the properties of the metal. There are inherent risks involved with the use of chelators. The chelator-metal complex must be excreted from the body without causing additional toxicity. In addition, chelators can bind to essential metals or cause the movement of metals from storage sites, thus increasing potential for toxicity. Chelators can move metals from innoc-

---

* The word chelate comes from a Greek word meaning "claw" (for example, the chelicerae or claw shaped mouthpart of *Crustacea*). A chelator acts as a claw to attach itself to the metal and hastens its removal from the organism.

TABLE 24.1
Chemical Characteristics and Methods of Detection of Some Metals

Metal	Chemical Symbol	At. #	At. Wt.	Appearance	Method of Detection	Clinical Sample
Antimony	Sb	51	121.76	Silvery-white, brittle crystalline metalloid	AAS, ESI-MS, GC-ICP-MS	Urine, blood
Arsenic	As	33	74.9216	Grey metalloid	AAS, ICP-AES, ICP-MS	Hair, nails, blood, urine
Asbestos	—	—	—	Mixture of minerals	PCM, TEM, Polarized light and x-ray diffraction	—
Cadmium	Cd	48	112.40	Silvery-white metal	GF-AAS, ICP-MS	Urine, blood
Copper	Cu	29	63.546	Brownish-red metal	ICP-MS, AAS	Blood
Iron	Fe	26	55.847	Silvery-white metal	AAS	Blood
Lead	Pb	82	207.2	Bluish-gray metal	GF-AAS, radiographic techniques, (lead lines)	Blood
Mercury	Hg	80	200.59	Silvery liquid metal	AAS, ICP-AES, ICP-MS	Hair, nails, blood, bone, urine
Selenium	Se	34	78.96	Brick red powder, red crystals, gray crystals, metalloid	AAS, GC, x-ray diffraction, NAA	Blood, urine, placenta, hair, nails
Zinc	Zn	30	65.38	Brittle bluish-white metal	AAS, ICP-AES, ICP-MS	Urine, blood, bone, hair

Note: **AAS**, atomic absorption spectroscopy; **ESI-MS**, electron spray ionization mass spectroscopy; **GC-ICP-MS**, gas chromatography – inductively coupled mass spectroscopy; **ICP-AES**, inductively coupled plasma atomic emission spectroscopy; **ICP-MS**, inductively coupled plasma mass spectroscopy; **GF-AAS**, graphite furnace AAS; **NAA**, neutron activation analysis; **PCM**, phase contrast microscopy; **TEM**, transmission electron microscopy.

uous locations in the body to more sensitive areas (e.g., lead trapped in bone released into the circulation by the chelator).

Some commonly used chelators are mentioned below. It is important to realize that chelators, depending on the metal and clinical situation, may increase toxicity.

24.2.2 DIMERCAPROL

Dimercaprol (2,3-dimercapto-1-propanol, British anti-Lewisite, BAL) is an effective chelating agent for heavy metals such as As, inorganic Hg, Bi, Cd, Cr, Co, Ni, Sb, and Au (see Table 24.1 for abbreviations).* These metals form strong bonds with sulfur atoms in this compound. Once the metal is chelated, it is unable to enter the cell and may be excreted from the body.

24.2.3 ETHYLENEDIAMINETETRAACETIC ACID (EDTA)

EDTA forms four or six bonds with metal ions and forms chelates with both transition-metal ions and main-group ions. The Ca salt of EDTA is the chelator of choice for Pb toxicity. EDTA is used as an anticoagulant for stored blood in blood banks; it prevents coagulation by sequestering the Ca ions required for clotting. As an antidote for Pb poisoning, Ca disodium EDTA exchanges its chelated Ca for Pb, and the resulting Pb chelate is rapidly excreted in the urine. The Ca salt of EDTA, administered i.v., is also used in the treatment of acute Cd and Fe poisoning. Because of its potential for nephrotoxicity, Ca EDTA should be administered only when necessary. EDTA can be used in combination with other chelators in an effort to reduce the toxic effects of either agent used individually.

24.2.4 PENICILLAMINE

Penicillamine (cuprimine) is a chelating agent for Hg, Pb, Fe, and Cu. It forms soluble complexes, thus decreasing toxic levels of the metal.** Penicillamine is well absorbed from the GI tract and excreted in urine. Food decreases the absorption of penicillamine over 50%. Since penicillamine is a hydrolytic product of penicillin, it should not be used in patients who are allergic to this antibiotic.

24.2.5 DEFEROXAMINE

Deferoxamine is an Al and Fe(II) chelator that has been used in the treatment of acute Fe poisoning and chronic Fe or aluminum overload. It is isolated from the bacteria *Streptomyces pilosus* and is one of the few chelators available for the treatment of secondary Fe overload. It is not effective orally and requires prolonged subcutaneous injection to achieve efficient Fe excretion. Deferoxamine appears to remove both free Fe and bound Fe from hemosiderin and ferritin but not from hemoglobin, transferrin, or cytochromes.

---

* Dimercaprol was originally employed to treat the toxic effects of an As-containing mustard gas (Lewisite, dichloro-(2-chlorovinyl) arsine) used in World War I.

** Penicillamine has been used in the treatment of Wilson's disease, a genetic disease that results in accumulation of Cu.

24.2.6 Succimer

Succimer (dimercaptosuccinic acid, DMSA) and sodium dimercaptopropane-sulfonate (DMPS) are used in the treatment of acute Pb poisoning to remove excess Pb from the body, especially in children. It is also under investigation as a treatment for Hg poisoning due to dental fillings. Succimer combines with Pb in the serum and is excreted by the kidneys. By removing the excess Pb, the chelator lessens damage to various organs and tissues of the body. In healthy individuals, approximately 20% of an oral dose of DMSA is absorbed from the GI tract. About 95% of circulating DMSA is bound to albumin. Most likely, one of the sulfhydryls (SH) in DMSA binds to a cysteine residue on albumin, leaving the other SH available to chelate metals.

24.3 ANTIMONY (Sb)

24.3.1 Chemical Characteristics

Antimony (Sb) displays both metallic and nonmetallic characteristics and is sometimes referred to as a metalloid. It is moderately flammable and presents somewhat of a fire hazard in the forms of dust and vapor when exposed to heat or flame. When heated or on contact with acid, it emits toxic fumes of stibine. Most antimonial salts have been known to cause toxicity.

24.3.2 Uses

Sb is used as solder, in sheet and pipe metal, storage battery casings, pewter, in paints, ceramics, and in enamels for plastics, metals and glass. Sb oxides have been added to clothing as a flame retardant. It has been used clinically for its antiinfective properties and in the treatment of parasitic infections such as leishmaniasis and schistosomiasis.

24.3.3 Mechanism of Toxicity

Like other metals, Sb produces its toxicity by the formation of ligands with cellular organic compounds and constituents. Once the metal-organic compound complex is formed, the molecules lose their ability to function properly, which leads to disruption or death of affected cells. The binding of metals to oxygen, sulfur, and nitrogen can inactivate essential enzymes or protein function.

24.3.4 Toxicokinetics

Sb is poorly absorbed following gastrointestinal ingestion or inhalation, and absorption is a function of the compound's solubility. GI absorption has been estimated to be < 10% in humans. Systemic distribution varies among species and is directly related to its valence state. Sb is not metabolized but binds to macromolecules and reacts covalently with SH and phosphate groups. Excretion occurs via the urine and feces. The absorption of Sb from the respiratory tract is dependent on particle size.

Pentavalent forms of Sb have been detected more frequently in the liver and spleen and trivalent forms with greater frequency in the thyroid gland. It accumulates in the skeletal system and in fur of mammals.

24.3.5 Signs and Symptoms of Acute Poisoning

In humans, acute poisoning has occurred as a result of accidental or suicidal ingestion of Sb compounds with death ensuing within several hours. Symptoms of severe Sb poisoning include vomiting, watery diarrhea, collapse, irregular respiration, and hypothermia. Toxicological effects of Sb in humans following inhalation or ingestion include: pneumoconiosis, altered ECG readings, increased blood pressure, dermatosis, ocular irritation, abdominal distress, headache, nausea, vomiting, jaundice, and anemia. Acute exposure to other forms may result in hair and weight loss, skin problems, and damage to heart, liver, and kidneys. Inhalation of Sb dust by factory workers produced GI irritation, probably as a result of Sb dust transported via the nasal mucosa. Information regarding the acute inhalation toxicity of Sb in humans is lacking.

24.3.6 Treatment of Acute Poisoning

Treatment for acute Sb poisoning is best accomplished by using DMPS, although chelation may not always be indicated. BAL may be the most effective treatment for trivalent Sb in the circulation, although this treatment has little effect following stibine gas exposure. Dialysis has been recommended for treatment of pentavalent Sb exposure. Dimercaprol has also been used in cases of Sb poisoning.

24.4 ARSENIC (As)

24.4.1 Chemical Characteristics

Arsenic (As) is a naturally occurring element that is not a true metal but a metalloid. Organic forms are usually considered to be less toxic than the inorganic forms. Some organic As compounds are gases or low-boiling liquids at normal temperatures. Burning of As, or contact with acid, results in production of arsine, a deadly gas. More than 21 As compounds are of concern based on their environmental presence.

24.4.2 Occurrence and Uses

Inorganic As is found in groundwater, surface water, and many foods such as rice and grains. Exposure is primarily through drinking water, but food is considered a significant source as well. As has been used clinically as an anticancer agent. Arsenic trioxide (As_2O_3) is a major ingredient of traditional Chinese medicine (TCM) and is used against acute promyelocytic leukemia. Fowler's solution (potassium arsenite) had been used as a treatment for patients with asthma. Inorganic As compounds are mainly used as wood preservatives, insecticides, herbicides, and in the production of metal alloys.

24.4.3 Mechanism of Toxicity

The toxicity of As is dependent upon the chemical form and the oxidation state at the time of exposure. The physical state (gas, solution, powder particle size), the rate of absorption into cells, elimination rate, and the nature of chemical substituents determine the toxic outcome. The mechanism of As toxicity may be related to the inactivation of key enzyme systems. Inorganic pentavalent As does not react with the active sites of enzymes directly, but first reduces to trivalent As before exerting toxic effects. Bonding of trivalent As to –SH and –OH groups interferes with enzyme activity. Inactivation of pyruvate dehydrogenase with trivalent As will prevent generation of adenosine-5-triphosphate (ATP). Arsenic inhibits succinic dehydrogenase activity and can uncouple oxidative phosphorylation, a process that results in disruption of all cellular functions. As targets and accumulates within mitochondria.

24.4.4 Toxicokinetics

Arsenate and arsenite are well absorbed by both oral and inhalation routes. As is methylated in the body by alternating reduction of pentavalent As to trivalent As, the latter of which is the more toxic form. Most mammals metabolize As to methylarsonic acid (MMA) and dimethylarsinic acid (DMA). MMA and DMA are readily excreted in the urine, and this acts as a detoxification mechanism. Increases in tissue concentrations result if As methylation is diminished. Glutathione and other thiols act as reducing agents in these reactions. In mammals, the liver is an important site of As methylation, especially following first passage through the liver. Arsenic is also methylated in other tissues such as testes, kidney, liver, and lung.

24.4.5 Signs and Symptoms of Acute Toxicity

Patients with acute exposure experience GI distress characterized by nausea, vomiting, abdominal pain, and profuse watery or bloody diarrhea. Death is common in patients that have ingested large doses. Serious respiratory effects such as pulmonary edema, hemorrhagic bronchitis, and respiratory distress are seen with acute oral poisoning. Hypotension, tachycardia, and complaint of a metallic taste in the mouth and garlic odor on the breath, as well as delirium, are often noted in patients with acute toxicity. Anemia and leukopenia are common effects of acute As poisoning in humans. Acute arsine gas exposure is characterized by headache, nausea, vomiting, diarrhea, and abdominal pain. Dyspnea and severe jaundice are frequent signs.

24.4.6 Signs and Symptoms of Chronic Toxicity

Chronic As toxicity is characterized by changes in skin pigmentation, plantar and palmar hyperkeratoses, GI symptoms, anemia, skin cancers, and liver disease. In patients treated with Fowler's solution, which contains potassium arsenite, nonchirrhotic portal hypertension has been seen. Bone marrow depression resulting in anemia and leukopenia, Raynaud's phenomena, and acrocyanosis may also occur. Peripheral neuropathies have also been reported. Nerve injury was associated with Swedish Cu smelter workers chronically exposed to As_2O_3.

24.4.7 Treatment of Acute Poisoning

Delay or prevention of As absorption in cases of high-dose oral exposure may be accomplished by consumption of large volumes of water, gastric lavage, or cathartics initiated within a few hours of exposure. Chelation therapy is indicated for acute As poisoning, including BAL and D-penicillamine. Patients who are minimally symptomatic and have chronic As poisoning may be removed from the source of their exposure without chelation therapy.

24.4.8 Carcinogenesis

There is convincing evidence from many epidemiological studies suggesting that inhalation exposure to inorganic As compounds increases the likelihood of developing lung cancer. Most cases involved inhalation of arsenic trioxide by workers at copper smelting plants, resulting in a significant increase in respiratory cancer mortality. The likelihood that ingestion of inorganic As results in increased risk of skin cancers and basal cell carcinomas have also been noted.

24.5 ASBESTOS

24.5.1 Chemical Characteristics

Asbestos is composed of a group of six different fibrous minerals (amosite, chrysotile, crocidolite, and the fibrous varieties of tremolite, actinolite, and anthophyllite) that occur naturally in the environment. There are two different silicate mineral groups in which asbestos belongs. Chrysotile belongs to the serpentine family of minerals, while the rest belong to the amphibole family. Chrysotile accounts for over 90% of the world's asbestos production. Of the five members of the amphibole group, crocidolite (blue asbestos) and amosite (brown asbestos) are widely used for commercial purposes.

24.5.2 Occurrence and Industrial Uses

The ancient Greeks spun and wove asbestos into cloth much like cotton. Until the late 1800s, when major deposits were discovered in Canada, asbestos was not widely available. Asbestos deposits are found throughout the world and are still mined in Australia, Canada, South Africa, and the former Soviet Union.

Asbestos was used to make thermal insulation for boilers, pipes, and for fireproofing and reinforcement material. The military used asbestos extensively in ships and other applications during World Wars I and II. Commercial uses in buildings increased greatly thereafter until the 1970s, when growing concerns about health risks led to voluntary reductions. Asbestos has been used in thousands of products, mainly because it is plentiful, readily available, inexpensive, strong, fire retardant, heat resistant, chemical corrosion resistant, and a poor conductor of electricity. Products and building materials made with asbestos are often referred to asbestos-containing materials (ACM) and asbestos-containing building materials (ACBM), respectively. Fibers mixed into asbestos cement, asphalt, and vinyl are usually firmly bound. Generally, when these materials are in good condition there is no cause for concern. Drilling, cutting, grinding, or sanding may release fibers.

24.5.3 MECHANISM OF TOXICITY

The exact mechanism of toxicity of asbestos fibers to lung cells and pleura has not been fully elucidated. The generation of oxidants by fiber uptake or cellular interaction appears to be involved in the cellular response to asbestos. Information about associated health risks have come from studies of individuals exposed to levels of asbestos fibers that are > 5 μm in length. Inhalation of asbestos fibers may lead to the development of a slow buildup of scarlike tissue in the lungs and the pleura, preventing proper expansion and contraction.

Lung cancer and mesothelioma are two cancers frequently associated with asbestos exposure. The mechanism is not precisely known, but studies have suggested that chromosomal alterations and generation of reactive oxygen species are critical.

24.5.4 TOXICOKINETICS

Following ingestion of asbestos, some of the fibers penetrate the GI epithelium and distribute to other tissues, such as the lymphatic or systemic circulation, resulting in widespread distribution. Macrophages are probably involved in the uptake and distribution process. Most of the asbestos fibers that are deposited in the lung during inhalation are transported by mucociliary action. Only a small fraction of inhaled fibers penetrate the epithelial layer of the lungs (the retention of asbestos fibers in the lungs of asbestos workers was estimated to have a clearance half-life of greater than 10 years).

24.5.5 SIGNS AND SYMPTOMS OF ACUTE TOXICITY

Temporary breathing difficulties have been reported in individuals exposed to high concentrations of asbestos dust, which may be accompanied by local inflammatory response in the terminal bronchioles. Progressive fibrosis followed within a few weeks of the first exposure to dust.

24.5.6 SIGNS AND SYMPTOMS OF CHRONIC TOXICITY

Long-term inhalation of asbestos fibers in humans results in chronic, progressive pneumoconiosis (*asbestosis*). The disease is common among occupational groups directly exposed to asbestos fibers, such as insulation workers, but also extends to those working near the application or removal of asbestos. A prolonged inflammatory response caused by the presence of fibers in the lungs is characterized by fibrosis of the lung parenchyma. This can be seen radiographically 10 years after the first exposure. The main clinical symptom is shortness of breath, often accompanied by abnormal chest sounds (rales) and cough. In severe cases, disruption of respiratory function may result ultimately in death.

24.6 CADMIUM (Cd)

24.6.1 OCCURRENCE AND USES

Cadmium (Cd) sulfate is used as an astringent. Cd sulfide (CdS, Cd yellow) and Cd selenide (CdSe) are important pigments. The latter metal is electrolytically deposited on Fe or steel and forms a chemically resistant coating. Cd lowers the melting point of metals with which it is alloyed, thus making it useful in the manufacture of fusible metals for automatic sprinkler systems, fire alarms, and electric fuses. Cd salts are also used in photography and in the manufacture of fireworks, rubber, fluorescent paints, glass, porcelain, and as shielding material in atomic energy plants. Cd sulfide is a component in photovoltaic cells and nickel-Cd batteries.

Most Cd enters the environment through coal burning, waste incineration, metal mining and smelting, disposal of metal-containing products, waste-site leakage, and from the use of phosphate fertilizers. Exposure to the general population occurs through cigarette smoke, food consumption, drinking water, and incidental ingestion of soil. For nonsmokers, food is the largest nonoccupational source of exposure. The U.S. EPA reports that average Cd levels in foods range from 2 to 40 ppb, with grain and cereal products, potatoes, leafy vegetables, and root vegetables containing the highest levels. On the average, each person ingests about 30 µg of Cd daily, while smokers absorb an additional 1 to 3 µg per day. Except in areas near Cd-emitting industries or incinerators, minimal exposure occurs through drinking water or ambient air.

24.6.2 MECHANISM OF TOXICITY

Liver is the primary target in acute Cd exposure. Investigations have revealed hepatocellular necrosis with infiltration by inflammatory cells. Although the underlying mechanism of Cd toxicity has not been elucidated, possible factors include oxidative stress or lipid peroxidation of cell membranes.

In 1993, Cd was classified as a human carcinogen. Occupational exposure is associated with lung and prostate cancers, although the carcinogenic mechanism is not known. Cd does not form stable DNA adducts but stimulates cell proliferation and inhibits DNA repair.

24.6.3 TOXICOKINETICS

Absorption of Cd varies considerably by the route of exposure. Only about 5% of an ingested dose of Cd is absorbed from the GI tract, while absorption from the lung is as high as 90%. Cd clears rapidly from the blood and concentrates in various tissues. Most of the absorbed Cd is found in the liver and kidney and may be related to the ability of these organs to produce large amounts of metallothionein (MT), a small metal-binding protein with a great affinity for Cd. Although binding with MT lessens the toxic effects of Cd, it also hinders its elimination.

24.6.4 SIGNS AND SYMPTOMS OF ACUTE TOXICITY

Heating of Cd and its compounds to high temperature produces Cd oxide fumes, which upon inhalation cause flu-like symptoms (*metal fume fever*). The condition is benign, and treatment is symptomatic. More severe exposures may cause lung damage and fatality. Cd oxide fume is a severe pulmonary irritant. Cd dust is a less potent irritant than Cd fume because of its larger particle size, which appears to be a more important determinant of toxicity.

Inhalation of fumes with a high Cd concentration has been responsible for fatalities, while nonfatal cases are seen at lower concentrations. Pulmonary symptoms and clinical signs reflect lesions ranging from nasopharyngeal and bronchial irritation to pulmonary edema and death. Other possible symptoms include, headache, chills, muscle aches, nausea, vomiting, and diarrhea. Respiratory symptoms linger for several weeks, and impairment of pulmonary function persists for months.

24.6.5 SIGNS AND SYMPTOMS OF CHRONIC TOXICITY

Chronic exposure to Cd affects the kidney, lungs, and bone. In kidney, chronic exposure is implicated in the development of cancer. In lungs, long-term inhalation results in decreased lung friction and emphysema. Even if absorption by ingestion is low, chronic exposure to high levels of Cd in food has caused bone disorders, including osteoporosis and osteomalacia.* Other consequences of Cd exposure are anemia, yellow discoloration of the teeth, rhinitis, occasional ulceration of the nasal septum, damage to the olfactory nerve, and loss of the sense of smell (anosmia).

24.7 COPPER (Cu)

24.7.1 OCCURRENCE AND USES

In ancient times, copper (Cu) was useful for its curative powers, largely due to its antibacterial and antifungal properties, in the treatment of wounds and skin diseases, and pulmonary diseases. Today, it is widely recognized for its effectiveness in the treatment of a number of internal diseases including anemia, cancer, rheumatoid arthritis, stroke, and heart disease. For instance, Cu complexes, such as Cu aspirinate and Cu tryptophanate, markedly increase the healing rate of ulcers and wounds. While studies have shown that nonsteroidal anti-inflammatory drugs, such as ibuprofen, suppress wound healing, Cu complexes of these drugs promote normal wound healing in addition to retaining anti-inflammatory activity.

24.7.2 PHYSIOLOGICAL ROLE

Cu is both a toxic and essential element for living systems. Cu occurs as part of the prosthetic group of proteins. As a cofactor for the enzyme Cu/Zn superoxide dismutase, Cu protects against free radical damage that may affect proteins, membrane lipids, and nucleic acids. It is necessary for enzymes involved in aerobic metabolism, such as cytochrome c oxidase in mitochondria, lysyl oxidase

---

* In a Japanese population, long-term ingestion of water and food contaminated with Cd was associated with a crippling condition, "*itai-itai*" (*ouch-ouch*) disease. The syndrome is characterized by pain in the back and joints, osteomalacia (adult rickets), bone fractures, and occasional renal failure. Women are more commonly affected.

in connective tissue, dopamine β-hydroxylase in the CNS, and ceruloplasmin, a Cu transport protein. Cu deficiencies have been linked to mental retardation, anemia, hypothermia, bone fragility, and impaired cardiac, neuronal, and immune functions.

24.7.3 MECHANISM OF TOXICITY

Although poorly understood, the mechanism of Cu toxicity is related to the dose and length of exposure (acute or chronic toxicity). Acute toxicity via oral ingestion of high doses of Cu results in nausea and vomiting. Acute Cu toxicity appears to be related to direct irritation of the stomach by Cu ions.

Similarly, the mechanism of chronic toxicity is not clearly defined. It has been postulated to participate in Fenton-type reactions and lysosomal lipid peroxidation leading to cell death.

24.7.4 TOXICOKINETICS

Ingested Cu is absorbed in the stomach, where low stomach pH frees bound Cu ions from partially digested food particles. Cu complexes and solubilizes with amino acids and organic acids in the intestinal tract. The largest portion of ingested Cu is absorbed by the duodenum and ileum through simple diffusion. Cu-transporting ATPases discharge Cu into the serosal capillaries where they bind to albumin and amino acids for transport to the liver. Circulating Cu may also combine with ceruloplasmin (a sialoglycoprotein) in the circulation and returned to the liver as ceruloplasmin-bound Cu.

Approximately one half of the Cu consumed is absorbed by the GI tract, two thirds of which is secreted into the bile and excreted in the feces. Small amounts of Cu are also excreted in the urine, hair, and sweat. Cu bioavailability is influenced by age and amount ingested.

Cu has a great affinity for metallothionein, a small cysteine-rich protein thought to be involved in its storage and transport. High Cu levels stimulate metallothionein synthesis. Glutathione, amino acids, ATP, and recently identified Cu metallochaperones have been shown to help in intracellular transport. Cu-binding ligands protect against toxicity by regulating its movement. The ligands transport Cu within the cell, making it available for intracellular enzymes.

24.7.5 SIGNS AND SYMPTOMS OF ACUTE TOXICITY

Most human cases of acute poisonings with high doses of Cu result from attempted suicides and accidental ingestion of contaminated food and beverages. Acute Cu toxicity is associated with bleeding and ulceration of the GI mucosa, acute hemolysis, and hemoglobinuria. Hepatic necrosis accompanied with jaundice, hypotension, tachycardia, tachypnea, nephropathy, and CNS manifestations, including dizziness, headache and convulsions, can result from acute exposure. The principal targets are the GI tract, liver, kidney, blood, CNS, and cardiovascular system. There are little known effects on the muscular, integumentary, or ocular systems.

24.7.6 Signs and Symptoms of Chronic Toxicity

The liver is the major target of chronic Cu toxicity. Liver disease due to chronic Cu exposure is well characterized in individuals with Wilson's disease, a genetic disorder that results in systemic accumulation of Cu. Chronic exposures have been reported, with high-dose Cu supplements and in drinking water, whose pathology resembles that seen in Wilson's disease. Chronic exposure has also resulted in CNS effects and hemolytic anemia. The anemia is secondary to hepatic necrosis that releases Cu into the circulation, resulting in red blood cell destruction.

24.7.7 Treatment of Acute Poisoning

Removal from Cu exposure is recommended and is often sufficient to resolve most symptoms associated with Cu toxicity. Drinking 4 to 8 ounces of milk or water prior to gastric lavage is recommended for acute poisonings. To prevent further absorption, activated charcoal is suggested. If symptoms persist, Ca disodium-EDTA or intramuscular dimercaprol is given, followed by penicillamine. Vigorous irrigation with water is used for ocular exposure. Application of topical corticosteroids is applied for cases of Cu dermatitis.

24.8 IRON (Fe)

24.8.1 Chemical Characteristics

Iron (Fe) forms ferrous (2^+) and ferric (3^+) compounds. Ferrous compounds are easily oxidized to ferric compounds. Ferrous sulfate (green vitriol or Cuas), the most important of the ferrous compounds, usually occurs as pale-green crystals. The ferrous and ferric ions combine with cyanides to form complex cyanide compounds.

24.8.2 Occurrence and Uses

Ferric ferrocyanide, a dark-blue, amorphous solid formed by the reaction of potassium ferrocyanide with a ferric salt (*Prussian blue*), is used as a pigment in paint and in laundry bluing. Potassium ferricyanide (*red prussiate of potash*) is obtained from ferrous ferricyanide (*Turnbull's blue*) and is used in processing blueprint paper. Fe compounds are also employed in the treatment of hypochromic or Fe-deficiency anemia.

24.8.3 Physiological Role

Fe is an essential metal for almost all living systems, due to its involvement in a number of Fe-containing enzymes and proteins. It is estimated that one third of the world's population suffers from anemia due to Fe deficiency. It is an important component of hemoglobin, myoglobin, and cytochrome enzymes.

The average adult human stores about 3.9 to 4.5 g of Fe. Of this, 65% is bound to hemoglobin, 20 to 30% is bound to the Fe storage proteins ferritin and hemosiderin, and the remaining 10% is a constituent of myoglobin, cytochromes, and

Fe-containing enzymes. Hemoglobin is required for oxygen and carbon dioxide transport. As a component of cytochromes and nonheme Fe proteins, Fe is required for oxidative phosphorylation. Myeloperoxidase, a lysosomal enzyme, requires Fe for proper phagocytosis and killing of bacteria by neutrophils. Fe deficiency results in anemia and decreased immune competence.

24.8.4 MECHANISM OF TOXICITY

Although Fe deficiency is a widespread concern, Fe toxicity, or Fe overload, still presents a significant problem. Organ and cell damage arising from chronic Fe overload affects the liver, heart, and pancreatic beta cells. Hemosiderosis is a rare condition caused by excess Fe intake or improper Fe metabolism. Cirrhosis and hepatoma account for a large number of premature deaths in individuals with the hereditary form of this disease, hematochromatosis.

Since Fe metabolism is important for the maintenance of homeostasis, Fe overload will likely have a negative effect on its regulation. Accumulation results in cell and organ damage. The precise mechanism of toxicity of overload remains unknown, but a number of possibilities have been explored. Metals such as Fe tend to amplify oxidant damage via the Fenton reaction. Subsequently, Fe overloads have been observed to target systems with very active mitochondria. The use of antioxidants effectively combats Fe-mediated oxidative damage. In addition, Fe accumulation within the cellular lysosomal compartment sensitizes lysosomes to damage and rupture. Release of lysosomal enzymes into the cytoplasm of the cell induces autophagocytosis, apoptosis or necrosis.

24.8.5 TOXICOKINETICS

Fe metabolism is unique in that it operates primarily as a closed system, with Fe stores being efficiently reused by the body. Fe losses are minimal (< 1 mg/day), but absorption is usually poor. The metal generally is present in foods in the ferric form, bound to proteins and organic acids. Release of Fe from these carriers is a prerequisite for Fe to be absorbed. While only 10% of Fe ingested in the diet is absorbed, severe deficiency increases absorption to about 30%.

Low pH in the stomach reduces the ferric form to the ferrous form, which is then absorbed by the intestinal mucosal cells. Under the influence of apoferritin, ferrous Fe is converted back to the ferric form and eventually enters the plasma. Transferrin transports Fe to the liver, where it is bound to ferritin and hemosiderin. Fe is transported via transferrin from the liver to the bone marrow for the production of hemoglobin and myoglobin, and to other tissues for the incorporation into cytochromes and nonheme Fe.

24.8.6 SIGNS AND SYMPTOMS OF ACUTE TOXICITY

Acute Fe poisoning has been well documented and is divided into 5 clinical stages: (1) GI toxicity, (2) relative stability, (3) shock and acidosis, (4) hepatotoxicity, and (5) GI scarring.

GI toxicity occurs within a few hours of ingestion. Symptoms include nausea, emesis, and diarrhea. These symptoms are often mistakenly interpreted as caustic damage to the gut but are instead a result of free radical generation. Approximately 6 to 12 h after ingestion there is a period of **relative stability** in severely poisoned patients. This stage must be differentiated from mild poisoning, and careful clinical assessment usually will identify some degree of hypovolemia and acidosis. **Shock and acidosis** may occur a few hours to 24 to 48 h after ingestion. Hypovolemic shock occurs in response to fluid and blood losses from the gut. Cardiogenic shock usually occurs 24 to 48 h after ingestion and represents a depressant effect of Fe upon myocardial cells. **Hepatotoxicity** occurs within 2 days of ingestion and is the second most common cause of death in Fe poisoning. The liver is at risk because its portal circulation exposes it to the highest concentrations of Fe. Liver cells have a high metabolic activity that favors production of free radicals. Finally, **GI scarring** occurs 2 to 4 weeks after ingestion. Patients present with partial or complete bowel obstruction as the initial injury to the gut lumen heals by scarring and stenosis.

24.8.7 Signs and Symptoms of Chronic Toxicity

Chronic Fe toxicity can be caused by hereditary hematochromatosis due to abnormal absorption of Fe from the intestinal tract, from excess dietary Fe, and from repeated blood transfusions for certain forms of anemia (transfusional siderosis). The symptoms of all three types are very similar and result in disturbances of liver function, diabetes mellitus, endocrine disturbances, and cardiovascular effects.

24.8.8 Treatment of Acute Poisoning

Treatment of acute poisoning is aimed toward removal of Fe from the GI tract by the induction of vomiting and gastric lavage. Deferoxamine is an Fe chelator and is the treatment of choice for acute Fe overload. Repeated phlebotomy has also been suggested, as it is effective in removing as much as 20 mg of Fe per treatment.

24.8.9 Clinical Monitoring

Calculation of percent transferrin saturation indirectly measures Fe stores (serum Fe and Fe binding capacity). The serum ferritin correlates well with Fe stores, but it can also be elevated with liver disease, inflammatory conditions, and malignant neoplasms. A complete blood count (CBC) is also an indirect measure of Fe stores, because the mean corpuscular volume (MCV) of the RBC is increased with Fe overload. The amount of storage Fe for erythropoiesis is quantified by performing an Fe stain on a bone marrow biopsy. Excessive Fe stores are determined by bone marrow and liver biopsies.

24.9 LEAD (Pb)

24.9.1 Occurrence and Uses

One of the oldest known metals, lead (Pb) was used by the ancient Babylonians, Egyptians, and the Romans to make water pipes and solder. Pb ranks 36th in abundance in the Earth's crust, is seldom found alone, and its compounds are widely distributed throughout the world. Three principal ores are galena (sulfide form), cerussite, and angelsite. The main use of Pb is in the production of storage batteries and in sheathing electric cables. It is also useful as protective shielding from x-rays and radiation from nuclear reactors.

Pb compounds are commonly used as pigments in paint, putty, and ceramic and as insecticides. It was incorporated as an "antiknock" agent in gasoline, until it was banned as an environmental pollutant.

24.9.2 MECHANISM OF TOXICITY

Pb toxicity affects virtually all organs and systems of the body. The proposed mechanism of Pb toxicity involves its ability to inhibit or mimic the action of calcium (Ca) and to interfere with vital proteins by binding to sulfhydryl, amine, phosphate, and carboxyl groups. Pb increases intracellular levels of Ca in brain capillaries, neurons, hepatocytes, and arteries that trigger smooth muscle contraction, thereby inducing hypertension.

Effects of Pb on blood have been extensively documented. Pb interferes with heme biosynthesis by interfering with ferrochelatase, ALAS (aminolevulinic acid synthetase), and ALAD (aminolevulinic acid dehydrase). Therefore, decreased hemoglobin and anemia result in individuals exposed to excessive Pb. Effects on heme synthesis impact renal and neurological parameters as well. In bone, Pb alters circulating levels of 1,25-dihydroxyvitamin D, affecting Ca homeostasis and bone cell function. In the nervous system, Pb substitutes for Ca as a secondary messenger in neurons, blocking voltage-gated Ca channels, inhibiting influx of Ca and subsequent release of neurotransmitter. The result is an inhibition of synaptic transmission. Pb inhibits glutamate uptake and glutamate synthetase activity in astroglia, thus inhibiting the regeneration of glutamate, a major excitatory neurotransmitter.

24.9.3 TOXICOKINETICS

The bioavailability of Pb is dependent on ingestion in the presence of food (10% or less) or after fasting (60 to 80%). Immediately following ingestion, Pb is distributed widely to plasma and soft tissue and redistributes and accumulates in bone. In children, bone Pb accounts for about 73% of the total body burden, while in adults it increases to 94% due to the slower turnover rate of bone with age.[*] The rate of disposition of inhaled inorganic Pb is about 30 to 50% but is largely dependent on the particle size and ventilation rate.

Pb not retained in the body is excreted primarily by the kidneys as soluble salts or through biliary clearance in the GI tract in the form of conjugates with organic compounds. Exhalation is also considered to be a major excretion route of organic Pb.

Distribution of Pb in humans has been well characterized. Blood Pb is found primarily in RBCs (99%); distribution occurs primarily to soft tissue. Liver, lung, spleen, and kidneys have the highest concentrations, with redistribution resulting in

---

[*] Pb absorption is dependent on nutritional status. In children, Fe deficiency correlates with higher blood Pb levels, suggesting that Fe may affect Pb absorption. A similar correlation was found with Ca levels.

high bone concentrations. Pb does not distribute routinely in bone, but will accumulate in those regions undergoing active calcification at the time of exposure.

Inorganic Pb is not metabolized or biotransformed, but forms complexes with a variety of protein and nonprotein ligands. Organic Pb is metabolized in the liver by an oxidative dealkylation reaction catalyzed by cytochrome P450.

24.9.4 SIGNS AND SYMPTOMS OF ACUTE TOXICITY

Exposure to excessive Pb, through the GI tract or by inhalation, usually results in cramping, colicky abdominal pain, and constipation. Severe abdominal pain is accompanied by nausea, vomiting, and bloody stools. Early symptoms of Pb exposure include fatigue, apathy, and vague GI pain. Arthralgias and myalgias of the extremities may also occur. Headache, confusion, stupor, coma, seizures, and optic neuritis are all manifestations of Pb neurotoxicity. Upon further exposure, central nervous system symptoms such as insomnia, confusion, impaired concentration, and memory problems become more pronounced. Lengthy exposure can present with a distal motor neuropathy, progressing to Pb encephalopathy with seizures and coma. Reproductive problems, such as infertility in men, spontaneous abortions, gouty arthritis, and renal failure, have been reported.

24.9.5 SIGNS AND SYMPTOMS OF CHRONIC TOXICITY

Chronically exposed individuals develop anemia and demonstrate pallor. Jaundice may be seen due to acute hemolysis. Examination of the gums may show a blue-gray pigmentation, or "lead-line."

24.9.6 TREATMENT OF ACUTE POISONING

Parenteral administration of chelating agents, dimercaprol and $CaNa_2$-EDTA, is used to reduce body burdens of absorbed Pb. Penicillamine has been used as an oral chelating agent, although it is not as effective as EDTA. In patients with kidney impairment, dimercaprol is recommended, since excretion is primarily in bile rather than urine. EDTA mobilizes Pb from bone to soft tissue and may aggravate acute toxicity if not given in conjunction with dimercaprol. DMSA (succimer) is the only FDA-approved orally administered chelating agent for treating children with Pb blood levels > 45 µg/dl.

24.9.7 CLINICAL MONITORING

Because Pb accumulates in RBCs rather than plasma, the method of choice for determination of Pb exposure was the erythrocyte protoporphyrin (EP). For two decades this assay was used to determine the accumulation of protoporphyrin in erythrocytes. The assay, however, proved to be insensitive to Pb levels in the 10 to 25 µg/dl range; it is not recommended for tracking childhood Pb poisonings. The evolution of more sensitive testing techniques has made measuring Pb in blood more feasible. Determinations can be made at concentrations as low as 1 µg/dl (Table

24.1). As Pb redistributes to bone, the use of radiographic techniques occasionally proves useful for the detection of "lead lines."

24.10 MERCURY (Hg)

24.10.1 CHEMICAL CHARACTERISTICS

There are three toxic forms of Hg: elemental, inorganic, and organic. Hg compounds are considered to be major pollutants of the biosphere, with organic mercurials as the most toxic forms.

24.10.2 OCCURRENCE AND USES

Two major sources of Hg deposition in the biosphere are the natural degassing of the earth's crust and the leaching of sediment. This natural source of contamination is estimated at 25,000 to 150,000 tons of Hg per year, which binds to organic or inorganic particles and to sediment that has a high sulfur content. Although discharges of Hg have been strictly regulated, some industrial activities still release substantial quantities of the metal. For example, fossil fuel contains as much as 1.0 ppm. Since 1973, approximately 5,000 to 10,000 tons of Hg per year has been discharged from burning coal, natural gas, and the refining of petroleum products, with one third of the atmospheric Hg due to industrial releases. Hg is used in a number of products including thermometers, barometers, electrical apparatus, paints, and pharmaceuticals.

Regardless of the source, both organic and inorganic Hg undergoes environmental transformation. Conversion of inorganic Hg to methyl Hg results in its release from sediment at a relatively fast rate and leads to its wider distribution. Inorganic Hg may be methylated and demethylated by microorganisms. Elemental Hg at ambient air temperatures volatilizes and is extremely dangerous.

24.10.3 OCCUPATIONAL AND ENVIRONMENTAL EXPOSURE

Methyl Hg released in the aqueous environment bioaccumulates in plankton, algae, and fish. In fish the absorption rate of methyl Hg is faster than that of inorganic Hg, and its clearance rate is slower, resulting in high methyl Hg concentrations. This is of interest since fish enter the food chain.

The pollution of the environment with Hg compounds has resulted in an increased level of neurotoxicity, referred to as Minamata disease, named after a historic outbreak of Hg poisoning in Japan. Two poisonings, one in Minamata Bay (1956–1975) and in Niigata (1964), occurred as a consequence of industrial releases of Hg compounds into Minamata Bay and the Agano River. An additional outbreak occurred in Iraq (1971–1972), resulting from eating bread made from seed grain coated with a methyl Hg fungicide.

Most human exposure to Hg is by inhalation, because it readily diffuses across the alveolar membrane due to its lipid solubility. Because of this property it has a high affinity for RBCs and the CNS.

24.10.4 MECHANISM OF TOXICITY

The mechanism of Hg toxicity is believed to be related to high-affinity binding of divalent mercuric ions to thiol or SH groups of proteins. Inactivation of various enzymes and structural proteins, and alterations of cell membrane permeability, are believed to contribute to the severe toxicologic effects. Increased oxidative stress, disruption of microtubule formation, interference with protein synthesis, DNA replication, and Ca homeostasis are purported pathways.

24.10.5 TOXICOKINETICS

Inhaled Hg vapor is efficiently absorbed (70 to 80%); absorption of liquid metallic Hg is considered insignificant. The absorption rate for inorganic mercuric salts varies greatly and is dependent largely on the chemical form. Oral absorption of organic Hg is nearly 100%.

For all forms of Hg, the highest accumulation is in kidney. Because of the high lipophilicity of metallic Hg, transfer through the placenta and the blood-brain barrier is complete. Inorganic Hg compounds have a lower lipophilicity and, although there is distribution to most organs, penetration is not as effective.

Metallic Hg is oxidized to the divalent form by the catalase pathway, and the divalent form is reduced to the metallic form. Elimination occurs via urine, feces, and expired air for metallic Hg. Inorganic Hg is eliminated in urine and feces, while organic Hg is eliminated primarily in the feces. Renal excretion of inorganic Hg increases with time. Both inorganic and organic forms are excreted in breast milk. A small fraction of Hg may be exhaled after exposure to Hg vapor. About 90% of methyl Hg is excreted in feces after acute or chronic exposure. Methyl Hg excretion however does not increase with time.

24.10.6 SIGNS AND SYMPTOMS OF ACUTE TOXICITY (INHALATION AND INGESTION)

Accidental acute exposure to high concentrations of metallic Hg vapor has resulted in human fatalities. The most commonly reported symptoms of acute inhalation exposure are cough, dyspnea, tightness, and burning pain in the chest. GI effects include acute inflammation of the oral cavity, abdominal pain, nausea, and vomiting. Increased heart rate and blood pressure are evidence of cardiovascular effects. Renal effects resulting in proteinuria, hematuria, and oliguria have been demonstrated, and severe neurotoxic effects resulting in behavioral, motor, and sensory disruptions are common.

Ingestion of inorganic mercurial salts causes severe GI irritation including pain, vomiting, diarrhea, and renal failure. Contact dermatitis, hyperkeratosis, acrodynia (*pink disease*), shock, and cardiovascular collapse are observed in patients with acute exposure to inorganic mercurial salts.

24.10.7 SUBACUTE OR CHRONIC POISONING

The major clinical symptoms of methyl Hg toxicity are neurologic and include, in order, paresthesia, ataxia, dysarthria, and deafness. There may be a latency period of weeks or months from the time of exposure until the development of symptoms. Some pathological features include degeneration and necrosis of neurons in focal areas of the occipital cortex and in the granular layer of the cerebellum. This particular distribution of lesions in the CNS is thought to reflect a propensity of Hg damage to small neurons in cerebellum and visual cortex.

24.10.8 CLINICAL MANAGEMENT OF HG POISONING

Treatments of Hg poisonings are considered to be experimental. Even prompt action and monitoring may result in fatality. For dermal or ocular exposure, washing of exposed areas is suggested. Reducing absorption from the GI tract refers mostly to inorganic forms. Oral administration of a protein solution has been suggested to reduce absorption, based on Hg's affinity for binding to SH groups. Administration of activated charcoal has been used in the case of acute high-dose situations. Gastric lavage and induction of emesis are also recommended, although emesis is contraindicated following ingestion of mercuric oxide, due to its caustic nature.

To reduce body burden, chelation therapy is the treatment of choice. The chelator used will depend on the form of Hg, route of exposure, and possible side effects that might be experienced. BAL is one of the more effective chelators for inorganic Hg salts, while D-penicillamine is marginally effective as a chelator for elemental and inorganic Hg.

24.11 SELENIUM (Se)

24.11.1 OCCURRENCE AND USES

Selenium (Se) closely resembles sulfur and is chemically related to tellurium. Like sulfur, it exists in several different forms. The burning of fossil fuels and coal accounts for much of the Se released into the environment. Se is used in photoelectric devices (Gray Se) and is used to impart a scarlet red color to glass and enamels (Red Se, sodium selenide) and as a decolorizer of glass. Sodium selenate is used as an insecticide, while Se sulfide is used clinically in the treatment of skin disorders such as dandruff, acne, eczema, and seborrheic dermatitis.

The amount of Se in food sources, whether consumed directly as plants or as meat from animals that have eaten the vegetation, varies according to soil levels. Most Se in foods is lost during processing, such as in the making of white rice or white flour. Many natural foods contain a much less toxic organic form of Se. Se is sometimes added to drinking water when deficient.

24.11.2 PHYSIOLOGICAL ROLE

Se, once classified solely as a toxic mineral, was recognized in the 1970s as an essential **trace** element. It is a component of the enzyme glutathione peroxidase, which accounts for its antioxidant function. It is also found in deiodinases, and thioredoxin reductase. Selenocysteine is the biologically active form of Se found in each of the above. The metal has a variety of properties ranging from anticancer and antioxidant to effects on the immune, reproductive, and nervous systems.

Two endemic diseases have been associated with Se deficiency. Keshan's disease is a form of heart disease characterized by cardiomegaly, congestive heart failure, abnormal ECG, and multifocal necrosis of the myocardium. The disease is prevalent in children and women of childbearing age and has been successfully treated with Se supplementation. Kashin-Beck disease is an osteoarthropathic disease characterized by atrophic necrosis and degeneration of the cartilage. Se has proven to be a successful treatment in this disease as well.

There is less than 1 mg of Se present in the average adult, most of it concentrated in liver, kidneys, pancreas, testes, and seminal vesicles. Men have a greater need for Se, which may function in sperm production and motility. Some Se is lost through the sperm as well as through the urine and feces. It is absorbed fairly well from the intestines, with an absorption rate of nearly 60%.

24.11.3 Mechanism of Toxicity

Long-term effects of excess Se on the hair, nails, skin, liver, and nervous system have been well documented; however the biochemical mechanisms by which Se exerts toxicity remain largely unknown.

Acute Se toxicity may be the result of inactivation of sulfhydryl enzymes that are necessary for cellular respiration. High Se concentrations have the ability to replace sulfur in biomolecules, especially under conditions of low sulfur, possibly resulting in toxicity. Replacement of selenomethionine for selenocysteine in protein synthesis is another purported mechanism of toxicity.

24.11.4 Toxicokinetics

Se compounds are absorbed by the GI route, ranging from 44 to 95% of ingested dose. Absorption depends on the physical state of the ingested form, the chemical form, and the dose, with soluble Se having greater absorption rates than solid. Se is also absorbed via inhalation. The metal distributes to all tissues, with the highest concentrations found in kidney, liver, spleen, and pancreas. Se also tends to concentrate in RBCs and is amenable to placental transfer.

Excessive amounts of Se are excreted primarily via the urinary system, leaving trace amounts of Se in the body. Excretion of Se occurs in feces, expired air, and sweat.

24.11.5 Signs and Symptoms of Acute Toxicity

Clinical signs of acute toxicity following ingestion of high doses of Se include excessive salivation, garlic odor to the breath, shallow breathing, and diarrhea. Pulmonary edema and lung lesions were observed in acute lethal doses. Tachycardia, abdominal pain, nausea, vomiting, and abnormal liver functions were seen in human acute *selenosis*. Inhalation of Se or its compounds results in irritation of the mucous membranes of the respiratory tract, dyspnea, bronchial spasms, bronchitis, and chemical pneumonias.

24.11.6 Signs and Symptoms of Chronic Toxicity

Clinical signs of chronic *selenosis* include loss of hair and fingernails, skin lesions, and clubbing of the fingers. Nervous system effects such as numbness, convulsions, paralysis, and motor disturbances have been described.

24.11.7 Clinical Management of Poisoning

There are no specific methods that are recommended for the treatment of acute high-dose exposure to Se via inhalation, and only supportive treatment has been recommended for oral overdose. Gastric lavage and induction of vomiting with emetics may reduce absorption, but because selenious acid is caustic, both procedures would be contraindicated. Chelators such as EDTA and BAL have not been successful treatments and, in fact, may increase its toxic effects.

24.12 ZINC (Zn)

24.12.1 Occurrence and Uses

Zinc (Zn) is used extensively as a protective coating or galvanizer for iron and steel. Its brass alloy is used as plates for dry cells and die casting. Clinically, Zn oxide has antiseptic and astringent properties. Zn salts have also been used in electroplating, for soldering, as rodenticides, herbicides, pigments, wood preservatives, and as solubilizing agents (zinc insulin suspensions).

24.12.2 Physiological Role

Zn is an essential metal required for proper functioning of a large number of metalloenzymes, including alcohol dehydrogenase, alkaline phosphatase, carbonic anhydrase, Zn-Cu superoxide dismutase, leucine peptidase, and DNA and RNA polymerase. Zn deficiency results in dermatitis, growth retardation, impaired immune function and congenital malformations. The metal has a role in the maintenance of nucleic acid structure of genes through the formation of "Zn finger" proteins.

Zn interacts with other physiologically important metals. Zn and Cu have a reciprocal relationship — i.e., large intake of Zn may result in Cu deficiency. The metal also interacts with Ca and is necessary for proper bone calcification. Cd competes with Zn in binding to sulfhydryl groups present on macromolecules. It also induces the metal-binding protein, metallothionein, which is involved in the absorption, metabolism, and storage of both essential and nonessential metals.

24.12.3 Mechanism of Toxicity

The mechanism of Zn toxicity has not been fully elucidated, although it enters cells via channels that are shared by Fe and Ca. This pathway may be a prerequisite for cell injury.

24.12.4 TOXICOKINETICS

Under normal physiologic conditions 20 to 30% of an ingested dose of Zn is absorbed via the GI route. Zn absorption is influenced by P, Ca, and dietary fiber, but once absorbed, it is widely distributed. The highest content is found in muscle, bone, GI tract, brain, skin, lung, heart, and pancreas. In blood, about two thirds of Zn is bound to albumin. The principal route of excretion is in the feces and, to a lesser extent, through the urinary system.

24.12.5 SIGNS AND SYMPTOMS OF ACUTE TOXICITY

Acute toxicity varies depending on the form ingested or inhaled. Metal fume fever, which is a result of inhalation of Zn oxides, causes chest pains, cough, and dyspnea. Zn chloride is more damaging and corrosive to the mucous membranes. Bilateral diffuse infiltrates, pneumothorax, and acute pneumonitis have been described. Oral ingestion of large doses of Zn sulfate has been associated with GI distress and alterations of GI tissue, including vomiting, burning in the throat, abdominal cramps, and diarrhea.

24.12.6 SIGNS AND SYMPTOMS OF CHRONIC TOXICITY

Hematological changes have been reported in patients with chronic exposure to Zn. Long-term administration of Zn supplements has been implicated in cases of anemia.

24.12.7 CLINICAL MANAGEMENT OF POISONING

General recommendations for management of excess Zn exposure include removal of the victim from the immediate area of exposure in the case of inhalation and irrigation with water for ocular and dermal exposure. For acute oral toxicity, administration of ipecac to induce vomiting is not recommended in the presence of caustic Zn compounds. Ingestion of large amounts of milk and cheese may reduce Zn absorption in the GI tract due to the high levels of phosphorus and Ca present in these products.

To reduce body burdens of Zn, administration of $CaNa_2$-EDTA is the treatment of choice, while dimercaprol has also been recommended.

REFERENCES

SUGGESTED READINGS

Agency for Toxic Substances and Disease Registry (ATSDR), Toxicological profiles for: arsenic (2000), asbestos (2001), cadmium (1999), lead (1999), mercury (1999), selenium (2001), and zinc (1994). U.S. Department of Health and Human Services, Public Health Service, Atlanta, GA.
Ellenhorn, M.J. and Barceloux, D.G., *Medical Toxicology. Diagnosis and Treatment of Human Poisoning*, Elsevier, New York, 1988.

Goldfrank, L.R., Flomenbaum, N.E., Lewin, N.A., et al., *Toxicologic Emergencies*, 7th ed., McGraw-Hill, New York, 2002.
Goyer, R.A. and Clarkson, T.W., Toxic effects of metals. in *Casarett and Doull's Toxicology: The Basic Science of Poisons*, 6th ed., Klaassen, C.D., Ed., McGraw-Hill, New York, 2001.
Hazardous Substances Data Bank, National Library of Medicine, Bethesda, MD, 2001.
Lewis, R.L., Metals, in *LaDou, J., Occupational and Environmental Medicine*, 2nd ed., Appleton and Lange, Stamford, CT, 1997, p. 405.
Linder, M. and Goode, C.A., *Biochemistry of Copper*, Plenum Press, New York, 1991.
Budavari, S., Ed., *The Merck Index*, 12th ed., Merck & Co., Inc, Rahway, NJ, 1996, p. 1455.
Stutz, D.R. and Janusz, S.J., *Hazardous Materials Injuries: A Handbook for Pre-Hospital Care*, 2nd ed., Bradford Communications Corporation, Beltsville, MD, 1988, p. 314.
Tiffany-Castiglioni, E., et al., Astroglia in lead neurotoxicity, in *The Role of Glia in Neurotoxicity*, Aschner M. and Kimelberg, H.K., Eds., CRC Press, Inc., Boca Raton, FL, 1996, p.175.

REVIEW ARTICLES

Aouad, F., et al., Evaluation of new iron chelators and their therapeutic potential, *Inorg. Chim. Acta.*, 339, 470, 2002.
Baldwin, D.R. and Marshall, W.J., Heavy metal poisoning and its laboratory investigation. *Ann. Clin. Biochem.*, 36, 267, 1999.
Brewer, G.J. and Yuxbasiyan-Gurkan, V., Wilson's disease, *Medicine*, 71, 139, 1992.
Carter, R.E. and Taylor, W.G., Identification of a particular amphibole asbestos fiber in tissues of persons exposed to a high oral intake of the mineral, *Environ. Res.*, 21, 85, 1980.
Dopp, E. and Schiffman, D., Analysis of chromosomal alterations induced by asbestos and ceramic fibers, *Toxicol. Lett.*, 96, 155, 1998.
Eaton, J.W. and Qian, M., Molecular bases of cellular Fe toxicity, *Free Rad. Bio. Med.*, 32, 833, 2002.
Hall, A.H., Chronic arsenic poisoning, *Toxicol. Lett.*, 128, 69, 2002.
Klaassen, C.D., Liu, J., and Choudhuri, S., Metallothionein: an intracellular protein to protect against cadmium toxicity, *Ann. Rev. Pharm. Tox.*, 39, 267, 1999.
Miller, A.L., Dimercaptosuccinic acid (DMSA), a nontoxic, water-soluble treatment for heavy metal toxicity, *Altern. Med. Rev.* 3, 199, 1998.
Rayman, M., The importance of selenium to human health, *Lancet*, 356, 233, 2000.
Tenenbein, M. Toxicokinetics and toxicodynamics of iron poisoning, *Toxicol. Lett.*, 102, 653, 1998.
Tossavainen, A., Karjaleinen, A. and Karhunen, P. J., Retention of asbestos fibers in the body, *Environ. Health Perspect.*, 102, 253, 1994.
Waalkes, M.P., Cadmium carcinogenesis in review, *J. In. Biochem.*, 79, 241, 2000.

25 Aliphatic and Aromatic Hydrocarbons

25.1 INTRODUCTION

25.1.1 ALIPHATIC AND ALICYCLIC HYDROCARBONS

Hydrocarbons (HCs) are composed of carbon and hydrogen molecules whose carbon–carbon (C–C) bonds are composed of either all single (*saturated*) bonds or combinations of single and multiple (*unsaturated*) bonds. Aliphatic HCs, the term usually pertaining to fats or oils, applies to straight, open chains of carbon atoms, rather than ring structures, the simplest of which are the saturated HCs (*alkanes*). In addition, alkanes exist as *unbranched* straight chains or *branched* (for butane or longer chains), depending on the structural isomerism. Multiple C–C bonds result when hydrogens are removed from the alkanes, yielding unsaturated HCs such as *alkenes* (double C–C bond) and *alkynes* (triple C–C bonds). Alicyclic HCs are saturated, ring structures consisting of three or more carbon atoms. Unlike the aromatic chemicals (below), cyclopropane, cyclobutane, cyclopentane and cyclohexane, for example, have three-, four-, five-, and six-membered rings, respectively, but do not exhibit double bonds within the rings.

25.1.2 AROMATIC HCs

Aromatic HCs are a special class of unsaturated HCs that contain one or more planar rings, such as a benzene ring. Benzene is the simplest aromatic molecule that can exist alone, attached as a substituent to other HCs (as a *phenyl* group), or as a substituted benzene (*halogenated* or *methylated* benzene). Benzene also exists as part of more complex aromatic systems consisting of a number of fused benzene rings, such as naphthalene or anthracene.

The vast majority of these compounds, however, are fundamental HCs but contain additional elements (*functional groups*) classifying them as **HC derivatives**, each of which possesses characteristic chemical properties. The functional groups consist of halogens (–X, such as F^-, Cl^-, Br^-, I^-), alcohols (–OH), ethers (–O–), aldehydes (–CO–H), ketones (–CO–), carboxylic acids (–COOH), esters (–CO–O–), and amines (–NH$_2$).[*]

---

[*] The formula –CO– represents a C=O double bond.

25.1.3 General Signs and Symptoms of Acute Toxicity

In general, exposure to HCs occurs primarily through inhalation, oral ingestion, and dermal routes. The ubiquitous nature of HC mixtures and their ready availability in consumer products render them easily accessible and a source of toxicity and fatality from accidental ingestion. In fact, in the U.S., 65,000 HC exposures were recorded in 2001 that required clinical intervention, 99% of which were accidental, and 65% involved children under 5 years of age. In addition, intentional inhalation is reported among adolescents and drug abusers, for the apparent euphoric effects. Deep inhalation of volatile HCs from cigarette lighter fluids (*sniffing*), paint adhesives (model airplane glue), and paint thinners, applied to the inside of a paper bag (*bagging*) or to a fabric (*huffing*), produces intended hallucinations and delusions. The effects, however, are accompanied by undesirable agitation, stupor, seizures, and increase the risk of cardiac arrhythmias.

Aliphatic and alicyclic HC gases and liquids are generally nontoxic or of low acute toxicity, with the majority of effects described as those for simple asphyxiants or pulmonary irritants (see Chapter 23, "Gases"). Aromatic and halogenated HCs are associated with acute, systemic, toxic potential, including hematological and hepatorenal toxicity, attributable in part to their volatility and viscosity. Some substances cause symptoms such as central nervous system (CNS) depression, narcosis, loss of consciousness, hallucination, stupor, and seizures. Gastrointestinal effects involve nausea and vomiting. Hematological consequences of HC toxicity result in mild hemolysis. Cardiovascular sensitization to circulating catecholamines, with the risk of arrhythmias, is a consequence of exposure to high concentrations of aromatics and chlorinated HCs.

Depending on the concentration of the chemical, dermal exposure produces thermal burns, requiring therapeutic intervention. Typical treatments for burn injuries, as well as use of HC ointments, such as Polysorbate 80, mineral oil, and petroleum jelly, are useful in managing the dermal trauma.

Although no antidote is available for HC poisoning, life-threatening toxicity is managed using supportive care. Because of the volatility of these chemicals, risk of aspiration pneumonitis increases with induction of vomiting, especially with administration of emetics, or with the use of gastric lavage.

25.2 PETROLEUM DISTILLATES

25.2.1 Occurrence and Uses

Petroleum and petroleum distillates represent an extremely valuable natural resource consisting of a complex mixture of thousands of aliphatic and aromatic compounds. Ninety percent of these petrochemicals are used for fuels for heating and transportation, as well as raw materials for the chemical industry. Thus, the derivatives of petroleum are used in the manufacturing of many common substances found in household products and in the industrial setting including, but not limited to, the production of oils, waxes, cements, fuels (gasoline, kerosene, lighter fluids), polymers (for plastics), paint and furniture products, and therapeutic agents (cod liver oil, mineral oil, laxatives).

25.2.2 MECHANISM OF TOXICITY

In general, toxicity and reactivity of aliphatic and alicyclic HCs are low. For instance, gaseous compounds have properties similar to pulmonary irritants or simple asphyxiants and usually produce anesthetic effects at very high ambient concentrations. Degree of cyclization or unsaturation does not correlate with toxicity. As with the simple asphyxiants, therefore, their toxicity is limited to the amount of substituted oxygen.

Aliphatic and alicyclic HCs are mostly flammable or combustible gases or liquids. Their ability to form explosive mixtures with air decreases as the carbon number increases above 13. Their ominous chemical nature appears to exaggerate their toxic potential, since most HCs are classified as nonpoisonous or have low acute toxicity upon exposure. Table 25.1 lists and summarizes the properties and toxicities of a variety of aliphatic and alicyclic HCs.

25.3 AROMATIC HYDROCARBONS

25.3.1 OCCURRENCE AND USES

Aromatic HCs consist of mononuclear or polynuclear benzene rings as part of their structure. They are widely distributed in petroleum and its products and are used as solvents and in the synthesis of organic chemicals.

25.3.2 MECHANISM OF TOXICITY

As with the aliphatic and alicyclic HCs, the toxicity of aromatic HCs is generally low.[*] At high concentrations, the substances affect the CNS, resulting in depression (narcosis), hallucinations, and stupor. Similarly, acute toxicity appears as minimal except in high concentrations. Common routes of exposure for liquids or solids include oral ingestion, inhalation, or dermal absorption. Aromatic HCs form explosive mixtures with air and are flammable with low flash points. They react with oxidizing agents, have moderate to strong aromatic odors, and are designated priority pollutants or hazardous waste by the U.S. Environmental Protection Agency (EPA). Table 25.2 lists and summarizes the properties and toxicities of some commonly encountered aromatic HCs possessing acute or chronic human toxicity. Other HCs have carcinogenic or mutagenic potential, primarily in animals, yet have not demonstrated acute or chronic toxicity in humans. These aromatic HCs are listed in Table 25.3.

---

[*] However, many of the polynuclear HCs are known or suspected human or animal carcinogens. The carcinogenic potential and clinical outcome of chronic exposure of these chemicals is addressed in Chapter 29, "Chemical Carcinogenesis and Mutagenesis."

TABLE 25.1
Properties, Sources, Uses, and Toxicity of Aliphatic and Alicyclic Hydrocarbons

Chemical	Properties	Source	Industrial[a] or Household Uses	Acute Human Toxic Effects
1,3-Butadiene	F colorless gas, aromatic odor	Petroleum distillate	Synthetic rubber, elastomers, food wrapping material	Asphyxiant; irritation, hallucinations; at high doses, narcosis; suspected carcinogen
Acetylene	F colorless gas	Petroleum distillate	Welding, illuminant, fuel, synthesis of acetylides	Simple asphyxiant; at high doses, headache, dyspnea, death
Cyclohexane	F colorless liq	Petroleum distillate	Solvent for paints & resins, organic synthesis	Low acute toxicity, CNS depression, pulmonary irritant
Cyclohexene	F colorless liq	Petroleum distillate, coal tar	Oil extraction, organic synthesis, gasoline stabilizer	Low acute toxicity, CNS depression, pulmonary irritant
Cyclopenta-diene	F colorless liq	Petroleum distillate	Resins, camphors, preparation of metals	Pulmonary irritant in rodents
Cyclopentane	F colorless liq	Petroleum distillate	Solvent, shoe industry, wax extraction	Low acute toxicity, CNS & respiratory depression, pulmonary irritant
Ethane	F odorless, colorless gas	Natural gas; petroleum cracking[b]	Fuel, refrigerant	Nonpoisonous, simple asphyxiant
Ethylene	F colorless gas	Petroleum distillate	Major starting material for organic synthesis; anesthetic	Simple asphyxiant; at high doses, narcosis & unconsciousness
Isobutane	F colorless gas	Natural gas; petroleum cracking	Liquid & motor fuels, organic synthesis	Simple asphyxiant; at high doses, narcosis

Isooctane	F colorless liq, gasoline odor	Petroleum distillate	Octane fuel reference for gasoline, solvent	Low acute toxicity, pulmonary irritant
Methane	F odorless, colorless gas	Natural gas from Earth's crust & landfills	Heating fuel, production of other gases	Nonpoisonous, simple asphyxiant
n-Butane	F colorless gas	Natural gas; petroleum cracking	Liquid & motor fuels, propellant, organic synthesis	Simple asphyxiant; at high doses, narcosis
n-Octane	F colorless liq	Petroleum cracking, gasoline	Solvent, organic synthesis	Low acute toxicity, CNS depression, pulmonary irritant
n-Pentane	F colorless liq, gasoline odor	Petroleum distillate	Solvent, plastics	Pulmonary irritant, narcosis
Propane	F colorless gas	Petroleum distillate	Fuel, refrigerant, organic synthesis	Simple asphyxiant; at high doses, narcosis
Propylene	F colorless gas (burns yellow)	Gasoline refining, Catalytic cracking of petroleum	Polypropylene (plastics)	Simple asphyxiant; at high doses, mild anesthetic

Note: F = flammable, liq = liquid.

[a] Used in manufacturing, synthesis, or as part of industrial processes.

[b] *Cracking* refers to the breaking of carbon-carbon bonds in the formation of smaller chemicals using pyrolysis (*thermal cracking*) or a catalyst (*catalytic cracking*).

TABLE 25.2
Properties, Sources, Uses, and Toxicity of Aromatic HCs

Chemical (or Common Name)	Properties	Source	Industrial[a] or Household Uses	Human Toxic Effects
Benzene	F colorless liq	Coal tar, landfills, petroleum	Solvent, dyes, paints, organic synthesis	**Acute**: pulmonary & dermal irritant; narcosis, convulsions; **chronic**: blood, BM, CNS, dermal, respiratory toxicity
Cumene (cumol)	F colorless liq	Petroleum, gasoline	Solvent, organic synthesis	**Acute**: pulmonary & dermal irritant; narcosis; **chronic**: unknown
Napthalene (tar camphor, mothballs)	White crystalline flakes	Petroleum, gasoline	Moth repellant, dyes, explosives, lubricants	**Acute**: pulmonary & dermal irritant; narcosis; hemolytic anemia (oral); **chronic**: ocular opacities
Styrene (cinnamol)	F yellow liq	Petroleum, gasoline	Polystyrene plastics, rubber, resins	**Acute**: pulmonary & dermal irritant; narcosis; **chronic**: unknown
Toluene (toluol)	F colorless liq	Coal tar, petroleum, gasoline	Production of benzene, TNT; solvent	**Acute**: similar to benzene; **chronic**: less toxic than benzene
Xylene (xylol)	F colorless liq	Petroleum, gasoline	Solvent, dyes, paints, organic synthesis	Similar to toluene

Note: BM = bone marrow, CNS = central nervous system, F = flammable, liq = liquid.

[a] Used in manufacturing, synthesis, or as part of industrial processes.

TABLE 25..3
Properties, Sources, and Effects of Aromatic HC with Low Suspicion of Human Toxicity

Chemical (or Common Name)	Properties	Source	Toxic Effects
Anthracene (green oil)	Greenish crystals	Dyes	Low toxicity; unknown carcinogenic potential
Benzo[a]-anthracene (tetraphene)	Greenish-yellow fluorescent crystals	Petroleum, gasoline	Lethal in mice (10 mg/kg, i.v. only); animal carcinogen
Benzo[a]pyrene	Yellowish crystals	Coal tar, petroleum, gasoline, tobacco smoke, smog	**Acute:** low; known mutagen, procarcinogen, teratogen in test species
Dibenz[a.h]-anthracene	Colorless crystals	Dyes	Similar to benzo[a]-anthracene
Phenanthrene	Blue fluorescent crystals	Dyes, explosives, pharmaceutical industry	**Acute:** low toxicity in humans; animal carcinogen
Pyrene	Colorless-yellowish crystals	Coal tar, petroleum, gasoline, tobacco smoke, smog	Pulmonary irritant in animals, no evidence of carcinogenicity or mutagenicity in animals

25.4 HALOGENATED HYDROCARBONS

25.4.1 OCCURRENCE AND USES

Halogenated aromatic or halogen-substituted aliphatic HCs (halocarbons) consist mostly of mononuclear benzene rings or straight, open chains of carbon atoms, respectively, whose hydrogen atoms are partially or fully replaced by halogen atoms (fluorine, chlorine, bromine and iodine). These liquids or solids are widely used as solvents, refrigerants, fire retardants, in organic synthesis of a variety of chemicals, and in the past, as general anesthetics.[*]

25.4.2 MECHANISM OF TOXICITY

Exposure to volatile liquid and gaseous halocarbons occurs primarily through inhalation, oral ingestion, and dermal exposure. As with the aliphatic, alicyclic, and aromatic HCs, the toxicity of halocarbons is generally low. At high concentrations, the volatile liquids and gases appear to affect the CNS and intestinal tract, resulting in anesthesia, drowsiness, incoordination, nausea, and vomiting. Hepatic, renal, and cardiac toxicity can prove fatal with inhalation at high concentrations. Some compounds are known animal and human carcinogens. Halocarbons range from noncombustible to highly flammable gases or liquids, the latter of which form explosive mixtures with air or when heated. Although the compounds are generally stable, they react violently with alkali metals and oxidizers. Table 25.4 lists and summarizes the properties and toxicities of common halocarbons with acute or chronic human toxicity.

25.5 METHODS OF DETECTION

Quantitative analysis of HCs is usually performed when sampling of ambient or contaminated areas is necessary. Identification of HC liquids is also performed in suspected forensic cases. Gas chromatographic (GC) techniques are sensitive to detecting HCs in air, soil, and biological samples. The volatility of the liquids renders them suitable for monitoring through a packed GC column (solid phase). For examining the composition of the flowing gas, a flame ionization or electron capture detector is required. Mass spectrometry (GC-MS) or nitrogen-specific detectors have been employed when absolute specificity is a principal requirement. These techniques have also been important in validating the other screening methods.

---

[*] Because of their toxicity, the use of chlorinated halocarbons as general anesthetics has been replaced by less toxic agents.

TABLE 25.4
Properties, Sources, Uses, and Toxicity of Halocarbons

Chemical	Properties	Industrial[a] or Household Uses	Human Toxic Effects
		Aliphatic Halocarbons	
1,2-Dibromoethane	NC colorless liq (sweet odor)	Fumigant, gasoline antiknock compound, solvent	**Acute:** CNS depression, pulmonary irritant, dermal, hepatic, renal; chronic: respiratory, depression, HA; AC, SHC
Carbon tetrachloride	NC colorless liq (characteristic odor)	Solvent, fire extinguishers, dry cleaning, aerosol propellants	Similar to chloroform
Chloroform	NC colorless liq (sweet odor)	Solvent for paints, degreaser, refrigerant (former anesthetic)	**Acute:** low–anesthesia, dizziness, hallucinations, HA, fatigue; **chronic:** hepatic, renal, CNS, cardiac toxicity; AC, SHC
Ethyl chloride (muriatic ether)	F colorless liq, gas (ether odor)	Solvent, refrigerant, topical anesthetic	**Acute:** anesthesia, narcosis, unconsciousness, respiratory irritation, cardiac arrest
Halothane (fluothane)	NC colorless liq (sweet odor)	General clinical anesthetic	**Acute:** CNS depression, anesthesia, cardiac, ocular irritation; **chronic:** hepatic
Methyl chloride	F colorless explosive gas (sweet odor)	Refrigerant, local anesthetic, organic synthesis	**Acute:** HA, nausea, vomiting, narcosis, convulsions, coma; **chronic:** ocular, hepatic, renal, BM toxicity
Methylene chloride	NC colorless liq	Solvent for paints, degreasing agent	**Acute:** low (inhalation)– irritation, fatigue, HA, narcosis; **chronic:** hepatic; AC, SHC
Trichloroethylene, tetrachloroethylene	NC colorless liq (chloroform, ether odor, respectively)	Solvent, dry cleaning, degreaser, anesthetic (limited)	**Acute:** CNS depression, narcosis; **chronic:** respiratory, cardiac failure; AC, SHC (metabolized to phosgene, trichloroethanol)
Vinyl chloride	F colorless gas	Resins, plastics, refrigerant	**Acute:** low–anesthesia, dizziness, narcosis; **chronic:** hepatic, renal; AC, known HC

(*continued*)

TABLE 25.4 (CONTINUED)
Properties, Sources, Uses, and Toxicity of Halocarbons

Chemical	Properties	Industrial[a] or Household Uses	Human Toxic Effects
Aromatic Halocarbons			
Benzyl chloride	NC colorless-yellowish liq	Dyes, solvents, resins, plastics, perfumes, lubricants	**Acute:** ocular, dermal, respiratory corrosive liq; pulmonary edema, CNS depression; AC
Chlorobenzene	F colorless-yellowish liq (almond-like odor)	Solvent, manufacture of phenol & aniline	**Acute:** low–anesthesia, dizziness, narcosis (in animals); AC
Hexachloro-naphthalene (halowax)	NC yellow solid	Electric wire insulation, lubricant	**Acute:** chloracne, dermatitis, nausea, confusion
Monohalogenated benzenes (fluoro-, chloro-, bromo-, iodo-benzene)	F liquids (aromatic odor)	Solvent, dyes, paints, organic synthesis	**Acute:** cardiac arrhythmias, anesthesia, pulmonary irritation, narcosis, convulsions; **chronic:** blood, BM, CNS, dermal, respiratory toxicity

Note: AC = known animal carcinogen, SHC = suspected human carcinogen, NC = noncombustible, BM = bone marrow, CNS = central nervous system, F = flammable, liq = liquid.

[a] Used in manufacturing, synthesis, or as part of industrial processes.

REFERENCES

SUGGESTED READINGS

Budavari, S., Ed., *The Merck Index*, 12th ed., Merck & Co., Inc., Whitehouse Station, NJ, 1996.

Chamberlain, J., Gas chromatography, in *The Analysis of Drugs in Biological Fluids,* 2nd ed., CRC Press, Inc., Boca Raton, FL, 1995, chap 6.

Patnaik, P., *Comprehensive Guide to Hazardous Properties of Chemical Substances*, Van Nostrand Reinhold, New York, 1992.

Sawyer, T.W., Cellular methods of genotoxity and carcinogenicity, in *Introduction to In Vitro Cytotoxicology: Mechanisms and Methods*, Barile, F.A., CRC Press, Boca Raton, FL, 1994, chap. 9.

REVIEW ARTICLES

Ahmed, F.E., Toxicology and human health effects following exposure to oxygenated or reformulated gasoline, *Toxicol. Lett.*, 123, 89, 2001.

Baudouin, C., et al. Environmental pollutants and skin cancer, *Cell Biol. Toxicol.*, 18, 341, 2002.

Cronkite, E.P., et al., Hematotoxicity and carcinogenicity of inhaled benzene, *Environ. Health Perspect.*, 82, 97, 1989.

De Rosa, C.T., et al., Public health implications of environmental exposures. *Environ. Health Perspect.*, 106, 369, 1998

Ferguson, L.R., Natural and human-made mutagens and carcinogens in the human diet, *Toxicology*, 181, 79, 2002.

Hughes, K., et al., 1,3-Butadiene: exposure estimation, hazard characterization, and exposure-response analysis, *J. Toxicol. Environ. Health B. Crit. Rev.*, 6, 55, 2003.

Linden, C.H., Volatile substances of abuse, *Emerg. Med. Clin. North Am.*, 8, 559, 1990.

Lock, E.A. and Smith, L.L., The role of mode of action studies in extrapolating to human risks in toxicology, *Toxicol. Lett.*, 140, 317, 2003.

Moore, M.R., et al., Trace organic compounds in the marine environment, *Mar. Pollut. Bull.*, 45, 62, 2002.

Mullin, L.S., et al., Toxicology update isoparaffinic hydrocarbons: a summary of physical properties, toxicity studies and human exposure data, *J. Appl. Toxicol.*, 10, 135, 1990.

Norton, W.N., Mattie, D.R., and Kearns, C.L., The cytopathologic effects of specific aromatic hydrocarbons, *Am. J. Pathol.*, 118, 387, 1985.

Periago, J.F., Zambudio, A., and Prado, C., Evaluation of environmental levels of aromatic hydrocarbons in gasoline service stations by gas chromatography, *J. Chromatogr. A.*, 778, 263, 1997.

Plaa, G.L., Chlorinated methanes and liver injury: highlights of the past 50 years, *Annu. Rev. Pharmacol. Toxicol.*, 40, 42, 2000.

Ritchie, G.D., et al., A review of the neurotoxicity risk of selected hydrocarbon fuels, *J. Toxicol. Environ. Health B. Crit. Rev.*, 4, 223, 2001.

Willes, R.F., et al., Scientific principles for evaluating the potential for adverse effects from chlorinated organic chemicals in the environment, *Regul. Toxicol. Pharmacol.*, 18, 313, 1993.

Yoon, B.I., et al., Mechanism of action of benzene toxicity: cell cycle suppression in hemopoietic progenitor cells (CFU-GM), *Exp. Hematol.*, 29, 278, 2001.

Zapponi, G.A., Attias, L., and Marcello, I., Risk assessment of complex mixtures: some considerations on polycyclic aromatic hydrocarbons in urban areas, *J. Environ. Pathol. Toxicol. Oncol.*, 16, 209, 1997.

26 Insecticides

26.1 INTRODUCTION

The U.S. accounts for approximately one-half million tons per year of pesticide consumption in general, of which 91,500 tons are insecticides, making it the largest consumer of these products worldwide.[*] Consequently, there are a significant number of nonfatal poisonings from general pesticide use, averaging about 5000 cases annually. These cases primarily result from inadvertent ingestion of insecticide applicators and solutions for home use, as well as dermal and respiratory exposure to industrial insecticides. Insecticides are responsible for production of acute dermal and respiratory inflammation. Chronically, these agents are implicated in the production of dermal neoplasms.

26.2 ORGANOPHOSPHORUS COMPOUNDS (ORGANOPHOSPHATES, OP)

26.2.1 CHEMICAL CHARACTERISTICS

The structural core of organophosphates (OP) contains a central phosphate nucleus to which are attached a variety of aliphatic side chains, according to the following formula:

$$O \text{ (or S)}$$
$$||$$
$$[R_1O]_2-P-O \text{ (or S)}-R_2$$

where R_1 is a methyl or ethyl group and R_2 is an aliphatic or aromatic hydrocarbon side chain. Most of these compounds are dense liquids (specific gravity above 1.25) or solids at room temperature, have low vapor pressure, and are slightly soluble or insoluble in water at 20°C. Table 26.1 outlines the physical characteristics and relative rodent toxicity of a variety of OP insecticides. The sulfur-containing compounds, such as dimethoate, require metabolic activation prior to binding to the enzymatic target.

26.2.2 OCCURRENCE AND USES

The OP insecticides were originally developed as nerve gases as possible chemical warfare agents during World War II, the first compound of which was tetraethyl

---

[*] The NCFAP (National Center for Food and Agricultural Policy) reported that over 131, 461, 183, and 210 million lbs of fungicide, herbicide, insecticide, and "other" pesticides, respectively, were applied to U.S. crops per year between 1992 and 1997.

TABLE 26.1

Names, Chemical Properties, and Rodent Toxicity of Organophosphorus Insecticides Arranged According to Rodent Oral LD_{50}

Common Name	Chemical Name or Synonym	Physical Characteristics	Median Oral Rodent LD_{50} (mg/kg)
TEPP	Tetraethyl pyrophosphate	Liq, agreeable odor, misc in water and org liq	1.1
Disulfoton	Phosphorodithioic acid O,O-diethyl ester	Colorless oil, immisc in water	2.3–6.8
Mevinphos	Phosdrin	Yellow liq, misc with water	3.7–6.1
Parathion ethyl	Paraphos, Thiophos	Pale yellow liq, practically insol in water	3.6–13
Azinophos methyl	Guthion	Crystalline solid, sol in alcohols and org liq	11
DDVP	Dichlorvos[a]	Non-flam liq, misc with alcohol and org liq	56–80
Chlorpyrifos	Dursban, Lorsban	White crystals, misc with alcohol and org liq	145
Dimethoate	Cygon, Roxion	S-containing crystals, ss in water	250
Malathion	Malamar 50, Cython	Brown-yellow liq, ss in water, misc in org liq	1000–1375
Ronnel	Fenchlorphos, Ectoral	White powder, insol in water, misc in org liq	1250–2630

Note: flam = flammable, insol = insoluble, liq = liquid, misc = miscible, org = organic, sol = soluble, ss = slightly soluble.

[a] Found in the commercial household product *No Pest Strip*®.

pyrophosphate (TEPP). The biological action of the nerve gases, such as sarin, tabun, and soman, is similar to, but more toxic than the OPs. Soman is not only the most toxic of the three but one of the most toxic compounds ever synthesized, with fatalities occurring with an oral dose of 10 μg/kg in humans (see Nerve Gases in Chapter 32, "Chemical and Biological Threats to Public Safety").

Currently, OPs are popular chemicals used as household and agricultural insecticides. Their wide distribution as industrial chemicals allows access to the general population. They are conveniently used for suicidal attempts and are found as crop contaminants* and in accidental occupational exposure. Consequently, in the U.S., they accounted for over 10,000 cases of exposure last year. About 1% of these cases resulted in fatalities in 2002, confirming their role as a public health hazard. As with

---

* *Orange-picker's flu* is a condition characterized by chronic low-level exposure to handling of fruits and vegetables that are sprayed with OP agents. The syndrome is common among farm workers in citrus states, such as Florida and California. Use of neoprene or nitrile gloves affords some protection from exposure. OPs penetrate latex and vinyl gloves, and do not provide enough barrier to exposure.

the organic hydrocarbons (Chapter 25), exposure routes include oral ingestion, inhalation, or dermal contact. The agents are most rapidly absorbed after inhalation, especially when delivered in aromatic hydrocarbon vehicle solvents.

26.2.3 MECHANISM OF TOXICITY

Acetylcholine (Ach) is a neurotransmitter found throughout the central (CNS), autonomic (sympathetic and parasympathetic), and somatic nervous systems. Specifically, Ach receptors are located at autonomic preganglionic sympathetic nicotinic and parasympathetic muscarinic synapses, autonomic postganglionic muscarinic parasympathetic synapses, somatic neuromuscular cholinergic synapses, and central cholinergic synapses. Ach activity is either terminated or potentiated by alteration of metabolism at cholinergic synapses, principally through interference with reuptake or enzymatic degradation. In the enzymatic pathway, acetylcholine esterase (**Ach-Σ**, *true* or *RBC* cholinesterase) is predominantly distributed among red blood cells (RBCs), central, somatic, and autonomic neurons, gray matter of the brain, spinal cord, lung, and spleen. Pseudocholinesterase (*plasma* cholinesterase) is located in serum, plasma, white matter, liver, pancreas and heart tissue.

Ach forms an ester link with the anionic site of the enzyme, and is subsequently hydrolyzed to inactive components according to the following **reversible** reactions:

1. Ach + Ach-Σ → Ach—Ach-Σ complex
2. Ach—Ach-Σ complex → choline + acetyl—Ach-Σ
3. acetyl—Ach-Σ + H_2O → acetic acid + Ach-Σ

The active enzyme is subsequently regenerated.

OPs inhibit the action of Ach-Σ by phosphorylating the active esteratic site, forming an **irreversible** OP—Ach-Σ complex, rendering it incapable of hydrolyzing Ach. Thus, inhibition of the enzyme results in an accumulation and overstimulation of Ach at autonomic and somatic receptors. The irreversible nature of the complex requires days to weeks for disassembly. In addition, phosphorylation prompts the enzyme to undergo an accelerated "aging" process, where it loses an alkyl group and prevents it from spontaneously regenerating. These circumstances account for the toxic manifestations of OP.

26.2.4 SIGNS AND SYMPTOMS OF ACUTE TOXICITY

Low doses of OP insecticides produce mild to moderate toxicity, depending on the remaining percentage of available Ach-Σ activity.* Acute initial toxic effects mimic exaggerated cholinergic muscarinic stimulation, including salivation, lacrimation, excessive sweating (diaphoresis), miosis, tachycardia, hypertension, and tightness of the chest (bronchoconstriction). Higher doses cause overstimulation of both nic-

---

* While 20 to 50% of enzyme activity remains with mild toxicity and 10 to 20% remains with moderate toxicity, RBC cholinesterase levels normally vary within the general population. Enzyme concentrations also vary in the presence of other conditions, such as malnutrition, cirrhosis, and pregnancy, making interpretation of the levels unreliable for diagnosis or management.

otinic and muscarinic receptors,* resulting in diarrhea, urinary incontinence, brady-cardia, muscle twitching, fatigue, hyperglycemia, bronchospasm, and bronchorrhea. Increased depolarization at nicotinic neuromuscular synapses results in muscle weakness and flaccid paralysis.

CNS cholinergic stimulation suppresses central medullary centers accounting for depressed respirations, headache, anxiety, restlessness, confusion, psychosis, seizures, and coma.** Death with OP poisoning is secondary to respiratory paralysis and cardiovascular collapse.

Acute pancreatitis, myocardial dysrhythmias, and hydrocarbon pneumonitis following aspiration of the solvent vehicle are complications of OP poisoning. Although chronic effects from OP toxicity are limited, some latent pathology may develop. OP-induced delayed neuropathy (OPIDN) is a delayed neurotoxicity that may develop 1 to 3 weeks after exposure. The syndrome is characterized by muscular weakness and paralysis of extremities, especially of hand and foot muscles, progressing to a persistent spastic spinal paresis. OPIDN is associated with inhibition of the neuronal enzyme, neurotoxic esterase, and Ach-Σ "aging." The syndrome is either slowly reversible over several months or irreversible. Intermediate syndrome (IMS) is also characterized by muscular paralysis inner-vated by cranial nerves. It is associated with excessive exposure to OPs and results in prolonged Ach-Σ inhibition at the neuromuscular junction. Prevention, or recov-ery from development, of IMS is mostly accomplished by early therapeutic inter-vention following OP exposure.

26.2.5 CLINICAL MANAGEMENT OF ACUTE POISONING

Decontamination, airway stabilization, and activated charcoal are important initial supportive measures for OP intoxication. Washing dermal areas with a mild soap, removal of contaminated clothes, and rinsing the eyes is necessary for dermal or ocular exposure. Atropine and pralidoxime (2-PAM) follow as specific OP antidotes.

Atropine is a competitive antimuscarinic cholinergic antagonist at central and peripheral autonomic receptors. It has no effect at neuromuscular or nicotinic recep-tors. In adults, atropine (1 to 2 mg i.v.) counteracts the excessive bronchial and autonomic secretions and normalizes heart rate. The dose is repeated every 5 to 10 min, depending on improvement of respiration.

2-PAM is a quaternary amine of the oxime class that reactivates Ach-Σ by severing the OP—Ach-Σ covalent bond at nicotinic, muscarinic, and central cholin-ergic sites. Pralidoxime is most effective when administered soon after exposure, before the poisoned enzyme complex has "aged" and becomes resistant to the effects of the antidote. The drug also scavenges remaining OP molecules, has few adverse reactions, and its action is synergistic with atropine. An initial dose of 1 to 2 g, by continuous i.v. infusion is followed by 500 mg/h for 24 h, in order to maintain effective therapeutic levels of 4 μg/l.

---

* Less than 10% of normal enzyme activity is available for degrading Ach.
** It is noteworthy that CNS depression is manifested more commonly in children than in adults.

26.3 CARBAMATES

26.3.1 CHEMICAL CHARACTERISTICS, OCCURRENCE, AND USES

As with the OP compounds, the carbamates are used as household and agricultural insecticides. The incidence of toxicity, routes of exposure, modes of encountering the agents, and distribution are similar to the OPs. Most carbamates display low dermal toxicity, except for aldicarb, which is highly toxic by both oral ingestion and dermal contact.

The mechanism of toxicity, however, differs slightly from that of the OP compounds. Table 26.2 summarizes the chemical properties and toxic animal data of some popular carbamate insecticides.

26.3.2 MECHANISM OF TOXICITY

Carbamates **reversibly** inhibit Ach-Σ by carbamoylation of the esteratic site, allowing the carbamate–enzyme complex to quickly and spontaneously dissociate (within minutes to hours). Thus, toxicity is limited as the enzyme is capable of rapid regeneration after binding.

26.3.3 SIGNS AND SYMPTOMS OF ACUTE TOXICITY

Because of the reversibility of the substrate–enzyme complex, the toxicity of the carbamates is proportionately of shorter duration and less intensity than OPs. Effects are limited to activation of muscarinic and nicotinic sites. In addition, poor penetration of the blood-brain barrier limits CNS toxicity of carbamates.

26.3.4 CLINICAL MANAGEMENT OF ACUTE POISONING

As with the OPs, treatment of carbamate poisoning is symptomatic. Atropine is indicated as an antidote. Since "aging" of the carbamoylated complex does not occur,

TABLE 26.2
Names, Chemical Properties, and Rodent Toxicity of Carbamate Insecticides Arranged According to Rodent Oral LD$_{50}$

Common Name	Chemical Name or Synonym	Physical Characteristics	Median Oral Rodent LD$_{50}$ (mg/kg)
Aldicarb	Temik	Crystalline solid, sol in water	~1.0
Carbofuran	Furadan	White crystalline solid, sol in water	2.0
Methiocarb	Mesurol	White crystalline solid, insol in water	60–70
Bufencarb	Bux	Yellow solid, sol in xylene and alc	61–97
Propoxur	Baygon	Crystalline solid, sol in alc and org liq	85
Carbaryl	Sevin	Crystalline solid, sol in water	250

Note: alc = alcohol, insol = insoluble, liq = liquid, org = organic, sol = soluble.

pralidoxime is not indicated and may actually increase toxicity. Practically, when prior medical history does not allow distinguishing OP from carbamate exposure, pralidoxime administration should not be withheld.

26.4 ORGANOCHLORINE (OC) INSECTICIDES

26.4.1 CHEMICAL CHARACTERISTICS

OC insecticides are low-molecular-weight, fat-soluble compounds with greater selectivity for lipid storage in insects. As a group, these polychlorinated cyclic compounds are structurally similar, especially the stereoisomers dieldrin and endrin. Table 26.3 summarizes the chemical properties and animal toxicological profiles of some popular OC insecticides.

26.4.2 OCCURRENCE AND USES

OC compounds have applications as insecticides in agriculture and as industrial and commercial pesticides, especially in mosquito abatement and red fire ant control. Because of their high lipid solubility, high carcinogenic potency, and their potential for low-level accumulation with chronic exposure, some of these agents are no longer produced in the U.S. (endrin, aldrin, dieldrin). DDT (dichlorodiphenyltrichloroethane, Table 26.3), developed during World War II for protection of armed forces against disease-carrying insects, is the best known of the chlorinated compounds. The persistence of DDT in the environment and the contribution of the insecticide to reduction of wildlife populations prompted the reevaluation of the utility of DDT and related chlorinated hydrocarbons. Heavy use of DDT in the U.S. before 1966 was probably responsible for a previously undetected epidemic of premature births. Studies since then on human reproductive effects have been suggestive of the human reproductive toxicity of DDT. The pesticide is still widely used and highly effective in areas where mosquito-borne malaria is a major public health problem.

Gamma (γ)-benzene hexachloride is currently used as a pediculocide, scabicide, and ectoparasiticide. It is available as a shampoo and lotion for the topical treatment of conditions due to itch mite (*Sarcoptes scabie*), lice (*Pediculus humanus* sp.), and tick (dog and deer tick) infestations in humans and animals. The preparation is applied once for several minutes, as a 1% lotion or shampoo, after which it is rinsed off. One reapplication may be required to eliminate the parasites.

26.4.3 MECHANISM OF TOXICITY

From 1990 to 2000, over 30,000 poisonings were reported in the U.S. resulting from OC exposure. Most of the human toxicity data associated with OC is derived from clinical case studies of excessive inadvertent application, overexposure, frequent reapplications, and accidental and intentional ingestion of lindane. Most exposures with lindane occur in infants, pregnant women, and nursing mothers. Overall, the OC compounds have proven to be selective neurotoxins. Toxic effects are greater in young victims, since they readily penetrate their immature skin. Prolonged contact

TABLE 26.3
Names, Chemical Properties, and Rodent Toxicity of Organochlorine Insecticides Arranged According to Rodent Oral LD$_{50}$

Common Name	Chemical Name or Synonym	Physical Characteristics	Toxicological Properties	Median Oral Rodent LD$_{50}$ (mg/kg)
Endrin[a]	Mendrin, Endrex	Colorless to light tan solid, mild odor, sol in org liq	Stereoisomer of dieldrin	7.5–18
Aldrin[a]	Aldrite, Aldrex	Tan-dark brown solid, sol in org liq	Metabolized to dieldrin	39–60
Dieldrin[a]	Octalox, Dieldrex	Light tan solid, mild odor, mod sol in org liq	Toxicity similar to aldrin	40–50
Lindane	γ-benzene hexachloride; Kwell®	White crystalline solid, insol in water	Used therapeutically as a pediculocide; CNS toxicity	80–90
Heptachlor	Heptamul	White or light tan waxy solid; camphor odor	Blood dyskrasias, liver necrosis	100–160
DDT	Dichlorodiphenyl-trichloroethane	Colorless to white solid, mild odor, sol in org liq	CNS toxicity	110–120
Chlordane	Toxichlor, Velsicol 1068, Corodane, Belt	Colorless or amber viscous liquid, sol in org liq	Highly toxic orally, dermally, and by inhalation in humans	340
Methoxychlor	Methoxy-DDT	Crystalline solid	Low toxicity, less than DDT	>5,000

Note: insol = insoluble, liq = liquid, org = organic, sol = soluble.

[a] Use has been discontinued in the U.S.

with the agent, compromised skin, or application over a wide surface area also increases chances for dermal absorption and systemic toxicity.

OCs alter membrane chloride ion permeability and interfere with normal GABA-ergic (γ-aminobutyric acid) neuronal transmission. The loss of this inhibitory neurotransmitter translates into the neurotoxic sequelae.

26.4.4 Signs and Symptoms of Acute Toxicity

Most of the toxic effects of OCs are due to CNS stimulation. Inhibition of GABA leads to motor, sensory, and behavioral changes, typically manifested as apprehension, irritability, confusion, sensory disturbances, dizziness, tremors, and seizures. The chemicals sensitize involuntary autonomic muscle activity to catecholamines. In particular, myocardial arrhythmias are promptly precipitated. In addition, respiratory failure and hepatic and renal damage are a consequence of large lindane ingestion. As with the aliphatic and aromatic hydrocarbons, aspiration pneumonia is possible after inhalation of the organic vehicle delivering the insecticides.

26.4.5 CLINICAL MANAGEMENT OF ACUTE POISONING

Treatment involves symptomatic and supportive management of the condition. Decontamination, gastric lavage, and administration of activated charcoal reduce toxicity after oral ingestion. Washing of the affected area may reduce absorption after dermal exposure. Myocardial arrhythmias are managed with antiarrhythmics such as lidocaine, while benzodiazepines are indicated for preventing or reducing development of seizures.

26.5 MISCELLANEOUS INSECTICIDES

26.5.1 PYRETHROID ESTERS

The pyrethroid insecticides are derived from the naturally occurring compound, pyrethrum, from the dried flower heads of the yellow flower *Chrysanthemum cineriaefolium.*[*] The synthetic acid-alcoholic esters are categorized into several classes of the active ingredients, namely pyrethrins types I and II.[**] Pyrethrum flowers have been used as insecticides for centuries, particularly by Caucasian tribesmen and Armenians. The powdered form was introduced into the U.S. in 1855, after which its importation expanded tremendously. Type I pyrethrins include allethrine, permethrin, and cismethrin; type II pyrethrins include fenvalerate, deltamethrin, and cypermethrin. The compounds (0.17 to 0.33%) are combined with piperonyl butoxide or n-octyl-dicycloheptane dicarboximide (2 to 4%) in therapeutic nonprescription pediculocide preparations for the treatment of lice, tick, and mite infestation.[***] Pyrethrins are noted for their quick "knock-down" effect of flying insects, particularly flies and mosquitoes. The products are available in lotions, sprays, and shampoos for skin or scalp applications, as well as for removal from furniture and bedding material.

Type I pyrethrins produce repetitive depolarization of axons by inhibiting inactivation of sodium channels. Type II pyrethrins have a similar mechanism, but longer duration of action, and also affect GABA receptor-mediated chloride channels. Most poisonings, however, are benign and limited to contact irritant dermatitis, allergic dermatitis, and rhinitis. Pulmonary asthmatic reactions may occur in sensitive individuals. Some cases of severe poisoning have been reported from massive oral ingestion that resulted in coma, convulsions, and death.

---

[*] *Chrysanthemum* is from the ancient Greek name meaning golden flower; *cineriaefolium* is from two Greek words meaning ash-colored leaves.

[**] Cinerin I or II, and jasmolin I or II, are synonyms.

[***] These agents, found in commercial products RID® and NIX®, inhibit enzyme deactivation of the pyrethrins, thereby producing a synergistic effect with the insecticide.

Treatment is symptomatic and limited to alleviation of the inflammatory response. Oral or topical corticosteroids and H_1-antihistamine blockers may be of use as anti-inflammatory agents.

26.5.2 NICOTINE

Nicotine is a pyridine alkaloid (1-methyl-2-[3-pyridyl] pyrrolidine) obtained from the cured and dried leaves of the tobacco plant, *Nicotiana* sp. The plant is indigenous to the southern U.S. and tropical South America (see Chapter 13, "Sympathomimetics," for a detailed description). Early American settlers in the nineteenth century recognized the insecticidal properties of nicotine as they dusted their vegetable crops with finely powdered tobacco leaves. The leaves contain from 0.6 to 9% of the alkaloid along with other nicotinic derivatives. The demand for nicotine as an insecticide declined with the advent of the organophosphate compounds.

Toxic effects of nicotine as a contact insecticide are identical to ingestion of large amounts of the compound in other commercial products. Nicotine stimulates nicotinic receptors of all sympathetic and parasympathetic ganglia, neuromuscular junction innervating skeletal muscle, and CNS pathways. Of the target organs affected by nicotine, the most significant is the cardiovascular system. Nicotine produces a characteristic bradycardia or tachycardia. Nicotine's action on the central nervous system results in stimulation, followed by predominance of parasympathetic overtone, i.e., salivation, lacrimation, urination, defecation, and vomiting. Continued exposure progresses to muscular weakness, tremors, hypotension, and dyspnea. Convulsions and respiratory paralysis are advanced complications of unattended nicotine toxicity. Treatment of poisoning is primarily symptomatic and involves decontamination, induction of emesis (depending on the time of onset of symptoms), and maintenance of vital signs.

26.5.3 BORIC ACID (H_3BO_3)

Boric acid has numerous traditional therapeutic and commercial uses as a topical astringent (for minor swelling), as an ophthalmic bacteriostatic agent (in over-the-counter eyewash solutions), and as a topical antiseptic, herbicide, and insecticide. As a commercial, nontherapeutic product, the substance is an effective detergent, cleaning aid, flame retardant, herbicide, and insecticide, primarily useful as an "ant and roach killer." The undiluted powder is mixed in water with more palatable substances, such as flour or granular sugar, in order to attract the bugs. Consequently, the easy availability, accessibility, and similarity to products such as infant formulas, has facilitated its ability to interchange with these substances. This ease of confusion with other products accounts for the persistent number of poisoning cases. It has also been inadvertently substituted in solution for epsom salts (magnesium sulfate powder), mistakenly used as a muscle relaxant.

Topically, concentrated solutions of boric acid precipitate the formation of a desquamating, erythematous rash (boiled lobster appearance), characterized by production of severe redness, pain, and blisters. The chemical readily penetrates abraded skin and, along with oral ingestion, has the potential for systemic toxicity.

Symptoms of systemic toxicity include lethargy, fever, and muscular weakness, with progression to development of tremors and convulsions. Individuals who develop hypotension, CNS depression, renal failure, jaundice, and cardiovascular collapse are at risk of death.

As with nicotine, treatment of boric acid poisoning is primarily symptomatic and involves decontamination, gastric lavage, and maintenance of vital signs. Washing the contaminated area with soap and water effectively neutralizes its acidic reaction. Induction of emesis, however, is not recommended since regurgitation of acidic material contributes to further esophageal corrosion.

26.5.4 ROTENONE

Rotenone (tubotoxin, derrin) is a colorless-to-red, odorless insecticidal principle derived from the *Derris* plant genus.* The plant is predominantly grown in the southern U.S. and tropical South America. Rotenone, and the chemically related rotenoids (toxicarol, tephrosin, sumatrol), are a series of naturally occurring cyclic aromatic hydrocarbons. The agents are widely employed in agriculture for controlling chewing and sucking insects, and are dusted or sprayed on garden plants and crops as well.

The action of rotenone parallels that of the pyrethrins in providing quick *knock-down* of flying insects. Although considered to possess generally low toxicity, respiratory, dermal, oral, or ocular exposure results in symptoms that mimic the chemical irritants (Chapter 25). Pulmonary and systemic toxicity leading to respiratory depression, seizures, and coma have been reported. Management of poisoning is supportive and symptomatic.

26.5.5 DIETHYLTOLUAMIDE (DEET)

DEET (*m*-isomer of *N,N*-diethyl-3-methylbenzamide) is a popular insect repellant available in topical preparations at 5 to 100% concentrations (OFF® Insect Repellant). About 5 to 10% of a dermal application is absorbed, due to its high lipid solubility, and stored in lipid compartments, resulting in a prolonged plasma half-life (2.5 h). Although generally considered a chemical with low toxicity, dermal reactions reflect excessive topical application of sprays, creams, lotions, or alcohol-soaked DEET-containing towelettes. Ocular or dermal irritation is generally limited to allergic reactions and is the most frequent complaint. Prolonged dermal contact with significant absorption, or oral ingestion, has precipitated CNS toxicity. This is manifested by the development of headache, lethargy, confusion, and tremors. Hypotension, seizures, and coma are rare.

Treatment is largely symptomatic and supportive and involves decontamination, gastric lavage, and maintenance of vital signs, if necessary. Washing the contaminated area with soap and water and induction of emesis is recommended if needed.

---

* *Derris* roots were used as fish poisons for centuries by native tribes of Central America and South America.

26.6 METHODS OF DETECTION

As with the aliphatic and aromatic hydrocarbons, quantitative analysis of insecticides is usually performed on samples from ambient or contaminated areas, including air, water, and soil. Gas chromatographic (GC) techniques are sensitive and specific depending on the internal and external standards used. Although most of the insecticides have low vapor pressures, the volatility of the liquids, coupled with a specific detector, renders them suitable for monitoring through a GC column (solid phase). Most of the solid insecticides are soluble in organic liquids, which also makes them amenable for GC analysis. Flame ionization, electron capture, mass spectrometry (GC-MS), or nitrogen-specific detectors have been employed for specific identification.

REFERENCES

SUGGESTED READINGS

Albertson, T.E. and Ferguson, T.J., Insecticides: chlorinated hydrocarbons, pyrethrins, and DEET, in *Toxicology Secrets*, Ling, L.J. et al., Eds., Hanley & Belfus, Inc., Philadelphia, 2001, chap. 46.

Budavari, S., Ed., *The Merck Index*, 12th ed., Merck & Co., Inc., Whitehouse Station, NJ, 1996.

Chomchai, S., Insecticides: organophosphates and carbamates, in *Toxicology Secrets*, Ling, L.J. et al., Eds., Hanley & Belfus, Inc., Philadelphia, 2001, chap. 45.

Leonard, P., Gianessi, L.P., and Marcelli, M.B., *Pesticide Use in U.S. Crop Production: 1997 National Summary Report*, National Center for Food and Agricultural Policy (NCFAP), Washington, DC, 2000.

Lide, D.R., Ed., *CRC Handbook of Chemistry & Physics,* 83rd ed., CRC Press, Boca Raton, FL, 2002.

Patnaik, P., *Comprehensive Guide to Hazardous Properties of Chemical Substances*, Van Nostrand Reinhold, New York, 1992.

REVIEW ARTICLES

Abu-Qare, A.W. and Abou-Donia, M.B., Combined exposure to DEET (N,N-diethyl-m-toluamide) and permethrin: pharmacokinetics and toxicological effects, *J. Toxicol. Environ. Health B. Crit. Rev.,* 6, 41, 2003.

Ahlborg, U.G., et al., Organochlorine compounds in relation to breast cancer, endometrial cancer, and endometriosis: an assessment of the biological and epidemiological evidence, *Crit. Rev. Toxicol.,* 25, 463, 1995.

Aks, S.E., et al., Acute accidental lindane ingestion in toddlers, *Ann. Emerg. Med.,* 26, 647, 1995.

Banerjee, B.D., The influence of various factors on immune toxicity assessment of pesticide chemicals, *Toxicol. Lett.,* 107, 21, 1999.

DeLorenzo, M.E., Scott, G.I., and Ross, P.E., Toxicity of pesticides to aquatic microorganisms: a review, *Environ. Toxicol. Chem.,* 20, 84, 2001.

He, F., Neurotoxic effects of insecticides — current and future research: a review, *Neurotoxicology,* 21, 829, 2000.

Karalliedde, L.D., Edwards, P., and Marrs, T.C., Variables influencing the toxic response to organophosphates in humans, *Food Chem. Toxicol.*, 41, 1, 2003.

Kassa, J., Review of oximes in the antidotal treatment of poisoning by organophosphorus nerve agents, *J. Toxicol. Clin. Toxicol.*, 40, 803, 2002.

Kwong, T.C., Organophosphate pesticides: biochemistry and clinical toxicology, *Ther. Drug Monit.*, 24, 144, 2002.

Lotti, M., Low-level exposures to organophosphorus esters and peripheral nerve function, *Muscle Nerve*, 25, 492, 2002.

Murphy, M.J., Rodenticides, *Vet. Clin. North Am. Small Anim. Pract.*, 32, 469, 2002.

O'Malley, M., Clinical evaluation of pesticide exposure and poisonings, *Lancet*, 349, 1161, 1997.

Ragoucy-Sengler, C., et al., Aldicarb poisoning, *Hum. Exp. Toxicol.*, 19, 657, 2000.

Ray, D.E. and Forshaw, P.J., Pyrethroid insecticides: poisoning syndromes, synergies, and therapy, *J. Toxicol. Clin. Toxicol.*, 38, 95, 2000.

Reigart, J.R. and Roberts, J.R., Pesticides in children, *Pediatr. Clin. North Am.*, 48, 1185, 2001.

Walker, B., Jr., and Nidiry, J., Current concepts: organophosphate toxicity, *Inhal. Toxicol.*, 14, 975, 2002.

27 Herbicides

27.1 INTRODUCTION

Herbicides constitute a wide variety of chemicals whose main classes include (1) the chlorphenoxy acids and their esters (2) triazines, (3) substituted ureas, (4) dipyridyl derivatives, and (5) mono or dinitro aromatics.

In the agricultural industry, the control of weeds and noxious vegetation is accomplished by the application of various contact herbicides that produce the rapid elimination of plant tissues for prolonged periods. Military use of defoliants, and commercial nonagricultural community and household use of herbicides along highways, commercial property, pedestrian walkways, parks, and lawns, accounted for 40% of the total herbicide consumption in the U.S. in 2001. Domestic maintenance of home lawns and gardens requires the use of selective herbicides that kill broadleaf vegetation without serious damage to the preferable grasses.

Although the acute and chronic toxicity of the herbicides are generally low, acute contact dermatitis and chronic exposure account for a substantial number of nonfatal poisonings from widespread application of the compounds. The number of cases average several hundred annually. As with the insecticides, herbicide poisonings result from inadvertent ingestion of herbicide applicators and solutions for home use, as well as dermal and respiratory exposure from industrial occupational exposure.

27.2 CHLORPHENOXY COMPOUNDS

27.2.1 CHEMICAL CHARACTERISTICS

Most of the chlorphenoxy compounds are odorless, colorless crystalline compounds with low vapor pressures. They are conveniently divided into selective and nonselective classes: (1) **selective** herbicides eliminate undesirable plant species but produce little deleterious effects on other plants in the contact area; and (2) **nonselective** herbicides destroy all plant life within the applied zone. Table 27.1 outlines the classes, chemical properties, and general human toxic characteristics of the chlorphenoxy herbicides.

27.2.2 OCCURRENCE AND USES

2,4-D (2,4-dichlorophenoxy acetic acid) was originally introduced in the 1940s as a plant growth stimulant (auxin-like compound), only later to retain the distinction as the first organic herbicide. Its residues have been detected in soil, sediments, groundwater, and marine estuaries. Similarly, 2,4,5-T (2,4,5-trichlorophenoxy acetic

TABLE 27.1
Names, Chemical Properties, and Human Toxicity of Chlorphenoxy and Bipyridyl Contact Herbicides Arranged According to Oral Rodent LD$_{50}$

Common Name	Chemical Name	Physical Characteristics	Toxicological Effects	Median Oral Rodent LD$_{50}$ (mg/kg)
		Chlorphenoxy Acids		
TCDD (dioxin)	2,3,4,8-tetrachloro-dibenzo-p-dioxin	Colorless to tan solid; banned by EPA	Dermal exposure: irritation, acne-like rash (chloracne, esp. with dioxin); respiratory exposure: NV, lethargy, stupor, weakness, somnolence, ataxia, hepatic, gastric disturbances, death from CV arrythmias	0.22–0.45
2,4-D	2,4-dichlorophenoxy acetic acid	White to yellow crystalline powder		100–500
2,4,5-T	2,4,5-trichlorophenoxy acetic acid	Colorless to tan solid; banned by EPA (1985)		300–500
Silvex	2-(2,4,5-trichlorophenoxy) propionic acid	Crystalline solid, banned by EPA (1985)		650
		Bipyridyl Derivatives		
Paraquat	1,1'-dimethyl-4,4'-bipyridinium	Colorless to yellow crystals	Ingestion, inhalation: respiratory irritant, pulmonary edema, interstitial fibrosis	100–125
Diquat (aquacide)	1,1'-ethylene-2,2'-bipyridilium	Colorless to yellow crystals	Low toxicity in humans	125–230
Picloram (amodon)	4-amino-3,5,6-trichloro-picolinic acid	White, crystalline powder	Mild toxicity in animals	>2500

acid) and its contaminant TCDD (2,3,4,8-tetrachloro-dibenzo-*p*-dioxin, dioxin) are potent, highly toxic agents, and more effective in eradicating woody plants.[*]

27.2.3 SIGNS AND SYMPTOMS AND MECHANISM OF ACUTE TOXICITY

Although the mechanism is not clear, toxicity of these compounds increases with decreasing phenoxy side chain length. Symptoms are similar for all chlorphenoxy compounds and are usually mild after a single exposure. There is no apparent compartmental accumulation. Toxic effects are related to their herbicidal action and depend on their translocation to all parts of the plants to which they are applied. Inorganic salts and aliphatic esters of 2,4-D ionize readily in aqueous solution and are not absorbed into the plant sap. Generally they remain on the leaf surface (*contact* herbicides), thus ensuring significant amounts for local human and mammalian contact. Alcoholic esters, however, penetrate the waxy cuticle surface and are translocated to the plant's conducting system (*translocated* herbicides). These agents are considered more efficient herbicides, and transfer less toxicity upon contact with humans or animals.

Toxicity from commercial applications is a direct result of dermal absorption, inhalation, or oral ingestion. Acute toxic effects from single oral ingestion are listed in Table 27.1 (oral ingestion of 4 to 6 g is potentially fatal in humans). Development of nausea, vomiting, muscular weakness, and hypotension are the most notable symptoms. Chloracne, a severe form of dermatitis, is characterized by small, black follicular papules on the arms, face, and neck of exposed individuals in contact with dioxin contaminants. In addition, toxicity from the petroleum distillate solvent vehicles is associated with significant toxicity (see Chapter 25, "Aliphatic and Aromatic Hydrocarbons").

27.2.4 CLINICAL MANAGEMENT OF ACUTE POISONING

Decontamination and washing exposed skin areas with mild soap neutralizes the acidic properties. Eye rinsing is important for ocular exposure. Airway stabilization and activated charcoal are important initial supportive measures, if necessary. Since the agents have generally low pKa (acidic) values, alkaline diuresis may enhance renal elimination.

27.3 BIPYRIDYL HERBICIDES

27.3.1 CHEMICAL CHARACTERISTICS, OCCURRENCE, AND USES

Paraquat (PQ) and diquat are nonselective bipyridyl herbicides used widely in agricultural, commercial, and residential applications (lawn maintenance) to eradicate

---

[*] In the late 1960s, over 11 million gallons of "Agent Orange" were used as a defoliant during the Vietnam War. The substance contained a mixture of 2,4-D and 2,4,5-T and, inadvertently, was contaminated with trace amounts of dioxin. Exposure to dioxin during the defoliation missions of the war (Operation Ranchland) prompted veterans exposed to the defoliant to file class action lawsuits in the 1970s against the U.S. government. The chemical demonstrated carcinogenic and teratogenic properties in animals upon chronic exposure. Epidemiological studies as to dioxin's chronic effects on human health are inconclusive.

broadleaf plants and shrubs. The chemicals inhibit plant photosynthesis by interfering with NADPH/NADP+ redox cycling. Their usefulness as contact herbicides resides in their ability to promote reseeding of lawns and gardens within 24 h after application. The two structurally similar compounds are often combined in commercial products, but the acute toxicity of diquat is lower in humans than PQ. Thus, most of the ensuing discussion focuses on PQ.

27.3.2 Toxicokinetics

PQ is poorly absorbed through skin and inhalation, although both contribute to significant accumulation via systemic absorption. Most of the compound remains at the site of exposure with dermal contact. About 10% is absorbed orally.

27.3.3 Mechanism of Toxicity

The toxicity of PQ was first recognized when U.S. Drug Enforcement Administration (DEA) programs were commissioned for the purpose of eradicating marijuana plants grown illicitly in the southwestern U.S. Using aerial reconnaissance, the herbicide was sprayed over fields suspected of devoting large areas to marijuana cultivation. Undaunted by the antidrug program, individuals who smoked surviving marijuana plants inhaled significant amounts of the herbicide. The associated pulmonary manifestations were categorically identified with PQ toxicity.

PQ is extremely toxic to humans and laboratory animals, the mechanism of which is illustrated in the reaction below. The oxidized [O] compound accumulates in lung and kidneys and undergoes redox cycling reactions (single electron reduction). It is metabolized by nicotinamide adenine dinucleotide phosphate (NADPH)-cytochrome P450-dependent reductase to the reduced [H] intermediate radical:

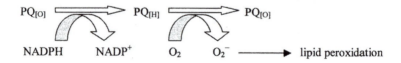

The reaction catalyzes the oxidation of NADPH to NADP+, resulting in a depletion of the reducing equivalent. With continued exposure, there is an eventual decrease in the NADPH/NADP+ ratio, thus depriving the cells of the protective role of reducing equivalents. The reduced intermediate ($PQ_{[H]}$) reacts with molecular oxygen to reform the oxidized PQ species (known as the *single electron reduction of oxygen*). The intracellular product of oxygen reduction is the superoxide anion radical (O_2^-). Through a subsequent series of catalyzed reactions, O_2^- may form hydroxyl radicals that are capable of causing lipid peroxidation and damage to vital cell membranes.

Glutathione (GSH) and superoxide dismutase also play a role as cellular defense factors against reactive oxygen species generated in tissues. GSH and superoxide dismutase depletion selectively enhance PQ-induced oxidative stress by further inhibiting the cell's ability to protect against damaging effects of free radical generation. In addition, dismutated oxygen (O·, singlet O_2) accumulates from O_2^-, producing an excess of hydroperoxides. This precipitates a series of potentiating reactions, undermining the stability of unsaturated lipids within cell membranes.

27.3.4 SIGNS AND SYMPTOMS OF ACUTE TOXICITY

Because of its interaction with pulmonary reactive tissue at the site of exposure, PQ selectively concentrates in alveolar type I and type II pneumocytes. PQ also concentrates in renal epithelial cells. The effect of the chemical is characterized as a "hit-and-run" event, since the redox cycling and free radical formation occur after the toxin is eliminated. Thus, three phases of PQ poisoning are described (outlined in Table 27.2) based on the dose and route of exposure. Although death is typically delayed for 2 to 3 weeks in phase II and up to 1 week in phase III, the majority of cases that reach these phases result in death. Acute alveolitis and pulmonary fibrosis, characterized by cough, dyspnea, tachypnea, edema, atalectasis, collagen deposition, and fibrotic development, are eventual consequences of phases II and III.

27.3.5 CLINICAL MANAGEMENT OF ACUTE POISONING

Development of pulmonary sequelae is associated with a poor prognosis. In general, PQ poisoning is managed aggressively with symptomatic and supportive care. Evaluation of esophageal erosion and determination of serum and gastric fluid levels of PQ are beneficial in predicting outcome. Activated charcoal, gastric lavage, and/or

TABLE 27.2
Phases of Paraquat Toxicity and Associated Clinical Effects

Phases of Toxicity	Time Range (days)	Minimum Dose (mg/kg)	Toxicological Effects	
			Oral Ingestion	Local Exposure
I. Asymptomatic or mild	1–5	20[a]	Nausea, vomiting, diarrhea; intestinal hemorrage, hemoptysis; oliguria	GI, dermal and ocular irritation
II. Moderate to severe	2–8	20–40	Vomiting, diarrhea; systemic accumulation, pulmonary fibrosis	Severe GI, dermal and ocular irritation, inflammation, and ulceration of skin and mucous membranes
III. Severe: acute fulminant toxicity	3–14	>40	Liver, kidney, cariac, pulmonary failure	Marked ulceration as with Phase II

Note: GI = gastrointestinal.

[a] Doses as low as 4 mg/kg have resulted in death.

TABLE 27.3
Names, Chemical Properties, and Human and Animal Toxicity of Triazines, Substituted Ureas, Nitroaromatic and Miscellaneous Contact Herbicides

Common Name	Chemical Name	Physical Characteristics	Toxicological Effects	Median Oral Rodent LD_{50} (mg/kg)
		Triazines		
Atrazine (Atranex, Primatol A)	2-chloro-4-ethylamino-6-isopropylamino-s-triazine	White, crystalline solid	Low toxicity in humans & animals: anemia, weakness, enteritis	1750
		Substituted Ureas		
Tribunil (methabenz-thiazuron)	1,3-dimethyl-3-(2-benzothiazolyl) urea	White, crystalline solid	Pulmonary congestion in animals	>2500
Monuron (monurex)	3-(4-chlorophenyl)-1,1-dimethyl urea	Crystalline solid, faint odor	Moderate toxicity, carcinogenic in lab animals	3700
		Mono- and Dinitro Aromatics		
Nitrofen (TOK)	2,4-dichloro-1-(4-nitrophenoxy) benzene	White, crystalline powder	Highly toxic in lab animals, carcinogenic in lab animals	0.6
Dinoseb (caldon)	2-sec-butyl-4,6-dinitrophenol	Orange-brown viscous liq	Used as herbicide & insecticide, highly toxic in lab animals	10–30
		Miscellaneous		
Alachlor (lazo)	2-chloro-2,6-diethyl-N-(methoxymethyl) acetanilide	Crystalline solid	Low toxicity in humans & animals, oncogenic in lab animals	1200

administration of a cathartic may prevent further absorption. Forced diuresis and hydration are effective only if intervention is attempted soon after ingestion and in the presence of lower doses of the herbicide. Although high-flow oxygen is generally used to counteract hypoxia, its use risks further acceleration of oxidative lung damage.

27.4 MISCELLANEOUS HERBICIDES

Table 27.3 summarizes the chemistry and toxicological properties of select herbicides. The triazines, substituted ureas, nitroaromatic, and miscellaneous classes are frequently used as contact, preemergence, and select herbicides. Their low to moderate toxicity to humans and animals make them suitable for agricultural, industrial, and household utility.

27.5 METHODS OF DETECTION

Gas chromatographic (GC) techniques are used to identify herbicides in air, soil, and biological samples. Most of the solids are soluble in organic liquids, which render them suitable for monitoring through a packed GC column (solid phase). Flame ionization, electron capture, or mass spectrometry (GC-MS) are specific detectors with sensitivities in the ppm range.

REFERENCES

SUGGESTED READINGS

Budavari, S., Ed., *The Merck Index*, 12th ed., Merck & Co., Inc., Whitehouse Station, NJ, 1996.
Ferguson, T.J. and Albertson, T.E., Herbicides, in *Toxicology Secrets*, Ling, L.J. et al., Eds., Hanley & Belfus, Inc., Philadelphia, 2001, chap. 48.

REVIEW ARTICLES

Bismuth, C., et al., Paraquat poisoning. An overview of the current status, *Drug Saf.,* 5, 243, 1990.
Bradberry, S.M., et al., Mechanisms of toxicity, clinical features, and management of acute chlorophenoxy herbicide poisoning: a review, *J. Toxicol. Clin. Toxicol.,* 38, 111, 2000.
Costa, L.G., Basic toxicology of pesticides, *Occup. Med.,* 12, 251, 1997.
Curtis, C.F., Should DDT continue to be recommended for malaria vector control? *Med. Vet. Entomol.,* 8, 107, 1994.
Daniel, O., et al., Selected phenolic compounds in cultivated plants: ecologic functions, health implications, and modulation by pesticides, *Environ. Health Perspect.,* 107, 109, 1999.
Eriksson, P. and Talts, U., Neonatal exposure to neurotoxic pesticides increases adult susceptibility: a review of current findings, *Neurotoxicology*, 21, 37, 2000.
Garabrant, D.H. and Philbert, M.A., Review of 2,4-dichlorophenoxyacetic acid (2,4-D) epidemiology and toxicology, *Crit. Rev. Toxicol.,* 32, 233, 2002.

Jones, G.M. and Vale, J.A., Mechanisms of toxicity, clinical features, and management of diquat poisoning: a review, *J. Toxicol. Clin. Toxicol.,* 38, 123, 2000.

Landrigan, P. et al., Paraquat and marijuana: epidemiological assessment, *Am. J. Public Health,* 73, 784, 1983.

Narahashi, T., Nerve membrane ion channels as the target site of insecticides, *Mini. Rev. Med. Chem.,* 2, 419, 2002.

Roeder, R.A., Garber, M.J., and Schelling, G.T., Assessment of dioxins in foods from animal origins, *J. Anim. Sci.,* 76, 142, 1998.

Sathiakumar, N. and Delzell, E., A review of epidemiologic studies of triazine herbicides and cancer, *Crit. Rev. Toxicol.,* 27, 599, 1997.

Spindler, M., DDT: health aspects in relation to man and risk/benefit assessment based thereupon, *Residue Rev.,* 90, 1, 1983.

Suntres, Z.E., Role of antioxidants in paraquat toxicity, *Toxicology,* 180, 65, 2002.

Vale, J.A., Meredith, T.J., and Buckley, B.M., Paraquat poisoning: clinical features and immediate general management, *Human Toxicol.,* 6, 41, 1987.

28 Rodenticides

28.1 INTRODUCTION

Rodenticides are a diverse group of chemically and structurally **unrelated** compounds. Unlike the herbicides and insecticides whose toxicity is uniformly categorized according to their chemical classification, the rodenticides are functionally organized according to their general category and their toxicity in rodents (LD_{50}), as outlined in Table 28.1. In addition, the substances differ in their mechanisms of action, clinical toxicity, effective doses, structural formulas, sources, and other uses.

Over $1.1 billion of commercial, industrial, and household rodenticide-containing products were produced and consumed in the U.S. in 2001, exceeding that of all other countries combined. Although these products are most familiar for their use in extermination of mice and rats, they are also employed in the elimination of small mammals (squirrels, chipmunks), snakes, and frogs. Table 28.1 outlines some properties of popular rodenticides still commercially available. The substances are further discussed individually below.[*]

Acute and chronic toxic profiles of the rodenticides differ significantly from each other in severity and mechanism. Exposure from ready accessibility of the compounds accounts for a substantial number of nonfatal poisonings, averaging several hundred cases annually. As with the herbicides and insecticides, these cases result from inadvertent ingestion of commercial packages for home use, as well as dermal and respiratory exposure as occupational hazards.

28.2 ANTICOAGULANTS

28.2.1 CHEMICAL CHARACTERISTICS

The warfarins (the carbon-3 substituted 4-hydroxycoumarin derivatives) and "super-warfarins" (brodifacoum, indanediones) are popular rodenticides, whose properties were originally isolated from the sweet clover plant.[**] By 1950, the warfarins achieved international notoriety as the most useful rodenticides. The clinical feasibility of oral anticoagulants became known soon after with the realization of their relatively low toxicity.

---

[*] The toxicity of strychnine, a popular rodent poison, is discussed extensively in Chapter 13, "Sympathomimetics." The toxicity of some metals, such as arsenic and zinc, are outlined in Chapter 24, "Metals."

[**] Sweet clover (*Melilotus species*), long popular as food for grazing animals, contains various substances in the coumarin family. The plant has been used in the treatment of varicose veins and venous insufficiency. The name *Melilotus* originates from the Greek word for honey, *meli*, and a term for clover-like plants, *lotos*.

TABLE 28.1
Names, Chemical Properties, and Toxicity of Common Rodenticides

Common Name	Chemical Symbol, Name, or Synonym	Physical Characteristics	Toxicological Properties or Mechanism	Median Oral Rodent LD_{50} (mg/kg)
Metals				
Arsensic	As	Brilliant gray metal, insol in water	Human carcinogen; binds to sulfur-containing enzymes	15–40 (trivalent salts)
Barium	Ba	Yellow-white malleable metal, salts sol in water	Hypokalemia, skeletal and cardiac muscle toxicity	20
Phosphorus (P)	Elemental, white P	White (also black, or red) solid, ss in water	Nonspecific enzyme inhibitor; irritant	<5
Thallium	Tl	Blue-white soft metal, salts usually sol in water	Inhibits sulfhydril-containing enzymes	25 (sulfate)
Zinc Phosphide	Zn_3P_2	Gray crystals, insol in water	Nonspecific enzyme inhibitor; irritant	40–45
Anticoagulants				
Brodifacoum	Talon, Ratak+	Off-white powder, insol in water	Inhibits vitamin K synthesis	0.27
Norbromide	Raticate, Shoxin	White crystals, insol in water		5.3
Warfarin (4-hydroxycoumarin derivative)	Coumadin® (sodium salt)	Crystals, salts sol in water		8–100
Miscellaneous				
Strychnine	Strychnidin-10-one	White, crystalline powder, sol in water	Inhibits glycine, an inhibitory amino acid neurotransmitter	5 (sulfate)
Red Squill (*Liliacea* plant)	Scillaren A, B; sea onion	Bulbs of the red variety, granular, bitter powder, ss in water	Digoxin-like toxicity	1–10

Note: insol = insoluble, sol = soluble, ss = slightly soluble.

28.2.2 Commercial and Clinical Use

Today, warfarins are incorporated in rodent powder bait formulas and in rodent drinking water from 0.025 to 0.5% concentrations. Clinically, the oral anticoagulants are used for the treatment and prevention of thromboembolic-related disorders including myocardial infarction, cerebrovascular disease, venous thrombosis, pulmonary embolism, and other intravascular coagulation disorders. When directed for use as rodenticides or in the clinical management of coagulative disorders, the desirable or toxic effects of oral anticoagulants differ only quantitatively.

28.2.3 Toxicokinetics

Warfarins are rapidly and completely absorbed, reaching peak plasma concentrations within 1 h. In circulation, warfarins are almost completely bound to plasma albumin (97 to 99%), localize to lipid and protein compartments ($V_d = 0.15$ l/kg), and have a long half-life (35 h).*

28.2.4 Mechanism of Toxicity

Warfarins are vitamin K antagonists that inhibit vitamin K-dependent newly synthesized precursor coagulation factor proteins. Warfarins inhibit the carboxylation of glutamate residues (Glu) to γ-carboxyglutamate (Gla) in the conversion of descarboxyprothrombin to prothrombin (clotting factor II). The site of action of warfarin is illustrated in Figure 28.1. Thus, the anticoagulant effect is not demonstrated until vitamin K plasma and liver storage are depleted (prothrombin levels must fall below 25% of baseline values). This criterion affects the kinetics of accumulation of the drug but not its biological effect. Thus, the earliest onset of toxicity or clinical activity is not obvious until at least 21 to 72 h after exposure or therapeutic administration, respectively. In addition, to be effective rodenticides, the traditional warfarins require a minimum of 21 days of several feedings. Alternatively, the surperwarfarins are lethal after only one or two feedings, making them correspondingly more toxic.

28.2.5 Signs and Symptoms of Acute Toxicity

Accidental exposure from ingested rodent bait mostly involves children, whereas intentional ingestion is associated with attempted suicides or in attempts to feign illness. Mild to moderate adverse effects are often seen during routine therapeutic management of coagulative disorders. Single exposures are rare but involve acute, high dose ingestion. Consequently, signs and symptoms usually appear with repeated ingestion or following an initial therapeutic course.

Gingival bleeding, epistaxis, joint and muscle pain, easy bruising, and an abnormal PT time** are among the initial features of anticoagulant overdose. Intentional

---

* The racemic forms, levorotatory or S-(−)-enantiomorphs, are active warfarin isomers, while the more potent superwarfarins have longer half-lives (156 h), higher lipid solubility, and are more selective for hepatic enzymes.

** Prothrombin.

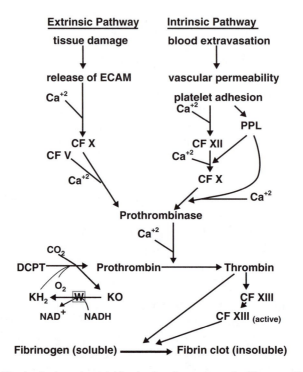

FIGURE 28.1 The intrinsic and extrinsic clotting factor cascade. The cascades illustrate the roles tissue damage or blood extravasation (exposure to collagen fibers) have in precipitating the formation of the fibrin clot. Warfarin (W) inhibits the enzymatic reduction of vitamin K epoxide (KO) to the reduced hydroquinone (KH_2) derivative. [CF II = prothrombin, CF III = thrombin, CF V = proaccelerin, CF X = Start-Prower factor, CF XII = Hageman factor, CF XIII = fibrin-stabilizing factor; DCPT = descarboxyprothrombin, KH_2 = vitamin K hydroquinone (reduced form), KO = vitamin K epoxide (oxidized).]

ingestion of high doses, or chronic repeated administrations are associated with severe coagulopathies, including hematuria, bloody stools, intracranial hemorrhage, and shock.

28.2.6 CLINICAL MANAGEMENT OF ACUTE POISONING

Replacement of blood loss and reversal of the anticoagulant effects are the primary goals of therapy. A unit of fresh frozen plasma* replenishes lost multiple clotting factors and restores blood volume. Chronic anticoagulant management necessitates the administration of vitamin K_1 (phytonadione). Subcutaneous or i.v. administration of this active form of vitamin K** rapidly corrects PT within 24 h. Maintenance with the oral dosage form may be continued for several weeks as needed.

---

* One unit of 300 ml of fresh frozen plasma (FFP) is prepared from whole blood within 6 h of collection and stored at −18°C. FFP is also used for the treatment of immunoglobulin deficiencies, burn trauma, and complement dysfunction.

** Other vitamin K derivatives, K_3 (menadione) and K_4 (menadiol), are therapeutically ineffective.

28.3 PHOSPHORUS (P)

28.3.1 CHEMICAL CHARACTERISTICS, OCCURRENCE, AND USES

A large class of irritating, corrosive, and asphyxiating phosphorus-containing compounds includes some broad categories of derivatives, namely: (1) tri- and pentavalent halide, sulfide, and oxide derivatives, (2) phosphine gas, (3) organic phosphate, phosphoric and phosphorus acid esters, and (4) organophosphorus insecticides. Only the more commonly encountered agents are discussed below (organophosphorus insecticides are thoroughly discussed in Chapter 26, "Insecticides").

White (elemental) phosphorus is a white or colorless, spontaneously flammable, highly toxic solid. It readily combines with oxidizing agents to form explosive mixtures. It is used in inorganic analytical chemistry and as a rodenticide. Its practical commercial application allows it to be spread on food (especially cheese) to attract mice and rats. Red phosphorus is less toxic and a less reactive but flammable compound, yet its fumes are highly irritating upon ignition. Red P is used to make safety matches, smoke bombs (for law enforcement), as a reactant for the manufacturing of pyrotechnic substances, fertilizers, P halides, and rodenticides. Phosphine is a flammable, highly toxic, colorless gas with a characteristic fish odor. It is used as a fumigant rodenticide and insecticide, and in the production of electronic components.

28.3.2 TOXICOKINETICS

Exposure to P and its derivatives is by oral ingestion or through inhalation of the flammable gases. Dermal, gastrointestinal, and respiratory irritation are hallmarks of P poisoning.

28.3.3 MECHANISM AND SIGNS AND SYMPTOMS OF ACUTE TOXICITY

Halides, oxides, and sulfides of P act as pulmonary irritants and dermal corrosive compounds. They are capable of spontaneous ignition, producing flames and fumes. They can combine with moist air or oxidizing agents to generate irritating or corrosive acidic conditions.

Phosphate esters (organic phosphates such as triethyl phosphate) inhibit acetyl cholinesterase. Oral ingestion, therefore, produces neurotoxicity, muscular weakness, and paralysis not unlike the organophosphate insecticides (see Chapter 26, "Insecticides").* Ingestion of elemental white P is associated with nausea, vomiting, diarrhea, and phosphorescent vomitus and stools (known as the *smoking stool syndrome*). Mucousal burning, abdominal pain, and a characteristic "garlic odor" to the breath, are frequent complaints from gastrointestinal irritation. Tremors, convulsions, jaundice, liver and cardiovascular failure, and coma develop following severe intox-

---

* It is important to note that not all organic phosphate esters are responsible for the development of neurotoxicity. In fact, the toxicity of trimethyl phosphate is related to its carcinogenic effect, while triphenyl phosphate lacks the neurotoxicity.

ication. Mortality rates of approximately 25 to 75% are noted from complications of systemic toxicity.

Phosphine gas is generated when solid rodenticides, such as zinc or aluminum phosphides, contact oxidizing agents or weak acids. The liberation and inhalation of the gas imparts a characteristic "fish odor" breath, especially when the powder mixes with stomach acid. Exposure produces signs and symptoms similar to pulmonary irritants and toxic products of combustion (see Chapter 23, "Gases"). Inhalation of phosphine vapors and fumes induces upper and lower respiratory tract injury (URT and LRT, respectively). Upper airway and ophthalmic injury is distinguished by local inflammation and irritation of ocular, oral, and nasal mucous membranes, including conjunctivitis, lacrimation, rhinitis, and pharyngitis. LRT symptoms include cough, wheezing, and tightness of chest with painful breathing. Early symptoms include nausea, fatigue, tremors, dizziness, and hypotension, followed by pulmonary edema, cardiogenic shock, central nervous system depression, convulsions, and coma.

Because of its proclivity for bone matrix, chronic, low-dose exposure to phosphates risks its accumulation in the skeleton. Peculiar symptoms develop such as tooth pain, sore mandible (classic *phossy jaw*), and nonspecific nutritional imbalances.

28.3.4 CLINICAL MANAGEMENT OF ACUTE POISONING

Treatment of phosphate poisoning is primarily supportive and symptomatic, and necessitates the use of gastric lavage, as well as administration of activated charcoal and sodium bicarbonate to reduce absorption and neutralize acidity, respectively. Treatment and decontamination should be instituted soon after exposure or upon dermal contact. Induction of vomiting is generally not recommended, due to phosphate's potentially corrosive nature. Cardiopulmonary support, renal perfusion, prevention of circulatory collapse, and oxygenation may be required.

28.4 RED SQUILL

28.4.1 CHEMICAL CHARACTERISTICS, OCCURRENCE, AND USES

Red squill* consists of the bulb of the red variety of *Urginea maritime* (Mediterranean squill, *Liliacea* family), most of which is imported for use as a rodenticide. More recently, less expensive importation of *Urginea indica* (Indian squill) has made this variety commercially more popular.

Squill contains many digoxin-like cardioactive glycosides, of which scillaren A and B make up most of the glycoside fraction. The compounds possess emetic, cardiotonic, and diuretic properties and were at one time ingredients of cough preparations (Cosanyl®). Scillaren and other cardioactive glycosides (strophanthin) were officially recognized for years and were considered efficacious, but their unreliable therapeutic stability and variable effects relinquished their clinical utility to the digitalis derivatives. Poisoning due to accidental or intentional ingestion of rodenticides containing scillaren compounds are uncommon.

Scilla is from the Greek meaning split, and refers to the separating scales of the plant. It is indigenous to the Mediterranean coasts of Spain, France, Italy, and Greece.

28.4.2 MECHANISM AND SIGNS AND SYMPTOMS OF ACUTE TOXICITY

The toxicity of red squill is similar to that of digoxin. Initial symptoms appear as blurred vision, arrhythmias, convulsions, and coma (interestingly rodents do not possess a vomiting reflex and consequently succumb to cardiac arrest, respiratory failure, and convulsions).

28.4.3 CLINICAL MANAGEMENT OF ACUTE POISONING

Clinical management requires intervention similar to that described for digoxin overdose (see Chapter 18, "Cardiovascular Drugs").

28.5 METALS: THALLIUM, BARIUM*

28.5.1 THALLIUM (Tl)

As with many potent compounds of metallic or botanical origin whose toxicity was yet to be recognized, Tl was used among the ancient civilizations for the treatment of syphilis, dysentery, tuberculosis, ringworm, and as a depilatory agent. Today the odorless and tasteless metal is incorporated in photoelectric cells, in semiconductor components, and rarely, as a rodenticide.

Tl inhibits oxidative phosphorylation through its ability to interfere with sulf-hydril-containing enzymes. Acute ingestion induces nausea, vomiting, diarrhea, and tremors.** Neurologically, Tl precipitates a syndrome resembling Guillain-Barré — i.e., acute febrile polyneuritis. The condition is characterized by agitation, confusion, pain, paresthesias, and weakness of the extremities radiating from the face and arms to the thorax and trunk. The syndrome is generally associated with repeated viral infections and eventually progresses to respiratory and cardiovascular collapse, convulsions, coma, and death.

Treatment of Tl intoxication is symptomatic and supportive. Chelation therapy is generally ineffective, although Prussian blue (potassium ferricyanoferrate) has shown some ability to decrease Tl absorption by forming insoluble complexes with the metal. Potassium chloride administration also prevents renal Tl reabsorption, thereby reducing blood Tl levels.

28.5.2 BARIUM (Ba)

Barium and its salts are used in the production of electronic components, paints, ceramics, lubricating oils, textiles, as a contrast agent in radiology (sulfate salt), and in analytical chemistry. Ba interferes with K^+ efflux from cells, thereby causing a reduction in extracellular K^+. Consequently, signs and symptoms of Ba poisoning

---

* Although arsenic is an active ingredient of some rodenticides, its toxicity is discussed in Chapter 24, "Metals."
** Alopecia is a classic pathognomonic sign of Tl toxicity. Unlike arsenic poisoning, however, Tl is not deposited in hair follicles.

are related to the production of (1) hypokalemia and (2) skeletal and cardiac muscle abnormalities (Table 28.1). Myoclonus, muscular rigidity, ventricular arrhythmias, vomiting, and diarrhea are secondary to the above effects.

Treatment of Ba exposure is symptomatic and supportive and requires the correction of the K^+ imbalance. K^+ administration, therefore, remains the most effective means of counteracting Ba-induced toxicity.

REFERENCES

Suggested Readings

Blumenthal, M., Ed., *The Complete German Commission E Monographs: Therapeutic Guide to Herbal Medicines*, American Botanical Council, Austin, TX, 1999, p. 218.

Review Articles

Bosse, G.M. and Matyunas, N.J., Delayed toxidromes, *J. Emerg. Med.*, 17, 679, 1999.

Costa, L.G., Basic toxicology of pesticides, *Occup. Med.*, 12, 251, 1997.

Cruickshank, J., Ragg, M., and Eddey D., Warfarin toxicity in the emergency department: recommendations for management, *Emerg. Med. (Fremantle)*, 13, 91, 2001.

Dorman, D.C., Toxicology of selected pesticides, drugs, and chemicals. Anticoagulant, cholecalciferol, and bromethalin-based rodenticides, *Vet. Clin. North Am. Small Anim. Pract.*, 20, 339, 1990.

el Bahri, L., Djegham, M. and Makhlouf, M., *Urginea maritima* L (squill): a poisonous plant of North Africa, *Vet. Hum. Toxicol.*, 42, 108, 2000.

Galvan-Arzate, S. and Santamaria, A., Thallium toxicity, *Toxicol. Lett.*, 99, 1, 1998.

Leonard, A. and Gerber, G.B., Mutagenicity, carcinogenicity and teratogenicity of thallium compounds, *Mutat. Res.*, 387, 47, 1997.

Moore, D., House, I., and Dixon, A., Thallium poisoning. Diagnosis may be elusive but alopecia is the clue, *B.M.J.*, 306, 1527, 1993.

Murphy, M.J., Rodenticides, *Vet. Clin. North Am. Small Anim. Pract.*, 32, 469, 2002.

Petterino, C. and Paolo, B., Toxicology of various anticoagulant rodenticides in animals, *Vet. Hum. Toxicol.*, 43, 353, 2001.

Rodenberg, H.D., Chang, C.C., and Watson, W.A., Zinc phosphide ingestion: a case report and review, *Vet. Hum. Toxicol.*, 31, 559, 1989.

Stone, W.B., Okoniewski, J.C., and Stedelin, J.R., Anticoagulant rodenticides and raptors: recent findings from New York, 1998-2001, *Bull. Environ. Contam. Toxicol.*, 70, 34, 2003.

Sutcliffe, F.A., MacNicoll, A.D., and Gibson, G.G., Aspects of anticoagulant action: a review of the pharmacology, metabolism and toxicology of warfarin and congeners, *Rev. Drug Metab. Drug. Interact.*, 5, 225, 1987.

Weiner, M.L. et al., Toxicological review of inorganic phosphates, *Food Chem. Toxicol.*, 39, 759, 2001.

29 Chemical Carcinogenesis and Mutagenesis

Yunbo Li, Zhuoxiao Cao, and Michael A. Trush

29.1 INTRODUCTION

Cancer remains a leading cause of morbidity and mortality in the human population, and the costs to society of this dreaded disease are prodigious. Cancer is a group of diseases in which there is an uncontrolled proliferation of cells that express varying degrees of fidelity to their precursor cell of origin. It has been proposed that cancer has six hallmarks: (1) self-sufficiency in growth signals, (2) insensitivity to anti-growth signals, (3) evasion of apoptosis, (4) tissue invasion and metastasis, (5) sustained angiogenesis, and (6) limitless replicative potential. The induction of a neoplasm is a multistage process that occurs over a long period of time, decades in humans. These stages have been experimentally defined as initiation, promotion, and progression. The causes of most human cancers remain unidentified; however, considerable evidence suggests that environmental and lifestyle factors, especially chemical agents, are important contributors. For example, tobacco smoking appears to be responsible for approximately 30% of all cancer deaths in developed countries. The notion that environmental agents are the principal causes of human cancers is largely derived from a series of epidemiological observations:

1. Although overall cancer incidence is reasonably constant between countries, incidences of specific tumor types can vary up to several hundred-fold.
2. There are large differences in cancer incidence within populations of a single country.
3. Migrant populations assume the cancer incidence of their new environment within one to two generations.
4. Cancer incidence within a population can change rapidly.

In addition to environmental agents, endogenous chemicals, such as estrogens have also been shown to contribute to the development of certain types of human cancers. Thus, understanding the molecular and cellular process underlying chemical carcinogenesis is of critical importance for carcinogenic risk assessment as well as development of mechanistically-based chemopreventive and therapeutic strategies for the management of human cancers.

TABLE 29.1
A Historical Overview of Chemical Carcinogenesis

1700	Ramazzini
	Noted that nuns exhibited a higher incidence of breast cancer than other women; attributed it to celibate life
1761	Hill
	Associated the use of tobacco snuff with induction of cancer of the nasal passage
1775	Pott
	Described the occurrence of soot-related scrotal cancer in chimney sweeps
1895	Rehn
	Associated occupational exposure to aromatic amine dyes with induction of bladder cancer
1915	Yamagawa and Ichikawa
	First experimental production of skin neoplasms by application of coal tar to ears of rabbits
1935	Sasaki and Yoshida
	First experimental production of liver neoplasms by administration of 3-dimethyl-4-aminoazobenzene in the diet to rats

29.2 HISTORY AND DEVELOPMENT

The evidence for the involvement of chemical agents in the induction of cancer was first noted in humans several centuries ago (Table 29.1). In 1700 Ramazzini observed a higher incidence of breast cancer in nuns, which he related to the celibate life of nuns. It is now known that the endogenous female hormone, estrogen, is an important contributor to breast cancer. The initial evidence of environmental chemical induction of cancer in humans was provided by Hill in 1761. He noted the association of the use of tobacco snuff with the induction of cancer of the nasal passage. Subsequently, Pott in 1775 described the occurrence of scrotal cancer in a number of patients with a history of employment as chimney sweeps during their childhood. These "climbing boys" were heavily and continuously exposed to the soot of the chimney due to poor hygiene. With remarkable insight, Pott attributed the induction of scrotal cancer to the occupation of the chimney sweeps, and suggested that the soot was causally related to the induction of scrotal cancer in these patients. During the nineteenth century, a number of chemicals were discovered and synthesized for various industrial uses. For example, the acrylamines, benzidine, and 2-naphthylamine were discovered and subsequently synthesized and utilized to produce various chemical species of pigments for coloring materials. The increased incidence of bladder cancer in workers employed in the aniline dye industry was first noted by Rehn in 1895. Subsequently, epidemiological studies conclusively implicated a number of acrylamines, including benzidine, 2-naphthylamine, and 4-aminobiphenol, in the induction of bladder cancer in workers in textile dye and rubber tire industries.

Although chemical induction of cancer in humans was noted centuries ago, utilizing experimental animals to examine chemical induction of cancer only began in the early twentieth century. In 1915, Yamagawa and Ichikawa described for the first time the induction of skin neoplasms (both benign and malignant) upon repetitive applications of coal tar to the ears of rabbits. Later in 1935, Sasaki and Yoshida further demonstrated that administration of the azo dye, 3-dimethyl-4-aminoazobenzene, in the diet to rats for extended periods of time led to the development of liver neoplasms. This was the first experiment demonstrating that a chemical can cause cancer at a site remote from its exposure. Since then, experimental animals, especially rats and mice, have been extensively used to study the chemical induction of cancer. Various intact animal assays, including the chronic rodent 2-year carcinogenesis bioassay, and transgenic and gene-knock-out mouse models have been developed for the identification of carcinogenic agents as well as for mechanistic studies. Studies with these animal models have resulted in a greater understanding of the biochemical and molecular processes underlying chemical carcinogenesis.

29.3 MECHANISMS OF CHEMICAL CARCINOGENESIS

29.3.1 METABOLISM

It is now widely appreciated that some carcinogenic agents, such as heavy metals, can directly cause carcinogenesis, whereas many organic chemicals need to first undergo metabolism to form reactive intermediates to induce carcinogenesis. Current understanding of the role of metabolism in chemical carcinogenesis has largely come from the pioneering studies by Elizabeth and James Miller several decades ago. Based on their studies with carcinogenic chemicals, including azo dyes and benzo(a)pyrene, the Millers proposed that chemical carcinogens can be converted through metabolism to electrophilic intermediates. These electrophilic metabolites exert their carcinogenic effects by covalent binding to cellular macromolecules. Accordingly, chemical carcinogens that require metabolic activation to exert their carcinogenic effects are termed procarcinogens, whereas their highly reactive metabolites are designated ultimate carcinogens. Metabolic intermediates between procarcinogens and ultimate carcinogens are called proximate carcinogens. The above terms are best illustrated by the metabolic pathway of benzo(a)pyrene, a widely distributed chemical carcinogen (Figure 29.1).

Both phase 1 and phase 2 enzymes are involved in the metabolism of chemicals, including carcinogens. Metabolism of carcinogens by phase 1 enzymes such as cytochrome P450 usually results in the formation of reactive metabolites, which can subsequently undergo phase 2 enzyme-catalyzed reactions, leading to detoxification and excretion. As such, induction of phase 2 enzymes via pharmacological agents has been demonstrated to be an effective approach to protecting against chemical carcinogenesis. The most extensively studied phase 2 enzymes in detoxifying carcinogens include glutathione S-transferases, UDP-glucuronsyltransferases, and NADPH:quinone oxidoreductases. Recently, transgenic and/or gene knockout animal models have become available for certain phase 1 and phase 2 enzymes. Use of these animal models has dramatically advanced understanding of the role of biotransformation in chemical carcinogenesis.

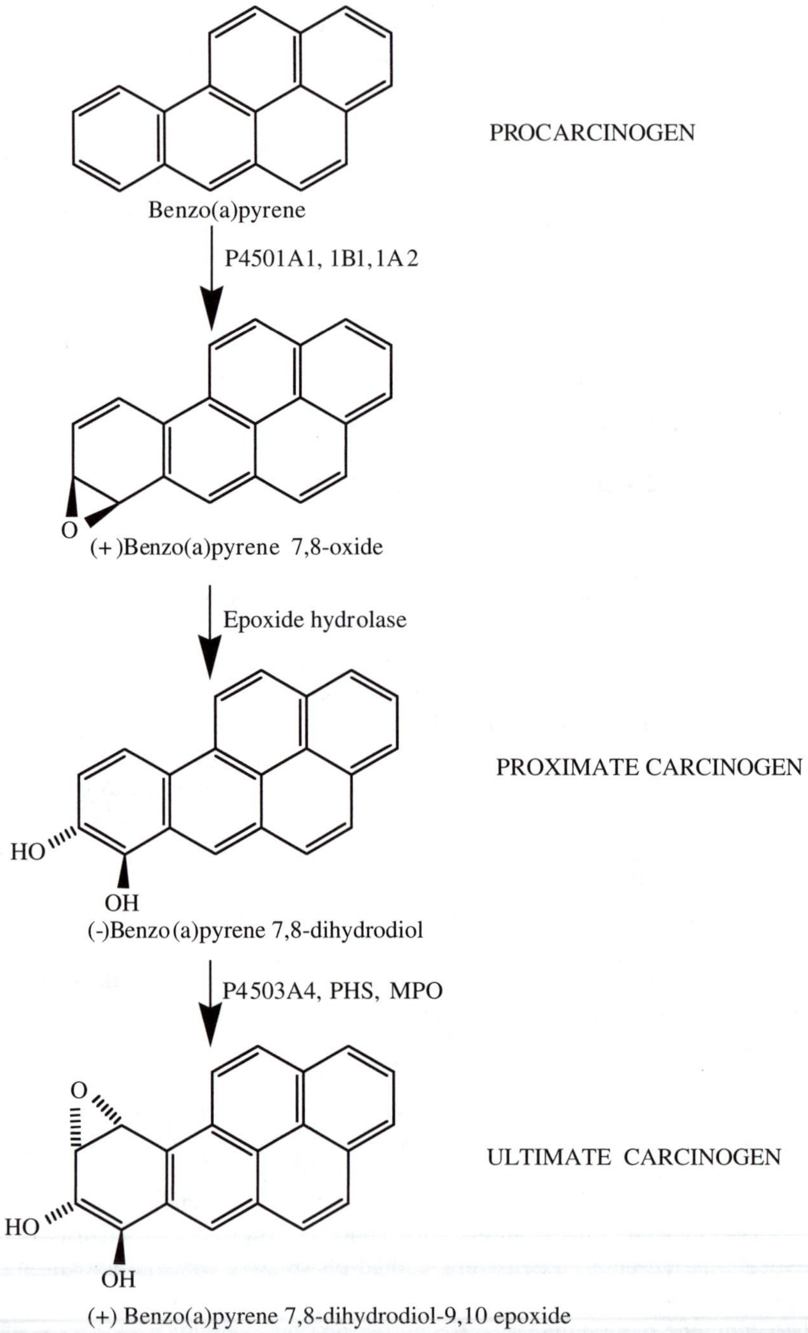

PROCARCINOGEN

Benzo(a)pyrene

P4501A1, 1B1, 1A2

(+)Benzo(a)pyrene 7,8-oxide

Epoxide hydrolase

PROXIMATE CARCINOGEN

HO''''

OH
(-)Benzo(a)pyrene 7,8-dihydrodiol

P4503A4, PHS, MPO

O''''

ULTIMATE CARCINOGEN

HO''''

OH
(+) Benzo(a)pyrene 7,8-dihydrodiol-9,10 epoxide

FIGURE 29.1 Metabolic activation of benzo(a)pyrene to form the proximate and ultimate carcinogens. MPO: myeloperoxidase; PHS, prostaglandin H synthase.

29.3.2 CHEMISTRY

Examining the relationship between chemical structures and carcinogenic activity is of critical importance for identification of potential chemical carcinogens and for understanding the mechanisms underlying their carcinogenic effects. In this regard, using the results of carcinogenesis bioassays of over 500 different chemicals, Ashby and Paton have investigated the influence of chemical structures on both the extent and the target tissue specificity of carcinogenesis for these chemical agents, and developed a list of chemical structures that exhibit a high correlation with the carcinogenicity in rodent bioassays. Among these chemical structures ("alerts") are aromatic nitro groups, aromatic ring N-oxides, aromatic mono- and dialkylamino groups, and aliphatic and aromatic epoxides. These structural "alerts" are apparently useful for carcinogenic risk assessment. Chemicals with these structural "alerts" should be avoided in the development of new pharmaceuticals.

29.3.3 FREE RADICALS AND REACTIVE OXYGEN SPECIES

Substantial studies have demonstrated that bioactivation of a number of chemical carcinogens also results in the formation of free radicals and reactive oxygen species (ROS). In addition to xenobiotic metabolism, free radicals and ROS can be generated from ionizing radiation, ultraviolet light, and a variety of cellular sources. Free radicals and ROS are reactive chemical species, which can cause oxidative damage to biomolecules, including nucleic acids, proteins, and lipids. Free radicals and ROS are also capable of reacting with DNA, leading to the formation of DNA adducts. Accumulating evidence over the past two decades suggests that free radicals and ROS are critically involved in carcinogenesis. As mentioned above, free radicals and ROS can cause direct damage to DNA, which may lead to the activation of protooncogenes/oncogenes and/or the inactivation of tumor suppressor genes. Free radicals and ROS are also able to interact with cell signaling molecules, including transcription factors and protein kinase cascades, resulting in altered cell signal transduction and gene expression. The ability of these agents to both elicit DNA mutations and cause dysregulated cell signaling has been proposed to contribute to the multistage carcinogenesis (Figure 29.2). The significance of free radicals and ROS in carcinogenesis has been further strengthened by the observations that a number of natural and synthetic antioxidative compounds exert anti-cancer effects both in animals and humans.

29.3.4 MUTAGENESIS

In a broad sense, carcinogenic agents may be classified into genotoxic and non-genotoxic carcinogens. A genotoxic carcinogen is able to interact with DNA directly, leading to mutations. The induction of mutations is due primarily to chemical or physical alterations in the structure of DNA that result in inaccurate replication of that region of the genome. The process of mutagenesis includes two major steps: structural DNA alteration, and cell proliferation that leads to the fixation of the DNA alteration. Interaction of reactive intermediates derived from

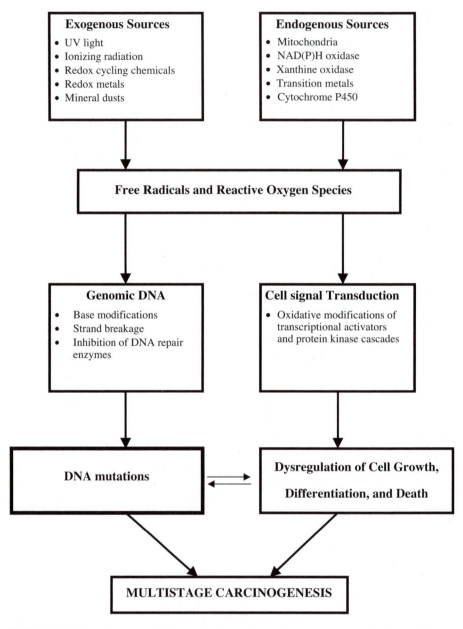

FIGURE 29.2 Involvement of free radicals and reactive oxygen species in multistage carcinogenesis.

the bioactivation of carcinogens with DNA can result in the formation of DNA adducts, DNA strand breaks, and DNA-protein cross-links. Among these alterations, formation of carcinogen-DNA adducts has been most extensively investigated. Carcinogens that result in the formation of bulky DNA adducts often specifically react with sites in the purine ring. In fact, the N7 position of guanine is the most nucleophilic site in DNA, at which many ultimate carcinogens form covalent adducts. Direct alkylation of DNA bases by several alkylating carcinogenic agents has also been demonstrated. Another common DNA modification is the hydroxylation of DNA bases, often caused by ROS. Such changes have been found in all four bases, but the most extensively investigated is the formation of 8-hydroxy-2'-deoxyguanosine. It should also be kept in mind that the interaction of carcinogens with DNA not only produces adducts on DNA bases, but also on the sugar and phosphate backbone. The covalent modifications of DNA by carcinogenic agents have been shown by many studies to result in mutations, which may ultimately lead to the development of cancer. Although the modifications of DNA by carcinogens described above are critically involved in the induction of DNA mutations, the mutagenesis process is also greatly affected by various DNA repair mechanisms.

29.3.5 DNA Repair

As stated above, the interaction of ultimate carcinogens with DNA results in the formation of various DNA adducts. Once the DNA adduct is formed, its continued presence in the DNA of the cell is largely determined by the cellular machinery to repair the structural alteration in the DNA. It is estimated that more than one hundred genes are dedicated to DNA repair. Because of the existence of this DNA repair machinery, the structural damage induced by carcinogens may be effectively repaired, and thus mutagenesis can be prevented. On the other hand, the persistence of DNA-carcinogen adducts is indicative of the insufficiency of DNA repair.

29.3.6 Epigenetic Carcinogenesis

As discussed above, direct interaction between reactive electrophilic metabolites and DNA, leading to mutations is an important mechanism of carcinogenesis induced by many carcinogens. These carcinogens are thus termed genotoxic carcinogens. On the other hand, there are many other chemicals that can cause cancer but do not directly affect DNA. These carcinogens are designated nongenotoxic (or epigenetic) carcinogens. For example, a study conducted by the National Toxicology Program on chemical carcinogenicity using the rodent bioassay revealed that 53% of the 301 chemicals analyzed were positive; 40% of those were classified as nongenotoxic carcinogens, with the most common target organ of cancer induction being the liver. Nongenotoxic carcinogens exhibit the following general characteristics: (1) they are nonmutagenic; (2) they show no evidence of direct chemical reactivity with DNA; (3) there are no common chemical structural features between these chemicals; (4) they exhibit a clear dose-threshold effect; and (5) their carcinogenic potential is generally lower than that of genotoxic carcinogens. While DNA damage can be described as a general mechanism of the carcinogenic effect of genotoxic carcinogens, nongenotoxic mechanisms are far more heterogeneous. Proposed mechanisms of nongenotoxic carcinogenesis are summarized in Table 29.2.

TABLE 29.2
Proposed Major Mechanisms of Nongenotoxic Carcinogenesis

- Prolonged stimulation of cell proliferation via chronic cytotoxicity or increased secretion of trophic hormones
- Inhibition of apoptosis in cells with DNA damage
- Impairment of DNA-replication fidelity and DNA-repairing machinery
- Disruption of gap-junctional intercellular communication
- Dysregulated cell signaling and gene expression via receptor- or nonreceptor-mediated pathways
- Altered DNA methylation status in the genes that control cell growth and differentiation
- Persistent immunosuppression, leading to compromised immunosurveillance

29.4   MULTISTAGE NATURE OF CHEMICAL INDUCTION OF CANCER

It is recognized that the process of carcinogenesis involves a variety of biological changes that, to a great extent, reflect the structural and functional alterations in the genome of the affected cell. As stated above, the process of carcinogenesis consists of three experimentally defined stages beginning with initiation, followed by the intermediate step of promotion, from which evolves the stage of progression (Figure 29.3).

29.4.1   INITIATION

Initiation is a phenomenon of gene alteration, which may result from the interaction of ultimate carcinogens with DNA in the target cell. Chemicals capable of initiating

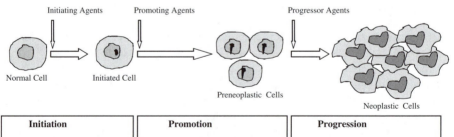

Initiation	Promotion	Progression
• Results from DNA mutations	• Results from clonal expansion of initiated cells	• Results from additional genomic structural alterations due to karyotypic instability
• Mutations may occur in oncogenes, protooncogenes, or tumor suppressor genes	• Cell signaling and gene expression are altered, leading to increased cell mitogensis and/or reduced apoptosis	• Leads to the formation of benign or malignant neoplasms
• Initiated cells may remain 'dormant', and rarely become neoplastic cells without undergoing promotion and progression	• Leads to the formation of preneoplastic cells	• Cells may acquire malignant phenotypes, such as invasiveness, angiogenesis and/or metastasis
• Irreversible	• Long duration and reversible, especially at earlier stage	• Irreversible

FIGURE 29.3 A schematic illustration of the three stages of chemical carcinogenesis.

cells are called initiating agents. Initiation without the following steps, promotion and progression, rarely yields malignant neoplasms. The following steps are critically involved in the initiation process by carcinogenic chemicals: (1) conversion of a chemical to a DNA-reactive metabolite (an ultimate carcinogen), (2) interaction of the ultimate carcinogen with DNA, leading to DNA structural alteration, (3) DNA repair that may reverse the structural damage, and (4) cell proliferation leading to the fixation of the DNA damage. Mutations of protooncogenes/oncogenes, such as the ras genes may result in their activation, leading to neoplastic transformation. On the other hand, mutations in tumor suppressor genes, such as the p53 gene, may cause their inactivation. Inactivation of the p53 tumor suppressor gene via point mutations has been implicated in the induction of cancer by various agents, including benzo(a)pyrene and aflatoxin B1. In fact, p53 is the most commonly mutated gene found in human cancers. One of the characteristics of the stage of initiation is its irreversibility, in the sense that the genotype/phenotype of the initiated cell is established at the time of initiation.

29.4.2 PROMOTION

In multistage carcinogenesis, the term promotion refers to a phenomenon of gene activation in which the latent altered phenotype of the initiated cell becomes expressed through selection and clonal expansion. The agents capable of inducing tumor promotion are thus termed tumor promoters. Typical tumor-promoting agents include tetradecanoyl phorbol acetate (TPA), phenobarbital, 2,3,7,8-tetracholorodibenzo-*p*-dioxin (TCDD), and cholic acid. In contrast to initiating agents, tumor promoters do not directly interact with DNA. The intermediate stage of promotion does not appear to involve direct structural changes in the cell but rather depends on an altered expression of genes. In fact, many tumor-promoting agents are able to modulate a variety of cell signaling pathways, resulting in altered gene expression. One distinct characteristic of promotion, in contrast to initiation and progression, is the reversible nature of this stage. In this regard, the existence of the promoted cell population (preneoplastic lesion) is dependent on the continued administration of the promoting agents. The regression of preneoplastic lesions upon withdrawal of the promoters may be due to increased cell death via apoptosis. This notion is supported by the observation that many tumor-promoting agents appear to inhibit apoptosis in the preneoplastic lesions. For most tumor-promoting agents, the dose-response relationships exhibit sigmoid-like curves with an apparent threshold and maximal effect. Another important aspect of tumor promotion is its long duration, which can be decades in humans. Because of its long duration and reversibility, tumor promotion is considered a preferred target for cancer chemoprevention. Evidence that tumor promotion occurs in human cancer development is demonstrated by the reduction of risk for developing lung cancer in individuals who quit smoking.

29.4.3 PROGRESSION

Progression is the last irreversible stage of multistage carcinogenesis, which usually develops from the cells in the stage of promotion. Progression results from continuing evolution of a basically unstable karyotype, leading to morphologically discernible alteration in cellular genomic structure. Either benign or malignant neoplasms are observed in this stage. Agents that only cause the transition of a cell from the stage of promotion to that of progression are termed progressor agents. Putative progressor agents may include hydrogen peroxide, arsenic salts, hydroxyurea, and organic peroxides, such as benzoyl peroxide. The progressor agents may have the ability to induce chromosomal aberrations and, in some cases, enhance the clastogenesis associated with evolving karyotypic instability. Mechanisms that underlie karyotypic instability are numerous and may include disruption of the mitotic machinery, dysregulated telomerase function, altered DNA methylation status, DNA recombination, gene amplification, and gene transposition. Due to significant genetic alterations, cells in the progression stage may gain the ability to undergo invasiveness and metastasis to eventually lead to the formation of a clinical cancer (Figure 29.3).

29.5 CARCINOGENIC AGENTS

It is widely appreciated that cancer can be induced by exposure to various agents, including both endogenous and exogenous substances. A carcinogen may be defined as an agent whose administration to previously untreated animals leads to a statistically significant increased incidence of malignant neoplasms as compared with that in appropriate untreated control animals. Carcinogens can be chemicals, physical agents (such as ultraviolet light and gamma radiation), and biological agents (such as viruses). Chemical carcinogens are the most commonly investigated carcinogenic agents.

29.5.1 CLASSIFICATION

There are a number of ways to classify chemical carcinogens. Chemical carcinogens may be classified based on their chemical nature into (1) organic chemical carcinogens, such as benzo(a)pyrene, aflatoxin B1, and benzene; (2) inorganic chemical carcinogens, including arsenic, cadmium, chromium, and nickel; and (3) hormonal carcinogens, typified by estrogens. Based on the reactivity with DNA, chemical carcinogens can be classified into genotoxic carcinogens and nongenotoxic (epigenetic) carcinogens. Based on the evidence of carcinogenicity in animals and humans, carcinogens may be classified as animal carcinogens and/or human carcinogens. In the evaluation of carcinogenicity for humans, the International Association for Research on Cancer (IARC) has categorized carcinogens into five groups:

1. **Group 1.** Agents in this group have sufficient evidence of carcinogenicity in humans and, as such, are called known human carcinogens. Arsenic, aflatoxin B1, benzene, estrogens, vinyl chloride, nickel, and chromium belong to this group.
2. **Group 2A.** Agents in this group possess sufficient evidence of carcinogenicity in animals, but have limited evidence of carcinogenicity in humans.

These agents are thus probably carcinogenic to humans. Within this group are benz(a)anthracene, polychlorinated biphenols, and styrene oxide.

3. **Group 2B.** Agents in this group possess either limited evidence of carcinogenicity in humans, or have sufficient evidence of carcinogenicity in animals and inadequate evidence of carcinogenicity in humans. Class 2B agents are possibly carcinogenic to humans. Examples of Group 2B agents are styrene and urethane.

4. **Group 3.** Agents in this group are not classifiable as to carcinogenicity.

5. **Group 4.** Agents in this group possess inadequate evidence of carcinogenicity in both animals and humans and, thus, are probably not carcinogenic to humans.

29.5.2 Occurrence

Chemical carcinogens are widely distributed and encountered in many human activities. They are found as pollutants in workplaces (Table 29.3), environmental chemicals, therapeutic drugs, dietary factors, and components in tobacco smoke (see Section 29.6).

29.5.3 Identification

Identification of carcinogenic agents is a critical step in carcinogenic risk assessment. Epidemiological studies provide the most definitive means of establishing carcinogenicity to humans from exposure to an agent. Because most epidemio-

---

TABLE 29.3
Some Established Human Carcinogenic Chemicals Found in Various Workplaces

Chemical Agents	Workplace	Cancer Induction
Arsenic	Copper mining and smelting	Cancer of the skin, lung, or liver
Cadmium	Smelting, battery making, welding	Bronchial carcinoma
Chromium and chromates	Tanning, pigment manufacturing	Cancer of nasal sinus and bronchus
Nickel	Nickel refining	Cancer of nasal sinus and bronchus
Benzidine and β-naphthylamine	Dye, textile and rubber tire industry	Bladder cancer
Para-aminodiphenyl	Manufacturing	Bladder cancer
Polycyclic aromatic hydrocarbons	Steel manufacturing, roofing	Skin or lung cancer
Benzene	Manufacturing, petroleum refining	Leukemia
Vinyl chloride	Chemical manufacturing	Liver angiosarcoma

logical studies are performed (or the conclusions are drawn) after exposure to an agent has occurred, they are not protective of human health. In addition, epidemiological studies have limited sensitivity for identification of carcinogens. Thus, various experimental methods have been developed to be used for identification of potential carcinogens. These experimental methods have been classified into three major groups:

1. Short-term assays, which include various mutagenesis assays and neoplastic transformation in cell culture. These assays last from several weeks up to 3 months.
2. Medium-term assays for qualitative and quantitative analysis of preneoplasia. These assays are carried out in animals and last for 2 to 8 months.
3. Long-term animal bioassays, with a time frame of 18 to 24 months.

Today, the "gold standard" for identification of potential carcinogenic chemicals is through the use of the chronic 2-year bioassay for carcinogenicity in rodents. This assay involves test groups of 50 rats and mice of both sexes and at two or three dose levels of the test agent. B6C3F1 mouse and F334 rat are the two strains typically used in the U.S. by regulatory agencies. Animals at about 8 weeks of age are placed on the test agent at the various doses for another 96 weeks of their life span. A variety of pretest analyses are conducted for determination of acute toxicity as well as the maximum tolerated dose (MTD), which will be used as the highest dose level in the subsequent 2-year bioassay. MTD is the dose which, in a 3-month study, causes no more than a 10% weight decrement, as compared to appropriate control groups, and does not produce mortality, clinical signs of toxicity, or pathological lesions other than those that may be related to a neoplastic response. Regarding the route of administration, the agent is administered by the route through which human exposure is believed to occur or will occur. This is often an oral route through gavage or dietary administration.

29.5.4 Carcinogenic Potential

It is obvious that not all carcinogenic chemicals are equally effective in inducing neoplasia; i.e., they exhibit different carcinogenic potencies. The carcinogenic potential of a chemical may be defined simply as the slope of the dose-response curve for induction of neoplasms. However, such a definition has generally not been the basis for estimating carcinogenic potential based on data from chronic carcinogenesis bioassays. Over the last several decades, a number of methods/equations have been developed to measure the carcinogenic potential. Among them, the tumorigenesis dose rate 50 (TD50) value has been widely used to estimate the carcinogenic potential for a number of chemical carcinogens. TD50 refers to the dose rate (mg/kg body weight/day) of the carcinogenic chemical, which, if administered chronically for a standard period, would induce neoplasms in half of the test animals at the end of the test adjusting for spontaneous neoplasms. Determination of carcinogenic potential is an important component of carcinogenic risk assessment.

29.5.5 CARCINOGENIC RISK ASSESSMENT

Carcinogenic risk assessment is a very complex and controversial process. A number of steps are involved in carcinogenic risk assessment. They are (1) identification of carcinogen and evaluation of carcinogenic potential, (2) mechanism elucidation, (3) exposure assessment, (4) dose-response assessment, and (5) qualitative and quantitative estimation of carcinogenic risk in human beings. As stated above, due to the nonprotective feature and limited sensitivity of epidemiological studies, various laboratory experimental methods, including both the *in vitro* and *in vivo* bioassays are extensively used for identification of carcinogens and evaluation of carcinogenic potential. As might be expected, a number of problems (or controversies) are involved in the scientific and practical application of the information derived from laboratory bioassays to the estimation of human risk. Obviously, one problem is the extrapolation of carcinogenic data obtained from laboratory testing to humans for estimating the carcinogenic risk. Another significant problem is the dose-response relationship. As discussed above, high doses (such as the use of MTD) of a test agent are used in the 2-year animal bioassay for identification of carcinogenicity. The actual levels of human exposure to a particular potential carcinogenic chemical are generally much lower than those used in laboratory animal experiments. Therefore, a problem arises when one tries to apply the carcinogenic data obtained in animals with high doses of a test agent to estimating the carcinogenic potential in humans whose exposure to that agent is considerably lower. The extrapolation from high dose to low dose in carcinogenic risk assessment is further complicated by the debate on the existence of a threshold for genotoxic carcinogens. Clearly, further understanding of the molecular mechanisms underlying chemical carcinogensis will improve the ability to assess carcinogenic risk to humans.

Another consideration in determination of carcinogenic risk in humans is whether or not the estimation is qualitative or quantitative. Qualitative risk estimation is much easier to develop based on qualitative analysis of the information obtained from various bioassays. In contrast, the quantitative risk estimation is much more difficult, and subject to great variations. Nevertheless, quantitative risk analysis with the utilization of various "safe" doses of carcinogenic agents and a variety of other factors as well as the integration of biological data, including toxicokinetic and toxicodynamic parameters, has been and is being applied to human risk situations of specific carcinogenic chemicals or mixtures. In this context, various mathematical and biomathematical models have been developed and utilized for the quantitative estimation of carcinogenic risk in humans. Among them are the one-hit (linear) model, multihit (k-hit) model, multistage model, extreme value model, log-probit model, and the MKV biomathematic model, and biologically based cancer modeling. Some of the above models have been proposed by regulatory agencies, such as U.S. Environmental Protection Agency (EPA) for quantitative analysis of carcinogenic risk.

29.6   TOBACCO SMOKE AS A SOURCE OF CHEMICAL CARCINOGENS

29.6.1   EPIDEMIOLOGY

Approximately 30% of all cancer deaths in developed countries are caused by cigarette smoking. This includes 87% of lung cancer, 60% of upper aerodigestive cancer, and 8% of other cancers. In the latter group, cigarette smoking is a recognized cause of cancers of the urinary bladder, pancreas, kidney, liver, and colon. Cigarette smoking has also been suggested as a risk factor in the development of leukemia, gallbladder cancer, cervical cancer, sinonasal cancer, and cancers in the adrenal gland. The linkage between cigarette smoking and breast cancer in females is plausible, but has been difficult to establish. Cigarette smoking as an important cause of human cancers is consistent with the demonstration that cigarette smoke contains many chemical carcinogens.

29.6.2   CARCINOGENS IN TOBACCO SMOKE

Tobacco smoke contains over 4000 characterized compounds, of which over 60 are carcinogens for which there is sufficient evidence of carcinogenicity in either laboratory animals or humans, according to evaluations by the IARC. These carcinogens belong to the following classes of chemicals: (1) polycyclic aromatic hydrocarbons, (2) aza-arenes, (3) N-nitrosamines, (4) aromatic amines, (5) heterocyclic aromatic amines, (6) aldehydes, and (7) miscellaneous organic and inorganic compounds, such as benzene and cadmium. Among these carcinogenic chemicals, polycyclic aromatic hydrocarbons and the tobacco-specific nitrosamine 4-(methylnitrosamine)-1-(3-pyridyl)-1-butanone (NNK) have been suggested to play major roles in tobacco smoke-induced carcinogenesis, especially lung cancer.

29.6.3   MECHANISM OF TOBACCO CARCINOGENESIS

It is well established that the carcinogenic chemicals existing in tobacco smoke are responsible for the induction of various cancers. Because of the great diversity of the carcinogenic agents in cigarette smoke, there is no single mechanism of tobacco-induced carcinogenesis. Moreover, most carcinogens in cigarette smoke require metabolic activation to exert their carcinogenic effects. Based on currently available data, Hecht proposed the major molecular and cellular events underlying cigarette smoke-induced carcinogenesis. Carcinogens form the link between nicotine addiction and lung cancer. While nicotine is considered not to be carcinogenic, nicotine addiction is the reason that the smokers continue to smoke, thereby leading to continuous exposure to tobacco-derived carcinogens. Carcinogens from cigarette smoke can be taken directly through inhalation and may be also absorbed into the systemic circulation and then distributed throughout the body. Many carcinogenic chemicals from tobacco are converted to reactive electrophilic metabolites by phase 1 enzymes, particularly the cytochrome P450 system. These electrophilic metabolites, if not completely detoxified by the subsequent phase 2 enzyme-mediated conjugation reactions, will bind covalently with DNA to form DNA adducts. In addition, free radicals and ROS derived from cigarette smoke also cause oxidative DNA damage, such as DNA strand breaks and base modifications. If the structural DNA damage escapes cellular repair mechanisms, it could persist and may cause mutations. Certain mutations could trigger the activation of a protooncogene/oncogene or the deactivation of a tumor suppressor gene. In this regard, substantial evidence suggests a crucial role for mutation-induced activation of the oncogene K-ras and inactivation of tumor suppressor gene p53 in tobacco smoke-induced lung carcinogenesis.

Cigarette smoke also contains a variety of tumor-promoting agents, which have been suggested to critically contribute to cigarette smoke-induced carcinogenesis. Epidemiological studies have convincingly demonstrated that smoking cessation leads to a great reduction of the cancer risk, further supporting the tumor-promoting activity of tobacco smoke.

29.6.4 INTERVENTION OF TOBACCO SMOKE-INDUCED CARCINOGENESIS

Largely due to the nature of the tumor-promoting activity of tobacco smoke, smoking cessation is probably the most effective way to reduce the tobacco smoking-induced cancer risk in cigarette smokers. While a minority (about 3%) of tobacco users achieve permanent abstinence in an initial attempt to quit, most continue to use tobacco for many years and typically cycle through multiple periods of relapse and remission. The success rate of quitting cigarette smoking can be increased to 15 to 30% with treatment for nicotine dependence. Pharmacological management of tobacco dependence includes five first-line drugs: (1) sustained-release bupropion hydrochloride, an atypical antidepressant, (2) nicotine chewing gum, (3) nicotine inhalers, (4) nicotine nasal sprays, and (5) nicotine patches. Two second-line drugs have been suggested in the U.S. if the first-line pharmacotherapies are not effective. They are clonidine hydrochloride and nortriptyline hydrochloride.

29.7 CANCER CHEMOPREVENTION

29.7.1 GENERAL CONSIDERATIONS

Generally, there are two complementary strategies for preventing cancer: (1) avoidance of exposure to cancer-inducing agents, such as chemical carcinogens, and (2) modulation of the host defense against carcinogenesis through dietary and/or pharmacological interventions, which is known as cancer chemoprevention. Cancer chemoprevention may be defined as the use of natural or synthetic pharmacological agents to prevent, arrest, or reverse carcinogenesis at its earliest stages. Because carcinogenesis is a multistage process and often has a latency of many years to decades, there is considerable opportunity for intervention via chemoprevention. Indeed, cancer chemoprevention has been successfully achieved in numerous animal experiments over the last two decades, and has been validated in several major clinical trials.

29.7.2 Cancer Chemopreventive Agents

Due to increased understanding of the molecular and cellular mechanisms underlying carcinogenesis, a number of potential targets for cancer chemoprevention have recently been identified and/or suggested, which greatly aid in the development of more effective chemopreventive agents. Many classes of agents, either natural or synthetic compounds have shown a great deal of promise in chemoprevention of human cancers. These chemopreventive agents may be classified into: (1) selective estrogen receptor modulators, such as tamoxifen and raloxifene, (2) anti-inflammatory agents, including aspirin and celecoxib, (3) antioxidants and phase 2 enzyme-inducers, such as antioxidant vitamins, isothiocyanates, and dithiolethiones, and (4) agents that selectively modulate other cellular receptors and signal transduction, such as retinoids and vitamin D analogs.

29.7.3 Mechanisms Underlying Cancer Chemoprevention

It is essential not only to evaluate the efficacy of chemopreventive agents in preclinical models and clinical trials, but also to understand the mechanisms involved. Such knowledge will provide a rationale for using pharmacological agents and dietary factors for preventive purposes and will be important for development of new selective and effective chemopreventive agents. Although there is a great understanding of the mechanisms by which some agents, such as tamoxifen, prevent (or protect against) carcinogenesis, for many other potential chemopreventive agents the mechanisms remain to be elucidated. This is partially due to the complex nature of the multistage carcinogenesis. In addition, different mechanisms may contribute to the protective effects of a particular agent. Nevertheless, for chemoprevention of chemical carcinogenesis, the following two mechanisms may be operative for many, if not most, agents: (1) mechanisms leading to alteration of toxicokinetics of carcinogens, and (2) mechanisms resulting in the inhibition of the multistages of carcinogenesis. In terms of altering carcinogen toxicokinetics, chemopreventive agents may work through either inhibiting the absorption of carcinogens or increasing their detoxification, primarily by induction of phase 2 and antioxidative enzymes. On the other hand, chemopreventive agents may inhibit the three stages of carcinogenesis, i.e., initiation, promotion, and progression, by modulating a number of cellular mechanisms/processes, such as: (1) stimulation of DNA repair, (2) induction of apoptosis and inhibition of cell proliferation, (3) stimulation of immune system, and (4) inhibition of neovascularization. Among the above listed potential mechanisms of cancer chemoprevention, the induction of phase 2 and antioxidative enzymes by chemopreventive agents, including dithiolethiones, isothiocyanates, and a number of phenolic compounds has recently received great attention and shown a great deal of promise.

Extensive studies over the last several years have resulted in a great understanding of the molecular events leading to the induction of antioxidative and phase 2 enzymes by chemopreventive agents. It is widely recognized that induction of cellular antioxidative and phase 2 enzymes by these cancer chemopreventive agents is regulated at the transcriptional level and is mediated by a specific response

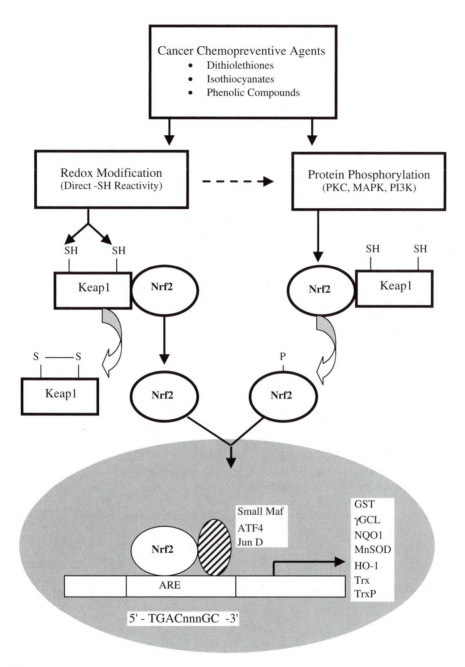

FIGURE 29.4 A schematic illustration of the major molecular pathways involved in the induction of antioxidative and phase 2 enzymes by cancer chemopreventive agents. PKC, protein kinase C; MAPK, mitogen-activated protein kinase; PI3K, phosphoinositide 3-kinase; GST, glutathione S-transferase; γGCL, gamma-glutamylcysteine ligase; MnSOD, manganese superoxide dismutase; HO-1, heme oxygenase-1; Trx, thioredoxin; TrxP, thioredoxin peroxidase.

element, the antioxidant response element (ARE), found in the promoter of the enzyme's gene. More recently, compelling evidence has been obtained from *in vitro* and *in vivo* studies suggesting that the bZIP transcription factor Nrf2 is the central protein that interacts with the ARE to activate antioxidative and phase 2 gene expression in response to the cancer chemopreventive agents. Several signaling pathways, including protein phosphorylation and sulfhydryl redox regulation, have been implicated in the activation of Nrf2 to lead to the stimulation of the ARE-driven gene transcription. The molecular pathways based on currently available data, by which cancer chemoprotective agents induce antioxidative and phase 2 gene expression through ARE, are outlined in Figure 29.4.

REFERENCES

SUGGESTED READINGS

Klaassen, C.D., Ed., *Casarett and Doull's Toxicology: The Basic Science of Poisons,* 6th ed., McGraw-Hill, New York, 2001, chap.8.

REVIEW ARTICLES

Gonzalez, F.J. and Kimura, S., Study of P450 function using gene knockout and transgenic mice, *Arch Biochem. Biophys.,* 409, 153, 2003.

Guengerich, F.P., Forging the links between metabolism and carcinogenesis, *Mutat. Res.,* 488, 195, 2001.

Hengstler, J. et al., Challenging dogma: thresholds for genotoxic chemicals? The case of vinyl acetate, *Annu. Rev. Pharmacol. Toxicol.,* 43, 485, 2003.

Kuper, H., Boffetta, P., and Adami, H.O., Tobacco use and cancer causation: association by tumour type, *J. Intern. Med.,* 252, 206, 2002.

Nguyen, T., Sherratt, P.J., and Pickett, C.B., Regulatory mechanisms controlling gene expression mediated by the antioxidant response element, *Annu. Rev. Pharmacol. Toxicol.,* 43, 233, 2003.

Preston, R.J., Quantitation of molecular endpoints for the dose-response component of cancer risk assessment, *Toxicol. Pathol.,* 30, 112, 2002.

Sporn, M.B. and Suh, N., Chemoprevention: An essential approach to controlling cancer, *Nature Rev. Cancer,* 2, 537, 2002.

30 Reproductive and Developmental Toxicity

30.1 INTRODUCTION

Drugs or chemicals that induce structural malformations, physical dysfunction, behavioral alterations, or genetic deficiencies in the fetus, or impair fertility, are referred to as **teratogens**. The expression of the teratogenic response — i.e., the embryotoxic effect of a compound on the growth and development of the fetus — is usually manifested at birth or in the immediate postnatal period. In addition, reproductive toxicity of a chemical may interfere early on in the reproductive cycle (first trimester), by impairing fertilization or interfering with implantation. These initial interactions between the fertilized ovum and the chemical in question may result in the inability to establish pregnancy or may cause spontaneous termination of pregnancy.

Drug use during pregnancy has increased dramatically in recent years. Studies indicate that about 90% of women have ingested one or more medications while pregnant (FDA, 1995). Excluding the commonly prescribed prenatal vitamins, iron supplements, and tocolytic* drugs, on average, women under 35 years of age take three prescriptions during the course of their pregnancies; in women over 35, this number rose to five. Some of the drugs used most extensively during pregnancy include antibiotics, analgesics, and narcotics, followed by antiepileptics, antihypertensives, antinauseants, psychotherapeutic agents, and respiratory medications. For most of these drugs, no well-controlled studies have been conducted in pregnant women. In spite of the current lack of information on the safety of drug products during pregnancy, there appears to be little reluctance to prescribe.

These studies, although initially alarming, are evidence for the complacency and lack of knowledge, both in the community and within the medical profession, about the insidious dangers of drug use during pregnancy. In addition, the well-intended practice of prescribing lower doses of drugs for pregnant women to minimize exposure to the fetus is misguided. The complicating factor lies in the ubiquitous availability and distribution of therapeutic drugs, as well as environmental chemicals and herbal products, that necessarily infiltrate the maternal/fetal environment. Although most therapeutic drugs are screened for their embryotoxic or teratogenic potential in animal reproductive studies, the majority of chemicals are not. In fact, U.S. federal regulations do not impose extensive requirements on pharmaceutical and chemical companies to provide such information. Also, most drug development programs do not routinely incorporate

---

* Any drug used to suppress premature labor.

screening or follow-up of drugs for potential embryotoxic effects in pregnant women during preclinical and clinical phases, or in the postmarketing period. Finally, chemicals not destined to be used clinically, but found in abundance throughout the environment (pesticides, solvents, metals), are generally devoid of any teratogenic testing. This leaves a multitude of chemicals used in the marketplace without human embryotoxic data.

30.2 HISTORY AND DEVELOPMENT

The thalidomide disaster of 1961 initiated a significant effort to establish a program for teratogenicity testing. Developed as a sedative/hypnotic with no particular advantage over drugs of the same class, thalidomide was initially shown to lack teratogenic effects in all species tested, except in the rabbit. Soon after its introduction to the European market, the drug was linked to the development of a relatively rare birth defect, known as *phoecomelia*. The epidemic proportions of the teratogenic effect prompted the passage of the Harris-Kefauver Amendment in 1962, one of the many additions since to the Federal Pure Food and Drug Act. The amendment requires extensive pharmacological and toxicological preclinical research before a therapeutic compound can be marketed.*

30.3 SUMMARY OF MATERNAL-FETAL PHYSIOLOGY

30.3.1 DEFINITIONS

Fetal development involves the gradual establishment and modification of anatomical structures from its beginning at fertilization (conception) to maturity. More precisely, the first 10 weeks roughly correspond to the first trimester. This phase is characterized as the period of time for *embryological development*, where differentiation of precursor stem cells progresses to the launching of fetal membranes and the embryonic disk. The remainder of the pregnancy (weeks 10 to 40) is dedicated to *fetal development*, where the established blueprints of organs and tissues undergo further growth and maturity. Together, the processes are referred to as *prenatal development*. Thus, in humans, the gestational period is normally of 9 months' duration (or 280 days from the first day of the last menstrual period, assuming a regular 28-day cycle). *Postnatal development* therefore begins at birth and progresses to maturity (i.e., for approximately 18 years).

30.3.2 FIRST TRIMESTER

The *first trimester* is the period corresponding to embryological and early fetal development. The main events occurring during the first trimester include:

---

* Interestingly, almost 40 years later, thalidomide has resurfaced (Thalomid®) and is used in the U.S. for the treatment of erythema nodosum leprosum. The package is painted within and without with red warning labels alerting the prescriber, pharmacist, and patient about the precaution against its use in women of childbearing potential.

a. **Cleavage** (days 1–6) — a series of cell divisions following fertilization of the ovum by the sperm cell, and terminating at the blastocyst stage.

b. **Implantation** (days 7–10) — adhesion, attachment and penetration of the uterine endometrial lining by the blastocyst; trophoblast, amniotic cavity, and inner cell mass form and expand during this stage; further development of the yolk sac, chorion, allantois, amnion, and embryonic disc (from the inner cell mass) ensues during weeks 3 and 4 (beginning of organogenesis).

c. **Placentation** (from weeks 2 to 10) — starting as early as day 10, blood vessels form around the periphery of the blastocyst to establish the presence of the placenta; the placenta is characterized by the formation of chorionic villi and appearance of fetal vessels.

d. **Embryogenesis** (also during weeks 5–10) — the process of differentiation and folding of the embryonic disc, producing a physically and developmentally distinct and recognizable embryo.

Because of the critical events occurring during this phase, the first trimester represents the most sensitive period of fetal development to external stimuli (especially drugs and chemicals).

30.3.3 SECOND AND THIRD TRIMESTERS

The *second trimester* corresponds to the third to sixth months of gestation and is characterized by rapid fetal development of organs and systems. The *third trimester* displays rapid growth and maturation of established organ systems in preparation for independent survival and function.

30.4 MECHANISMS OF DEVELOPMENTAL TOXICITY

30.4.1 SUSCEPTIBILITY

As noted above, the first 8 to 10 weeks of embryogenesis qualify as a sensitive period for the fetus to the presence of drugs or chemicals. For instance, exposure to exogenous compounds 21 days after fertilization have the potential for greatest embryotoxicity, resulting in death of the fetus. Whereas, exposure to compounds between the third and eighth weeks are potentially teratogenic, i.e., these agents may interfere with organogenesis. These effects are distinguished by the development of gross anatomic, metabolic, or functional defects and precipitation of spontaneous abortions.

Because the schematic for embryonic development is already established by the beginning of the second trimester, exposure to drugs or chemicals during the second or third trimesters are less likely to be teratogenic. However, they still may interfere with growth and maturation of critical organ systems, resulting in underdevelopment or alterations of normal organ function.

30.4.2 DOSE-RESPONSE AND THRESHOLD

Exchange of nutrients, gases, and waste material between the maternal and fetal circulations occurs starting from the fifth week after fertilization, with the initiation of the formation of the placenta. Maternal and fetal circulations do not mix. Instead, maternal blood enters intervillous spaces (sinuses) of the placenta through ruptured maternal arteries, then drains into uterine veins for return to the maternal circulation. Fetal blood enters the placenta by a pair of umbilical arteries and returns to the fetal circulation by the umbilical vein. The umbilical arteries branch into capillaries, are surrounded by the synctial trophoblast, forming the network of chorionic villi. Solutes, gases, and nutrients from the maternal circulation enter the sinuses, surround and bathe chorionic villi, and traverse the epithelium and connective tissues of the villi before penetrating the fetal capillary endothelial cells. The materials are then carried toward the embryo through the umbilical vein.

Chemicals enter the fetal circulation as with any other membrane barrier, i.e., the rate of exchange between maternal and fetal circulation depends on the established equilibrium across the placenta and the rate of penetration of the chemical through the endothelial/epithelial barriers. Lipid-soluble drugs and chemicals and dissolved gases readily infiltrate placental membranes, establishing high concentrations of the substance in venous cord blood. Thus, compounds may freely circulate around the embryo within 30 to 60 min of maternal administration. In addition, exogenous substances can alter dynamic tone of placental blood vessels, altering nutrient, gas, and waste exchange. In addition, they restrict oxygen transport to fetal tissues, change biochemical dynamics of the two circulations, and interfere with the endocrine function of the placenta.[*]

30.5 DRUGS AFFECTING EMBRYONIC AND FETAL DEVELOPMENT

30.5.1 CLASSIFICATION

The U.S. Food and Drug Administration (FDA) has established five categories of drug safety during pregnancy. Table 30.1 outlines the requirements for safety of prescribed drugs according to these criteria. The regulations act as guidelines for benefit-to-risk decisions for use of drugs during pregnancy. Drugs marketed in the U.S. bear a drug safety category designation.

30.5.2 DRUG CLASSES

Table 30.2, Table 30.3, and Table 30.4 categorize a variety of drug classes, their therapeutic uses, and some of their major adverse effects on the human fetus. The tables further distinguish agents whose teratogenicity is most frequently seen when administered during the critical first trimester (Table 30.2), during the second and third trimesters (Table 30.3), and agents whose complications are associated with undesirable or hazardous social habits and illicit drug use (Table 30.4).

---

[*] In its endocrine capacity, the placenta secretes human chorionic gonadotropin, placental prolactin, relaxin, estrogen, and progesterone. Also, the degree of chemical penetration of placental barriers relies less on the number and thickness of the layers and more on the dynamic physicochemical interactions between the drug and placenta.

TABLE 30.1
FDA-Established Drug Safety Categories during Pregnancy

Category	Description
A	Adequate, well-controlled studies in pregnant women have not shown an increased risk of fetal abnormalities.
B	Animal studies have revealed no evidence of harm to the fetus, however, there are no adequate and well-controlled studies in pregnant women. **or** Animal studies have shown an adverse effect, but adequate and well-controlled studies in pregnant women have failed to demonstrate a risk to the fetus.
C	Animal studies have shown an adverse effect and there are no adequate and well-controlled studies in pregnant women. **or** No animal studies have been conducted and there are no adequate and well-controlled studies in pregnant women.
D	Adequate well-controlled or observational studies in pregnant women have demonstrated a risk to the fetus. However, the benefits of therapy may outweigh the potential risk.
X	Adequate well-controlled or observational studies in animals or pregnant women have demonstrated positive evidence of fetal abnormalities. The use of the product is contraindicated in women who are, or may become, pregnant.

It is important to remember that, because embryonic tissues grow rapidly and have a high DNA turnover rate, they are vulnerable to many drugs which may not promote adverse reactions in children or adults. As explained above, the most sensitive period for embryonic development is within the first trimester of pregnancy, when the fetus is in the early stages of embryonic development. Some classes of agents require repeated, continuous, or high-dose exposure to elicit an untoward reaction. Other, more potent drugs, such as antineoplastic agents and synthetic retinoids, target rapidly proliferating cells and tissues. Their effects are significant and occur with higher frequency. In fact, the latter category carries a 25% risk of birth defects and anomalies. Some of the teratogenic risks estimated with specific classes of drugs are based on previous observations of effects with known teratogens.* Other teratogenic effects are based on clinical reports of women undergoing treatment for chronic conditions with anticonvulsants, thyroid medications, psychoactive drugs, and bacterial and fungal antibiotics. Finally, the complications surrounding multiple and illicit drug use (Table 30.4) and their effects on the human fetus are difficult to assign to individual drugs. Intravenous drug users are at greater risk of developing anemia, bacteremia, hepatitis, endocarditis, venereal disease, and

---

* The effects of sex hormones are based on the 1950s experience with the routine administration of diethylstilbestrol (DES) during pregnancy for the treatment of threatened or habitual abortions. Daughters of the mothers exposed *in utero* to DES displayed an increased incidence of clear cell adenocarcinoma of the vagina, menstrual dysfunction, spontaneous abortions, incompetent cervix, and preterm labor. In males, exposure to DES *in utero* resulted in meatal stenosis and hypospadias.

TABLE 30.2
Drug Classes That Affect Embryogenesis and Organogenesis in the Human Fetus (Primarily the First Trimester)

Drug Class[a]	Representative Drugs within This Class	Therapeutic Use	Some Adverse Effects on the Human Fetus
Antineoplastic agents	Methotrexate, 6-MP, cyclophosphamide, chlorambucil, busulfan	Treatment of cancers and neoplasms	Growth retardation, craniofacial hypoplasia, clubfoot
Synthetic retinoids (vitamin A)	Isotretinoin	Acne vulgaris	Cardiac defects, hydrocephalus, isolated mental retardation, spontaneous abortions
Androgenic, anabolic, progestational hormones	Synthetic androgens (testosterone derivatives), progestins, estrogens	Various indications (see Chapter 17)	Masculinization of female external genitalia, increased risk of reproductive developmental consequences later in life (see text footnotes on DES)
Anticonvulsants	Phenytoin, phenobarbital, carbamazepine	Epilepsy and related disorders	Cleft palate; cardiac, craniofacial, visceral abnormalities; mental retardation (effects are based on severity of condition, dose and concurrent use of anticonvulsants)
Vaccines	Rubella (other vaccines may be given depending on risk of infection)	Prevention of bacterial, viral infections	Placental & fetal infections
Thyroid drugs	I^{131}, T_3, methimazole, PTU	Hyper-, hypothyroidism	Fetal hypothyroidism, goiter, scalp defects (methimazole only)
Psychoactive agents	Lithium carbonate	Manic depression	Cardiovascular malformations (19% frequency)
Anticoagulants	Coumarins	Hypercoagulation disorders	"Fetal warfarin syndrome"[b]

Note: 6-MP = 6-mercatopurine, PTU = propylthiouracil, I^{131} = radioactive isotope iodine-131, T_3 = triiodothyronin.

[a] Drugs listed here have been shown to cause, or increase the risk for, human fetal abnormalities (pregnancy categories D and X). Compounds that have demonstrated animal teratogenicity, but not human fetal toxicity, are not included in this table (pregnancy categories A, B, and C). The toxic profiles of most of these agents are discussed in other chapters. Teratogenicity of these agents is generally associated with exposure early in pregnancy (i.e., during the first 12 weeks of gestation).

[b] "Fetal warfarin syndrome" is seen in 25% of fetuses exposed to coumarin anticoagulants during the first trimester and displays as mental retardation, bone stippling, and optic atrophy. Exposure during second and third trimesters is manifest as optic atrophy, cataracts, mental retardation, microcephaly, and microphthalmia.

TABLE 30.3

Drug Classes That Affect Human Fetal Development, Labor, Delivery, or Are Associated with Postnatal or Neonatal Complications

Drug Class[a]	Therapeutic Use	Representative Drugs within This Class	Some Adverse Effects in the Human Fetus
Opioids and related narcotics; salicylates	Analgesia	Any of the opioids	Narcotic withdrawal syndrome
		Salicylates, ASA	Fetal kernicterus, delayed onset of labor (large doses), neonatal bleeding
Neuroleptics, sedative/hypnotics	Psychoses	Diazepam (when given near term or during labor & delivery)	Perinatal: depression, irritability, tremors, hyperreflexia; Delivery: low Apgar scores, neurologic depression (no significant fetal risk associated with phenothiazines, tricyclics and most anxiolytics)
		Lithium carbonate	Perinatal effects: lethargy, hypotonia, goiter, poor feeding
Antibiotics	Bacterial, viral, fungal infections	Tetracyclines	Retardation of bone growth, permanent yellowish staining of teeth, ↓ resistance to dental caries
		Aminoglycosides	Ototoxicity
		Chloramphenicol	"Gray baby syndrome" (when administered near term)[b]
		Sulfonamides	Jaundice (when administered near term)
Cardiovascular drugs and diuretics	Cardiac disorders, hypertension	Propranolol	Bradycardia, hypoglycemia, growth retardation
		Thiazide diuretics	↓ fetal oxygenation, hyponatremia, hypokalemia, thrombocytopenia
		ACE inhibitors	Fetal renal failure, oligohydramnios sequence[c]
Oral hypoglycemics	Diabetes mellitus	Any of the oral hypoglycemics	Profound hypoglycemia in newborns
Drugs used during labor & delivery	Local anesthesia	Local anesthetics (lidocaine)	Maternal effects: CNS depression, bradycardia
	Caesarian delivery	Thiopental (barbiturates)	Concentration in fetal liver
	To arrest premature labor	Magnesium sulfate	Lethargy, hypotonia, respiratory depression

Note: ASA = acetylsalicylic acid (aspirin).

[a] Teratogenicity with these agents is associated with exposure later in pregnancy (i.e., during the second and third trimesters).

[b] "Gray baby syndrome" is associated with inability of the newborn to metabolize the drug, resulting in high blood levels. The syndrome is characterized by cardiovascular and circulatory collapse.

[c] Characterized by craniofacial deformities, limb contractures, and poor lung development, when administered primarily during second and third trimesters.

TABLE 30.4
Adverse Effects of Social Habits and Illicit Drugs on the Human Fetus

Social Habits and Illicit Drug Use[a]	Some Adverse Effects on the Human Fetus
Cigarette smoking[b]	Reduction in birth weight; ↑ risk for spontaneous abortions, placenta previa, premature rupture of membranes, congenital heart defects, orofacial clefts, SIDS; ↓ physical, intellectual and behavioral development[b]
Consumption of alcoholic beverages	Fetal alcohol syndrome: effects include spontaneous abortions, impairment of physical (CNS dysfunction, CV defects, growth retardation), intellectual (mental retardation), and behavioral development
Marijuana, opioids, amphetamines	Effects of individual agents are complicated by the unstable social, economic, and emotional environment of illicit and multiple drug use
Cocaine	Spontaneous abortions, fetal tissue hypoxia, intrauterine growth retardation, circulatory compromise, skeletal defects, hyperactivity, tremors
Caffeine	No apparent risk with moderate coffee drinking

[a] Teratogenicity with these agents is associated with exposure during any part of pregnancy. Cigarette smoking and alcohol consumption are the most common drug/behavioral addictions; alcohol is the leading teratogenic substance known among pregnant women.

[b] Effects of cigarette smoking on fetal development are mediated by the chronic hypoxic consequences of carbon monoxide and by the vasoconstrictor-stimulating effects of nicotine on fetal tissues.

AIDS.* Thus, children born of drug-addicted mothers are more likely to suffer the consequences of such complications rather than succumb to the effects of the direct action of the compound.

REFERENCES

SUGGESTED READINGS

Beers, M.H. and Berkow, R, Eds., High-risk pregnancy, in *The Merck Manual*, 17th ed., Merck Research Laboratories, Rahway, NJ, 1999, chap. 250.

Beers, M.H. and Berkow, R., Eds., Normal pregnancy, labor, and delivery, in *The Merck Manual*, 17th ed., Merck Research Laboratories, NJ, 1999, chap. 249.

Drug Facts and Comparisons, 56th ed., Facts and Comparisons, Wolters Kluwer Co., St. Louis, MO, 2002.

Women's Health Initiatives, Center for Drug Evaluation and Research, U.S. Food and Drug Administration, 2002.

* Acquired immune deficiency syndrome.

REVIEW ARTICLES

Barrow, P.C., Reproductive toxicology studies and immunotherapeutics, *Toxicology,* 185, 205, 2003.

Dencker, L. and Eriksson, P., Susceptibility *in utero* and upon neonatal exposure, *Food Addit. Contam.,* 15, 37, 1998.

Graeter, L.J. and Mortensen, M.E., Kids are different: developmental variability in toxicology, *Toxicology,* 111, 15, 1996.

Kelce, W.R. and Wilson, E.M., Environmental antiandrogens: developmental effects, molecular mechanisms, and clinical implications, *J. Mol. Med.,* 75, 198, 1997.

Mantovani, A. and Calamandrei, G., Delayed developmental effects following prenatal exposure to drugs, *Curr. Pharm. Des.,* 7, 859, 2001.

Mittendorf, R., Teratogen update: carcinogenesis and teratogenesis associated with exposure to diethylstilbestrol (DES) *in utero, Teratology,* 51, 435, 1995.

Nelson, B.K., Interactions in developmental toxicology: a literature review and terminology proposal, *Teratology,* 49, 33, 1994.

Riecke, K. and Stahlmann, R., Test systems to identify reproductive toxicants, *Andrologia,* 32, 209, 2000.

Rodier, P.M., Developing brain as a target of toxicity, *Environ. Health. Perspect.,* 103, 73, 1995.

Spielberg, S.P., Idiosyncratic drug reactions: interaction of development and genetics, *Semin. Perinatol.,* 16, 58, 1992.

Swan, S.H., Intrauterine exposure to diethylstilbestrol: long-term effects in humans, *APMIS,* 108, 793, 2000.

Ulbrich, B. and Palmer, A.K., Neurobehavioral aspects of developmental toxicity testing, *Environ. Health Perspect.,* 104, 407, 1996.

Wheeler, S.F., Substance abuse during pregnancy, *Prim. Care,* 20, 191, 1993.

31 Radiation Toxicity

31.1 PRINCIPLES OF RADIOACTIVITY

Radiation is a form of energy whose sources are synthetic and naturally occurring. Small quantities of radioactive materials occur naturally in the environment (atmosphere, water, and food) and are referred to as **internal** exposure. **External** exposure results from sunlight radiation and from synthetic and naturally occurring radioactive materials.

The observation by Becquerel in 1896 of the fogging of photographic plates by uranium salts prompted an intense search for an understanding of the phenomenon of radioactivity. The scientific experimental persistence of the Curies, Schmidt, Debierne, Rutherford, Bohr, and Soddy, lead to the discoveries of radioactive isotopes and identification of the types of radiation emitted by these elements. The landmark publication of Bohr's theory of atomic structure (1913) soon followed.[*] By 1942, Fermi prepared the schematics for the first nuclear reactor, 5 years after Rutherford's death. Rutherford's realization of the development of nuclear power until then remained unfulfilled. Since then, constructive research on the atomic nucleus has resulted in the means to harness this energy, not only for the production of electricity and nuclear weapons, but also for its application to the medical, pharmaceutical, chemical, and agricultural industries.

The electromagnetic spectrum consists of a wide range of wave-propagated energy, expressed as radiation energy. The spectrum is based on the photon (ρ) energy emitted from atomic sources, corresponding to frequency (cycles per second, Hz), which is inversely proportional to its wavelength (meters, λ) (Figure 31.1).

A proton is a particle of radiation energy, with a mass of 1836 m (mass units),[**] and possesses a charge of +1. Electrons and neutrons constitute the other basic components of atoms, both stable and radioactive (their charges equal −1 and 0, respectively). Radiation energy above the UV range (i.e., higher frequencies, left of UV in Figure 31.1) is called *ionizing radiation* because of the ability of photon energy to displace electrons off their atomic nuclei. Nonionizing radiation occurs at frequencies below the visible spectrum (lower frequencies and to the right of VIS in Figure 31.1). UV, X-rays, and γ-rays represent the most commonly encountered high-energy rays capable of inducing cellular damage.

---

[*] Bohr's theory of atomic structure was based upon Rutherford's nuclear theory and Planck's quantum theory.

[**] For simplicity, an electron registers at 1 m and, being the smallest of the three particles, inconveniently weighs in at 9.1019×10^{-28} g.

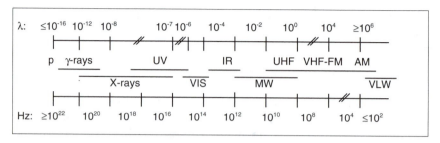

Frequency (Hz) and wavelength (λ, in meters) for the electromagnetic energy waves are approximate averages and may span wider ranges. Consequently the scales are not continuous.
Abbreviations: p = cosmic ray photons, γ-rays = gamma rays, AM = radio, IR = infrared, MW = microwave, UHF = ultrahigh frequency TV, UV = ultraviolet, VHF-FM = very high frequency TV and FM-radio, VIS = visible spectrum, VLW = very long waves (power).

FIGURE 31.1 The electromagnetic spectrum.

31.2 IONIZING RADIATION

31.2.1 BIOLOGICAL EFFECTS OF IONIZING RADIATION

Ionizing radiation induces somatic changes in cells and tissues by displacing electrons from their atomic nuclei, resulting in the intracellular ionization of molecules. Depending on the dose and length of exposure, the effects can be immediate, chronic, or delayed. Thus, reversible or irreversible DNA changes are induced, initiating a series of events that culminate in the production of a mutagenic response, a carcinogenic response, the inhibition of cell replication, or cell death. In addition, it is reasonable to expect that a change in DNA due to radiation exposure is inheritable and may result in genetic defects in the offspring. (For the mechanisms of carcinogenesis, see Chapter 29, "Chemical Carcinogenesis and Mutagenesis.")

31.2.2 SOURCES

Undesirable exposure to ionizing radiation emanates from a variety of isotope sources. High-energy diagnostic or therapeutic X-rays, used in the treatment of cancer, result in localized radiation injury (exposure to whole-body therapeutic irradiation is rare). Occupational exposure involves variable amounts of radioactivity from nuclear reactors, linear accelerators, and sealed cesium, americium, and cobalt sources used in therapeutic instruments and detectors. Radium and radon gas are naturally occurring hazardous isotopes embedded in the Earth's crust and often encountered in communities and households close to concentrated sources. Large amounts of radioactivity have also escaped from nuclear reactors, such as Three Mile Island in Pennsylvania (1979) and Chernobyl, Ukraine (1986).

The Chernobyl reactor accident of April 1986 provides the best-documented example of a massive radionuclide release in which large numbers of people across a broad geographical area were exposed acutely to radioiodines released into the atmosphere. The reactor accident resulted in massive releases of ^{131}I and other radioiodines. Approximately 4 years after the accident, a sharp increase in the incidence of thyroid cancer among children and adolescents in Belarus and Ukraine (areas covered by the radioactive plume) was observed. The most comprehensive and reliable data available describing the relationship between thyroid radiation dose and risk for thyroid cancer following an environmental release of ^{131}I were documented following this accident.*

31.2.3 CLINICAL MANIFESTATIONS

Total dose- and rate-dependent effects of radiation — i.e., radiation dose per unit of time — result most often in acute cell injury. A single rapid high dose of radiation may be less injurious if exposure occurs over weeks or months. Injury resulting from exposure also depends on the cumulative body surface area exposed, where acute exposure to high whole-body doses is fatal. In addition, rapidly proliferating cells are more susceptible to the effects of ionizing radiation than cells with lower turnover rate. Lymphoid, hematopoietic, gonadal, endothelial, osteogenic, and gastrointestinal and pulmonary epithelial cells are most sensitive. Consequently, it is reasonable to expect that the initial and persistent adverse reactions associated with cancer radiation therapy include hair loss, nausea, vomiting, diarrhea, bone marrow suppression, coughing, dyspnea, and dermal changes. Patients with bone marrow suppression have increased susceptibility to infection and bleeding disorders. Sloughing of the epithelial lining of the GI tract, resulting in vomiting and diarrhea, facilitates excessive fluid loss and precipitates electrolyte imbalances. In addition, acute or chronic occupational or accidental exposures to significant doses of ionizing radiation predictably produce skin cancers, leukemias, osteogenic sarcomas, and lung carcinomas.

Cell membrane disruption, resulting in swelling and erythema, occurs after initial exposure to low doses of radiation. At higher levels, acute reversible necrosis is possible. More persistent damage and chronic ischemia occurs with continuous radiation of slowly regenerating cells. Chronic effects are characterized by fibrosis and scarring of irradiated tissues. Irreversible necrosis, impaired wound healing, and inflammation of affected organs (dermatitis, cystitis, enteritis) are significant consequences of chronic radiation exposure. Table 31.1 categorizes and summarizes the clinical effects associated with acute and prolonged ionizing radiation. Regeneration of cells and tissues depends on dose and rate of irradiation and the commencement of supportive therapy.

The most useful and rapid method for clinical assessment of the degree of radiation exposure, especially ionizing radiation, is determination of the patient's total blood lymphocyte count. Serial determinations are performed every 6 h for at

---

* It is noteworthy that the thyroid radiation exposures after Chernobyl were virtually all **internal**, from radioiodines. Despite some degree of uncertainty in the doses received, it is reasonable to conclude that the contribution of external radiation was negligible for most individuals. Thus, the increase in thyroid cancer seen after Chernobyl is attributable to ingested or inhaled radioiodines. A comparable burden of excess thyroid cancers could conceivably accrue, should United States populations be similarly exposed in the event of a nuclear accident.

TABLE 31.1
Signs and Symptoms of Acute Radiation Syndromes

Syndrome	Radiation Dose[a]	Phase, Time-Dependent Reaction, or Target Organ	Toxic Effects
Cerebral syndrome	>30 Gy	Prodromal phase Listless phase Tremulous phase	Nausea, vomiting Apathy, drowsiness, prostration Ataxia, convulsions, death (within hours)
GI syndrome	≥4 Gy	Initial reaction Continuous or high dose exposure	NVD, dehydration, vascular collapse Progressive GI atrophy and necrosis, bacteremia, loss of plasma volume
Hematopoietic syndrome	2–10 Gy	Initial reaction Continuous or high dose exposure	Anorexia, apathy, NV; may subside Atrophy of lymph nodes, spleen, BM, immunosuppression; pancytopenia, bacterial infections, hemorrhage
Acute radiation sickness	Following radiation therapy ≤0.05 Gy	Initial reaction	NVD, anorexia, headache, malaise, tachycardia; usually subsides
Intermediate delayed effects	≤0.05 Gy	Prolonged, repeated exposure Higher doses or high localized exposure	Decreased fertility, libido; anemia, leukopenia Skin ulceration, atrophy, keratosis; alopecia; delayed (years) appearance of carcinomas, sarcomas
Extensive radiation therapy	≤0.05 Gy (prolonged or cumulative exposure to selected organs)	Kidneys Muscles Lungs Mediastinum Abdominal lymph nodes	Proteinuria, renal insufficiency, HT; ≥20 Gy <5 wks: fibrosis, renal failure Painful myopathy, atrophy Pulmonary fibrosis, pneumonitis (>30Gy) Pericarditis, myocarditis Ulceration, fibrosis, perforation of bowel
Late somatic-genetic defects	Variable	Somatic cells Germ cells	Leukemia, thyroid, skin, bone cancers ↑ risk of mutations and genetic defects

Note: GI = gastrointestinal; NVD = nausea, vomiting, diarrhea; BM = bone marrow; HT = hypertension.

[a] The gray (Gy) is the amount of energy absorbed by a tissue and applies to all types of radiation; the roentgen (R) is the amount of X- or γ-radiation in air; for X- or γ-radiation, the sievert (Sv) equals the Gy after factoring for its biological effect (one sievert = 100 rem).

least 48 h. A 50% fall in total lymphocytes every 24 h for 2 days is indicative of a potentially lethal injury.

31.2.4 NUCLEAR TERRORISM AND HEALTH EFFECTS

Although the U.S. Centers for Disease Control (CDC) has not been able to assess the level of threat of a terrorist nuclear attack, it has regularly participated in emergency-response drills. In cooperation with other federal, state, and local agencies, the CDC has developed, tested, and implemented extensive national radiological emergency response plans. The adverse health consequences of a terrorist nuclear attack vary according to the type of attack and the distance a person is from the radioactive emission. Potential terrorist attacks may include a small radioactive source with a limited range of impact, a nuclear detonation involving a wide area of impact, or an attack on a nuclear power plant. In any of these events, injury or death may occur because of the blast itself or as a result of debris thrown from the blast. In addition, individuals may experience external and/or internal exposure. Depending on the dose, type, route, and length of time of the exposure, the signs and symptoms are not unlike those of ionizing radiation.

The FDA has provided guidance documents and regulations in the event of a terrorist nuclear attack. A national emergency response plan would be activated and would include federal, state, and local agencies. In general, individuals can reduce the potential exposure and subsequent health consequences by limiting the time, increasing the distance, or keeping a physical barrier between them and the source. In addition, the FDA has determined that administration of potassium iodide (KI) is a safe and effective means of blocking uptake of radioiodines by the thyroid gland in a radiation emergency under certain specified conditions of use (*Federal Register* 1978, 1982).[*]

The effectiveness of KI as a specific blocker of thyroid radioiodine uptake is well established. The recommended dose is 130 mg per day for adults and children above 1 year of age, and 65 mg per day for children below 1 year of age. When administered at this level, KI is effective in reducing the risk of thyroid cancer in individuals or populations at risk for inhalation or ingestion of radioiodines. KI competes with radioactive iodine for uptake into the thyroid, thus preventing incorporation of the radioactive molecules into the gland. The radioactive compounds are subsequently excreted in the urine.

31.3 ULTRAVIOLET RADIATION (UV)

31.3.1 BIOLOGICAL EFFECTS OF ULTRAVIOLET RADIATION

UV rays are of lower frequency and longer wavelength than ionizing radiation (about 10^{-8} to 10^{-6} meters, Figure 31.1). Thus, the effects of UV radiation are less pene-

---

[*] The recommendations were formulated after reviewing studies relating radiation dose to thyroid disease risk. The FDA's evaluations relied on estimates of *external* thyroid irradiation after the nuclear detonations at Hiroshima and Nagasaki. It was concluded that the risks of short-term use of small quantities of KI were outweighed by the benefits of suppressing radioiodine-induced thyroid cancer.

trating and harmful. Unlike ionizing radiation, skin damage induced by UV rays (e.g., from sun exposure) is mediated principally by the generation of reactive oxygen species and the interruption of melanin production. Like ionizing radiation, however, cumulative or intense exposure to UV rays precipitates DNA mutations — i.e., base pair insertions, deletions, single-strand breaks, and DNA-protein cross-links. DNA repair mechanisms play an important role in correcting UV-induced DNA damage and preventing further consequences of excessive sunburn. Melanin production by melanocytes increases and the epidermis thickens in an attempt to prevent future damaging effects. The protective ability of antioxidant enzymes and DNA-repair pathways diminishes with age, thus setting the conditions for development of skin neoplasms later in life.

31.3.2 SOURCES

Radiation burn (*sunburn*) is commonly caused by prolonged or pristine exposure to the sun's UV rays. A recent fashionable phenomenon of obtaining a "tan" in tanning salons has resulted in excess exposure with tanning lamps, although these lamps produce more UVA than UVB.* Despite the availability of "sun blocking " products containing 5% PABA (ρ-aminobenzoic acid) that protect against the damaging effects of UV radiation, complications from sunburn still abound. The dissemination of public knowledge concerning the harmful effects of excessive exposure to the sun has not abated the development of its serious clinical effects, including production of acute reactions (sunburn), chronic changes (skin cancer), or photosensitivity.

31.3.3 CLINICAL MANIFESTATIONS

The extent of solar injury depends on the type of UV radiation, the duration and intensity of exposure, clothing, season, altitude and latitude, and the amount of melanin pigment present in the skin. In fact, individuals differ greatly in their response to sun. Fair-skinned persons have less melanin-producing cells. Consequently, they are more sensitive to UV rays than people of dark-skinned races, although the skin of the latter is still reactive and can become sunburned with prolonged exposure. In addition, harmful effects of UV rays are filtered out by glass, smog, and smoke, but enhanced by reflecting off snow and sand. The indiscriminate use of chlorofluorocarbons in aerosol propellants depletes the UV-blocking properties of ozone in the stratosphere, thus allowing for greater intensity of UV rays to penetrate through the protective upper atmospheric layers.

As with thermal, chemical, or electrical burns, severe solar radiation exposure is classified according to the severity and depth of the burn. *First-degree* burns are generally red, sensitive, and moist. The absence of blisters and blanching of the skin with application of light pressure are characteristic features. *Second-degree* burns are classified as superficial, intermediate, or deep, with partial skin loss. The presence of erythematous blisters with exudate is typical of *second-degree* burns. *Third-degree* burns involve deep dermal, whole skin loss. The skin appears black, charred, and

---

* The shorter wavelengths of the sunburn-producing UVB radiation (280–320 nm λ) are more damaging than UVA rays (320–400 nm λ).

TABLE 31.2
Chronic Effects of Sunlight and Photosensitivity Reactions

Reactions To Excessive Sunlight	Clinical Effects
General Dermatologic	Dermatoheliosis – aging of the skin due to chronic exposure to sunlight
	Elastosis – yellow discoloration of skin with accompanying small nodules
	Wrinkling, hyperpigmentation, atrophy and dermatitis
Actinic keratoses	Precancerous keratotic lesions, appear after many years of exposure to UV rays
Squamous/basal cell carcinoma	Occurs more commonly in light-skinned individuals exposed to extensive UV rays during adolescence
Malignant melanomas	Associated with increased, intense, prolonged exposure to UV light
Photosensitive reactions[a]	Erythema and erythema multiform lesions; urticaria, dermatitis, bullae; thickened, scaling patches

[a] See text for description of terms.

leathery. Subdermal vessels do not blanch with applied pressure and the areas exposed are generally anesthetic or insensitive to pain stimuli. Although generally not associated with sunburn, *fourth-degree* burns involve deep tissue and structure loss. Hypertrophic scars and chronic granulations develop unless skin grafting treatment is instituted.

Tap water compresses are effective in relieving symptoms of sunburn. Topical corticosteroids or astringent gels (such as aloe) may relieve the discomfort associated with extensive severe sunburn. Occlusive ointments or creams should not be applied to ruptured blisters or wounds.

Table 31.2 summarizes the chronic effects of sunlight and photosensitivity reactions. Actinic keratoses, described as precancerous keratotic lesions, result from years of sun exposure, especially in fair-skinned individuals. They present as pink, poorly marginated, scaly or crusted superficial growths on skin. Depending on the number of lesions present, they are usually treated with cryotherapy (freezing with liquid nitrogen) or with topical application of 5-fluorouracil (5-FU).

Photosensitive reactions involve the development of unusual responses to sunlight, sometimes exaggerated in the presence of a variety of precipitating, seemingly unrelated, circumstances. Erythema (redness) or dermatitis (inflammation of the skin or mucous membranes) is an acute response to direct UV light. It is mediated by dilation and congestion of superficial capillaries and type IV hypersensitivity cell-mediated reactions. In addition, macules, papules, nodules, and target ("bull's eye"-shaped) lesions are seen in the multiforme variation of erythematous reactions. Similarly, solar urticaria is a pruritic skin eruption characterized by transient wheals of varying shapes and sizes, with well-defined erythematous margins and pale centers. Development of urticaria is mediated by capillary dilation in the dermis in response to release of vasoactive amines (histamine and kinins) upon sun exposure. More severe photosensitivity reactions lead to the development of bullae, thin-walled blisters on the skin or mucous membranes greater than 1 cm in diameter and containing clear, serous fluid. Dehydration, scaling, scarring, fibrosis, and necrosis develop as the exposed areas heal.

Numerous factors contribute to the development of photosensitivity reactions. Xeroderma pigmentosum,* lupus erythematosus,** and porphyrias*** are among the pathologic conditions that are accompanied by photosensitivity reactions. Ingestion or application of antibacterial and antifungal antibiotics (sulfonamides, tetracyclines; griseofulvin, respectively) and thiazide diuretics are responsible for occasional photosensitive reactions. Contact with dermal products containing coal tar, salicylic acid, plant derivatives, and ingredients of colognes, perfumes, cosmetics and soaps, are also sources of the problem.

Preventive treatment and avoidance of sunlight (use of protective clothing, sunscreens, shaded areas) are generally helpful in averting skin reactions. Other therapies include use of topical or oral corticosteroids, H_1-blockers (antihistamines), antimalarial drugs (hydroxychloroquin), topical sunscreens with moisturizers, and psoralen UV light (PUVA).

31.4 NONIONIZING RADIATION

31.4.1 Sources

Nonionizing radiation emanates from sources with lower energy (low frequency) and longer wavelengths (right of the visible spectrum, Figure 31.1). Low frequency radiation, such as infrared light (IR), ultrasound, microwaves, and laser energy, are commonly encountered in the home and in the workplace. Televisions, radios, cellular phones, wireless devices, and microwave ovens are among the household sources. Plastic, wood, metal, and chemical industries account for occupational exposures. Medical applications (diathermy) are another source of exposure.

31.4.2 Biological Effects and Clinical Manifestations

In contrast to ionizing radiation, the lower energy of nonionizing radiation induces vibrational and rotational movements of intracellular atoms and molecules. Accordingly, burns and thermal injury are the most common consequences of exposure to direct low-energy rays. Deep penetration of dermal and subcutaneous tissue is observed when tissue intercepts the path of infrared or microwave rays. The latter are also capable of disrupting the normal function of electronic medical devices such as subcutaneously implanted cardiac pacemakers and monitors.

---

* A genetic disorder characterized by extreme photosensitivity and increased risk of skin cancer in sun-exposed skin. It is usually due to the lack of DNA repair enzymes in damaged skin.
** Systemic, inflammatory, multiorgan, autoimmune disease with characteristic development of rashes and joint pain.
*** Porphyria cutanea tarda is the most common form of porphyria. The syndrome is a sporadic, autosomal dominant condition characterized by skin fragility on the dorsal hands and forearms and facial hyperpigmentation.

REFERENCES

SUGGESTED READINGS

Beers, M.H. and Berkow, R., Eds., *The Merck Manual*, 17th ed., Merck Research Laboratories, Rahway, NJ, 1999, chap. 119.

Gavrilin, Y.I. et al., Chernobyl accident: reconstruction of thyroid dose for inhabitants of the republic of Belarus, *Health Phys.*, 76, 105, 1999.

Likhtarev, I.A. et al., Thyroid cancer in the Ukraine, *Nature*, 375, 365, 1995.

Robbins, J. and Schneider, A.B., Thyroid cancer following exposure to radioactive iodine, *Rev. Endoc. Metab. Dis.*, 1, 197, 2000.

Zvonova, I.A. and Balonov, M.I., Radioiodine dosimetry and prediction of consequences of thyroid exposure of the Russian population following the Chernobyl accident, in *The Chernobyl Papers. Doses to the Soviet Population and Early Health Effects Studies.* Volume I, Mervin, S.E. and Balonov, M.I., Eds., Research Enterprises Inc., Richland, WA, 1993, p. 71.

REVIEW ARTICLES

Baudouin, C. et al., Environmental pollutants and skin cancer, *Cell Biol. Toxicol.*, 18, 341, 2002.

Brent, R.L., Utilization of developmental basic science principles in the evaluation of reproductive risks from pre- and postconception environmental radiation exposures, *Teratology*, 59, 182, 1999.

Cardis, E., Richardson, D., and Kesminiene, A., Radiation risk estimates in the beginning of the 21st century, *Health Phys.*, 80, 349, 2001.

Dainiak, N., Hematologic consequences of exposure to ionizing radiation, *Exp. Hematol.*, 30, 513, 2002.

Hogan, D.E. and Kellison, T., Nuclear terrorism, *Am. J. Med. Sci.*, 323, 341, 2002.

Lomax, M.E., Gulston, M.K., and O'Neill, P., Chemical aspects of clustered DNA damage induction by ionising radiation, *Radiat. Prot. Dosimetry*, 99, 63, 2002.

Maisin, J.R., Chemical protection against ionizing radiation, *Adv. Space Res.*, 9, 205, 1989.

Mettler, F.A., Jr., and Voelz, G.L., Major radiation exposure — what to expect and how to respond, *N. Engl. J. Med.*, 346, 1554, 2002.

Moulder, J.E., Pharmacological intervention to prevent or ameliorate chronic radiation injuries, *Semin. Radiat. Oncol.*, 13, 73, 2003.

Moulder, J.E., Radiobiology of nuclear terrorism: report on an interagency workshop (Bethesda, MD, December 17–18, 2001), *Int. J. Radiat. Oncol. Biol. Phys.*, 54, 327, 2002.

Moysich, K.B., Menezes, R.J., and Michalek, A.M., Chernobyl-related ionising radiation exposure and cancer risk: an epidemiological review, *Lancet Oncol.*, 3, 269, 2002.

Muller, L. et al., Epidemiology and primary prevention of thyroid cancer, *Thyroid*, 12, 889, 2002.

Nohynek, G.J. and Schaefer, H., Benefit and risk of organic ultraviolet filters, *Regul. Toxicol. Pharmacol.*, 33, 285, 2001.

Pinnell, S.R., Cutaneous photodamage, oxidative stress, and topical antioxidant protection, *J. Am. Acad. Dermatol.*, 48, 1, 2003.

Rahu, M., Health effects of the Chernobyl accident: fears, rumours and the truth, *Eur. J. Cancer*, 39, 295, 2003.

Rosen, E.M. et al., Biological basis of radiation sensitivity. Part 1: Factors governing radiation tolerance, *Oncology (Huntington)*, 14, 543, 2000.

Skorga, P. et al., Caring for victims of nuclear and radiological terrorism, *Nurse Pract.*, 28, 24, 2003.

Urbach, F., Forbes, P.D., and Davies, R.E., Modification of photocarcinogenesis by chemical agents, *J. Natl. Cancer Inst.*, 69, 229, 1982.

32 Chemical and Biological Threats to Public Safety

32.1 INTRODUCTION

Terrorism is the threat or implementation of violent means to undermine, destabilize, inflict harm, or cause panic in a society. The threat of terrorism in the world, at any time and within any nation, is real. In the least, the induction of fear is a destabilizing force in a nation or state. The U.S. has only recently experienced serious terrorist threats with the events of September 11, 2001. Since then, the public's awareness of a variety of potential means that could be used as terrorist threats has prompted unprecedented political, military, biomedical, industrial, and community responses. Terrorist methods comprise the use of radiological, chemical, and biological agents capable of widespread, mass casualties and destruction. The ease of availability, the low cost of production, and the facility for wide dissemination of these means of destruction, makes them very attractive weapons.

Chemical and radiological toxicity have already been discussed throughout several chapters in this book (nerve gases, radiological toxicity). Therefore, only applicable classes of chemical and radiological agents are outlined below. Consequently, this chapter elaborates on the mechanisms of previously unclassified pathogenic agents and their toxic biological products, some of which only recently have been identified as potential toxic terrorist threats.

The U.S. Food and Drug Administration (FDA), together with other federal agencies, has prepared a series of working guidelines and information to help prepare against the threat of bioterrorism. The Office of Pediatric Drug Development and Program Initiatives (OPDDPI) also identifies and facilitates the development of drug products that may be used in the treatment of conditions caused by agents released in the event of a terrorist attack. These agents are of a pathogenic, radiological, or chemical nature. Table 32.1 compiles high-priority chemical and biological agents, and the syndromes resulting from their exposure, according to their potential as a bioterrorist threat.

Category A includes high-priority agents and pathogens rarely seen in the U.S. that pose a risk to national security. They are highly infectious and easy to disseminate, and the clinical effects from exposure result in high mortality rates. By their nature, Category A agents are capable of inciting public panic and disruption. In addition, they require special action for public health preparedness. Agents or the diseases in Category A include anthrax, botulism, plague, smallpox, tularemia, and organisms that induce viral hemorrhagic fevers. **Category B** lists the second highest priority agents. These organisms are moderately easy to disseminate, result in moderate morbidity and low mortality rates, and require specific enhancements of CDC's

TABLE 32.1
Chemical and Biological Agents with High Risk to National Security

Category	Category Description	Toxin or Disease	Causative Agent	Classification
A	Highly infectious, easily disseminated, high mortality rate	Anthrax	*Bacillus anthracis*	Spore-forming bacteria
		Botulism	*Clostridium botulinum*	Spore-forming bacteria
		Plague	*Yersinia pestis*	Enterobacteria
		Smallpox	Variola, vaccinia[a]	Poxvirus
		Tularemia	*Francisella tularensis*	Coccobacillus
		Hemorrhagic fever	Lassa, Junin, Machupo	Arenavirus
B	Moderate rates of infection, dissemination, morbidity and mortality	Brucellosis	*Brucella* sp.	Coccobacillus
		Epsilon toxin	*Clostridium perfringens*	Spore-forming bacteria
		Acute gastroenteritis	*Salmonella* sp., *Shigella* sp., *E. coli*	Enterobacteria
		Q fever	*Coxiella burnetii*	Obligate intracellular bacillus
		Ricin toxin	*Ricinus communis*	Castor beans
C	Highly infectious, ease of dissemination unknown	Hemorrhagic fever, ARDS	Hantavirus	Bunyaviridae
		Encephalitis	Bunyavirus	
		Encephalitis	Nipah virus	Paramyxoviridae

Note: ARDS = adult respiratory distress syndrome.

[a] Variola is the extinct human virus; vaccinia is the laboratory product used for smallpox vaccinations.

diagnostic capacity and enhanced disease surveillance. Other less identifiable substances in Category B (not discussed below) include: glanders *(Burkholderia mallei),* melioidosis *(Burkholderia pseudomallei),* psittacosis *(Chlamydia psittaci),* Staphylococcal enterotoxin B, typhus fever *(Rickettsia prowazekii),* and viral encephalitis (alphaviruses, such as equine encephalitis).

The third category of highest priority agents, **Category C**, includes pathogens that could be engineered for mass dissemination. Emerging threats, such as the Nipah virus and hantavirus, are available and easily produced and disseminated, provided there exists some technical knowledge of microbiology. Thus, they have the potential for high morbidity and mortality.

32.2 BIOLOGICAL PATHOGENIC TOXINS AS THREATS TO PUBLIC SAFETY

Naturally occurring or laboratory-derived biological pathogens and their products, released intentionally or accidentally, can result in disease or death. Human exposure to these agents may occur through inhalation, skin (cutaneous) exposure, or ingestion of contaminated food or water. Following exposure, physical symptoms may be delayed and sometimes confused with naturally occurring illnesses, thus contributing to the possible postponement in response. In addition, biological warfare agents may persist in the environment and cause problems long after their release.

The organisms discussed below fall into three major classes of microorganisms: bacteria,* rickettsia, and viruses. In addition, hazardous bacterial toxins are produced as by-products of their pathogenic metabolism. Incubation period, duration of illness, symptoms, means of transmission, treatment, and prognosis, are noted for each of the agents.

32.2.1 ANTHRAX (*BACILLUS ANTHRACIS*)

Anthrax is an infectious disease caused by the spore-forming bacterium, *Bacillus anthracis*. The organism is an obligate aerobe (cutaneous form) and facultative anaerobe (inhalation form). The highly resistant, prominent polypeptide capsule of the endospore renders *B. anthracis* immune to most methods of disinfection or natural processes of inactivation.** Thus, the organism may be present in the soil for decades, occasionally infecting grazing goats, sheep, and cattle. When ingested, the hibernating, dehydrated, protected spores release viable bacteria upon contact with gastrointestinal fluids. Human infection occurs by three routes of exposure to anthrax spores: cutaneous, gastrointestinal, and inhalation. Although human cases of anthrax are infrequent in North America, the U.S. military views anthrax as a potential biological terrorist threat because of its high resistance and ease of communicability through air.

The development of anthrax as a biological weapon by several foreign countries has been documented. Prior to the recent deliberate release of anthrax-laden letters throughout the U.S. in the fall of 2001, much of what is known about inhalation anthrax was learned from the accidental discharge of spores in 1979 in Sverdlovsk in the former Soviet Union. This accident resulted in 79 cases of anthrax and 68 deaths.

Cutaneous infection is the most common manifestation of anthrax in humans, accounting for 95% of cases. Inoculation through exposed skin results from contact with contaminated soil or animal products such as hair, hides, and wool. A painless papule at the site of inoculation progresses rapidly to an ulcer surrounded by vesicles, and then to a necrotic eschar. Systemic infection, complicated by massive edema and painful lymphadenopathy, is fatal in 20% of patients.***

Ingestion of undercooked or raw, infected meat causes the rare gastrointestinal infection. This is characterized by an acute inflammation of the intestinal tract. Initial

---

* Bacterial toxins are products of bacterial metabolism or components of their structures that stimulate immunologic responses or alter normal physiologic function.

** Interestingly, the capsule is observed in clinical specimens and is not synthesized *in vitro* unless special growth conditions are employed.

*** Since person-to-person transmission does not occur, there is no need to immunize or treat contacts, such as household family, friends, or coworkers, unless they also were exposed to the same source of infection.

signs of nausea, anorexia, vomiting, and fever are followed by abdominal pain, bloody vomitus, and severe diarrhea. As with the cutaneous form, systemic disease can progress rapidly.

Respiration of dried, airborne spores leads to inhalation anthrax (*wool-sorters' disease*). Initial symptoms of inhalation anthrax follow a prolonged, asymptomatic latent period (one week and up to two months) and present as fever, dyspnea, cough, headache, vomiting, chills, chest and abdominal pain. A progressive, dramatic worsening of the infection occurs after several days, to fever, pulmonary edema, and lymphadenopathy. Shock and death occur within 3 to 7 days of initial signs and symptoms.

The mortality rates from anthrax vary, depending on exposure and age, and are approximately 20% for cutaneous anthrax without antibiotics and 25–75% for gastrointestinal anthrax. Inhalation anthrax has a fatality rate that is 80% or higher. Anthrax is susceptible to an early antibiotic course of treatment with penicillin, doxycycline, and fluoroquinolones (an efficacy supplement for ciprofloxacin was approved by the FDA on August 30, 2000, for postexposure inhalation anthrax).

The anthrax vaccine is an effective control measure and was developed from an attenuated strain of *B. anthracis*. Clinical studies have calculated the efficacy level of the vaccine at about 92.5%. The vaccine derives from cell-free culture filtrates of this strain and, in its final formulation, is adsorbed onto an aluminum salt. The licensed anthrax vaccine, anthrax vaccine adsorbed (AVA),* is recommended for individuals at risk for occupational exposure and persons involved with diagnostic, clinical, or investigational activities with *B. anthracis* spores. Vaccination is not available to the general public and is not recommended to prevent disease.

32.2.2 BOTULISM

Botulism is cause by *Clostridium botulinum*, a Gram-positive, spore-forming anaerobic rod. Like *B. anthracis*, the bacterium lives in soil and intestines of animals. Besides botulism, production of protein toxins by the variety of clostridial species is associated with a range of diseases, including tetanus, gas gangrene, food poisoning, diarrhea, and pseudomembranous colitis.

Botulism is caused by the release of preformed botulinum toxin secreted by the organism in contaminated food. Interestingly, the organism's presence in the food or its existence in the victim's GI tract is not necessary for virulence. Anaerobic conditions favor the growth of the spores in contaminated meats, vegetables, and fish. The heat-resistant spores survive food processing and canning in sufficient numbers to cause toxicity upon release of the toxin.

The botulinum toxin is a neurotoxin capable of preventing the release of acetylcholine at peripheral cholinergic synapses (see Chapter 15, "Anticholinergic and Neuroleptic Drugs," for a description of the cholinergic system). Clinically, the disease has an onset of 12 to 36 h. Signs and symptoms are related to inhibition of skeletal muscle innervation and include flaccid muscular paralysis, blurred vision, difficulty swallowing, and respiratory paralysis. Striated muscle groups weaken as a result of the descending paralysis, eventually affecting the neck and extremities.

---

*To date, there is only a single anthrax vaccine licensed and manufactured in the U.S. (BioPort, Lansing, MI).

Supportive care and maintenance of vital functions, especially respirations, is of utmost importance in treatment. Specific antitoxin is available for some of the neurotoxin types (A, B, and E). With good supportive care and antitoxin administration, the mortality rate is reduced to 25%. Prolonged or permanent muscle paralysis may persist indefinitely.

32.2.3 PLAGUE (*YERSINIA PESTIS*)

Plague is an infectious disease of animals and humans caused by the bacterium *Yersinia pestis*. All yersinia infections are zoonotic, capable of spreading from rodents and their fleas (**urban plague**), as well as from squirrels, rabbits, field rats, and cats (**sylvatic plague**). Historically, pandemics resulting from yersinia infections have devastated human populations. The first of three urban plagues started in Egypt (541 AD) and spread through the Middle East, North Africa, Asia, and Europe, killing over 100 million persons. The Middle Ages (1320s) recorded a second pandemic that probably originated from Asia and spread through Europe, resulting in 25 million deaths in Europe. Recent history (1895) recorded a pandemic that began in Hong Kong and spread to Africa, India, Europe, and the Americas, leaving 10 million deaths in its wake over 20 years. The recognition of public health and maintenance of hygienic standards has essentially eradicated urban plague from most communities, although some cases are reported in the U.S. annually. Clinically, *Y. pestis* infections are manifested as bubonic plague and pneumonic plague.

The bite of an infected flea starts the incubation period of about 7 days for *Y. pestis*. The resulting clinical signs and symptoms of bubonic plague include the development of buboes (lymphadenopathy or swelling of the axillary or inguinal lymph nodes) and fever. In the absence of antibiotics, fatal bacteremia develops rapidly.

Aerosolized transmission of *Y. pestis* characterizes the highly infectious pneumonic plague.* A shorter incubation period results in fever, headache, malaise, and a cough accompanied by blood and mucus. Without early antibiotic intervention, the pneumonia progresses rapidly over 2 to 4 days to septic shock and death.

Early treatment with streptomycin, tetracycline, and chloramphenicol is effective in treating pneumonic plague. Prophylactic antibiotic treatment for 7 days will protect persons at risk for close (face-to-face) contact with infected patients. There is no vaccine against plague.**

32.2.4 BRUCELLOSIS (*BRUCELLA SUIS*)

Brucellosis is caused by the Gram-negative coccobacillus bacteria of the genus *Brucella*. Infections are generally zoonotic, with animal reservoirs maintained in sheep, goats, cattle, deer, elk, pigs, and dogs. Human infections are acquired by contact with infected animals and consumption of contaminated unpasteurized dairy products, and through improper laboratory handling (inhalation and cutaneous

---

* Person-to-person transmission occurs through close inhalation of infected respiratory droplets.
** Although gentamicin is not FDA approved for treatment of pneumonic plague, the Center for Civilian Biodefense Studies Working Group on Civilian Biodefense has recommended it along with streptomycin as a preferred therapy.

exposure).[*] Over 500,000 cases are reported worldwide annually. The disease is frequently a problem in countries that do not have good standardized and effective public health and domestic animal health programs. Areas currently listed as high risk are countries in the Mediterranean basin (Portugal, Spain, Southern France, Italy, Greece, Turkey, North Africa), South and Central America, Eastern Europe, Asia, Africa, the Caribbean, and the Middle East. Unpasteurized cheeses ("village cheeses") from these areas may present a particular risk for tourists. Close person-to-person transmission is rare. The incidence is lower in the U.S. (100 to 200 cases annually), and cases are most commonly reported from California, Texas, and residents and visitors from Mexico.

Depending on the species, human brucellosis causes a range of symptoms. Acute disease has an onset of 2 months. Initial symptoms are nonspecific and consist of fever,[**] sweating, headache, back pain, and malaise. Cutaneous, neurologic, and cardiovascular complications characterize severe infections. Chronic complications involve recurrent fevers, joint pain, and fatigue.

Because brucella species are slow growing upon initial laboratory isolation, diagnosis depends on serological identification in blood or bone marrow isolates. Treatment with doxycycline and rifampin in combination, for 6 weeks, prevents recurring infections. Timing of treatment and severity of illness dictates length of recovery, from several weeks to several months. Although the mortality rate is low (<2%) and is usually associated with the development of cardiovascular complications (endocarditis), the lack of an effective human vaccine is of concern as a bioterrorist threat. Adherence to recommended public hygiene guidelines is the most effective preventive measure against brucellosis.

32.2.5 SALMONELLOSIS (*SALMONELLA* SPECIES)

Salmonellosis is caused by infection with *Salmonella* species, a Gram-negative bacillus. It is a member of the Enterobacteriacea family that colonizes the GI tracts of many species of animals, including chickens, cattle, and reptiles. Because of the large number of reactions that salmonella display against human antibodies, over 2400 known serogroups have been classified into three pathological categories. These include:

1. Salmonella that are highly adapted to human hosts, such as *S. typhi* (Group D salmonella) and *S. paratyphi* (Group A), that produce typhoid fever and paratyphoid fever, respectively
2. Salmonella that are adapted to nonhuman hosts that cause disease almost exclusively in animals (with a few exceptions)
3. Salmonella that are not adapted to specific hosts and involve the majority of the 2200 serotypes, designated *S. enteritidis* (Group D nontyphoidal salmonella).

---

[*] Owners of dogs infected with *B. canis* (the species common in dogs) are not considered to be at risk of acquiring brucellosis, provided they are not exposed to infected secretions from untreated animals.
[**] In untreated patients, the fever is at times intermittent, from which is derived the name **undulant fever**.

Infections with species of *S. enteritidis* account for 85% of all salmonella infections in the U.S. (typhoid fever infections caused by *S. typhi* are rare, with only 400 to 500 cases reported annually). About 50% of salmonellosis cases are caused by *S. enteritidis* and *S. typhimurium*. Although the proportion of salmonellosis caused by these serotypes has decreased since 1996, an increasing number of isolates show resistance to multiple antimicrobial drugs. For instance, the incidence of a previously lesser known species, *S. newport*, has increased 32% from 1996 to 2001. It has thus become the third most frequent serotype, with many isolates resistant to more than nine antimicrobial drugs.

Approximately 1.4 million cases of salmonellosis infections occur in the U.S. annually, most of which are diagnosed as **gastroenteritis**. The disease results primarily from infection with group D nontyphoidal salmonella. Gastroenteritis usually starts 12 to 48 h after ingestion of the organisms, with nausea, mild to severe abdominal pain, followed by watery diarrhea, sudden fever, and sometimes vomiting and dehydration. Nontyphoidal salmonellosis is usually mild to moderate, is self-limiting, lasts 4 to 7 days, and has a mortality of less than 1%. A chronic carrier state is possible in nontyphoidal salmonellosis, but is more common with typhoid fever. In any event, chronic carriers shed organisms in the stools for at least a month, sometimes more than a year after disease. In addition, persistent shedding of organisms in the stool for more than 1 year occurs in only 0.2 to 0.6% of patients with nontyphoidal salmonellosis. Therefore, food handlers pose a serious epidemic risk.[*]

The mechanism of contraction of infection with group D nontyphoidal salmonella is similar to but more complicated than typhoid fever. Fecal-oral transmission occurs in individuals by direct or indirect contact with animals, foodstuffs, and excretions from infected animals or humans. As few as 100,000 organisms are required for human inoculation. Once ingested, the organisms that successfully escape the acidic stomach contents penetrate and pass through to the ileum and colon. The organism penetrates intact mucosal membrane barrier cells of the ileum or colon, multiplies within the mucosal cells, and activates an inflammatory response. The resulting pathology is mostly due to damage within the GI tract.

Occasionally, more severe, protracted illness and long-term consequences result from salmonella poisoning including: (1) enteric fever, (2) focal (localized) infections, and (3) bacteremia.

1. **Enteric fever** is a systemic syndrome manifested by fever, prostration, and bacteremia. Enteric fever is attributable primarily to group B, *S. typhi,* and with milder group A, *S. paratyphi*, referred to as parathyphoid fever (see below).
2. **Focal infections** of infected organs start in the GI tract and disseminate to the liver, gall bladder, and appendix. The organisms can proliferate to

---

[*] Gastroenteritis and bacteremia are common and more virulent among infants and children, elderly, and in immunocompromised individuals. Salmonellosis also occurs 20 times more often in patients with AIDS, sickle cell anemia, cirrhosis, and leukemia.

cause cardiac murmurs, pericarditis, pneumonia, rheumatoid-like arthritis, and osteomyelitis.

3. **Bacteremia,** characterized by sustained septicemia with *S. typhi, S. paratyphi, S. choleraesuis,* and *S. enteritidis,* is relatively uncommon in patients with gastroenteritis. However, salmonella from groups B and C1 can cause bacteremia lasting about 1 week.

Other routes of contagion include ingestion of poorly cooked meat and handling of raw, infected meat. Unsuspected ingestion of contaminated poorly cooked poultry, raw milk or eggs, and egg products, are often the perpetrators (the eggs may be contaminated both on their surface and within). Outbreaks are more common in summer months and are often related to contaminated egg or chicken salads.

Patients with nontyphoidal salmonellosis are at risk of developing a less common but significantly adverse disorder known as **Reiter's syndrome**. The postinfection sequelae are initiated by a bacterial-induced, aberrant, hyperactive immune response. The disease is characterized by arthritis, particularly affecting the knees, ankles, and feet. About 50% of patients experience prolonged recurrence of arthritis over several years.

Isolation of the organism from the stools, blood, pus, vomitus, and urine aids in the presumptive diagnosis. Identification is based on initial growth of the organism on appropriate culture media, followed by biochemical and serological confirmation.

There is no acceptable antibiotic cure for uncomplicated nontyphoidal salmonellosis. Gastroenteritis is treated symptomatically with fluids, electrolytes, and a bland diet (for dehydration and continuous fever). Antibiotics prolong excretion of the organism and are unwarranted in uncomplicated cases. Antibiotic resistance is more common with nontyphoidal salmonella than with *S. typhi.* In addition, antibiotics can prolong the shedding of organisms in the stools after the drug has been discontinued. Infections with *S. typhi* and *S. paratyphi* are treated with fluoroquinolones (e.g., ciprofloxacin), chloramphenicol, gentamicin, trimethoprim/sulfamethoxazole, or broad-spectrum cephalosporins.

As with brucellosis, the lack of an effective vaccine warrants concern that salmonella can be used as a possible bioterrorist tool. Epidemiologically, preventing contamination of foodstuffs by infected humans is paramount. Contaminated raw eggs may pass unrecognized in some foods such as homemade hollandaise sauce, caesar and other salad dressings, as well as homemade ice cream, mayonnaise, cookie dough, and frostings. Ready-to-eat food, raw food, fruits, vegetables, or prepared desserts must be properly cooked, handled, stored, and/or refrigerated. Hand washing is essential before handling any food and between different food items. It is easy to observe how direct deliberate or inadvertent contamination can occur in the absence of proper hygienic food handling measures.

32.2.6 TYPHOID FEVER

Typhoid fever is a less common but life-threatening infection caused by *Salmonella typhi.* About 400 cases occur each year in the U.S, of which 70% are acquired through international travel. In the developing world, it affects about 12.5 million persons each year. The organism is responsible for **enteric fever**. As with other salmonella, *S. typhi* penetrates intact intestinal mucous membranes after oral ingestion and remains viable within phagocytic macrophages. The immune cells migrate to liver, spleen, and bone marrow, transporting the organism to critical destinations. *S. typhi* eventually reactivates 10 to 14 days after ingestion. Gradually increasing nonspecific fever, headache, myalgias, malaise, and anorexia ensue and persist for about 1 week. Gastrointestinal symptoms resume. The cycle continues with bacteremia and colonization of the gallbladder, and with reinfection of the intestinal tract.

Humans are the natural host for *S. typhi*. Persons with typhoid fever, and about 1 to 5% of those who recover from the infection (carriers), maintain chronic colonization of the organism. The latter can carry the organism for more than one year after symptomatic disease, with the gallbladder acting as the physiologic incubator. Both are capable of shedding *S. typhi* in their feces.

As with other forms of salmonellosis, *S. typhi* is acquired through fecal-oral transmission. Typhoid fever is preventable by avoiding ingestion of poorly cooked, raw, or unwashed foods. Drinking bottled water or boiling potable water removes the risk of contamination. The disease is usually treated with antibiotics (ampicillin, trimethoprim-sulfamethoxazole, and fluoroquinolones), but vaccination is recommended especially for travelers to endemic areas. The vaccine is available for parenteral administration (ViCPS) and in capsule form (Ty21a) and requires 1 and 2 weeks for induction of adequate antibody titers, respectively. Complications of the untreated typhoid fever are associated with a 20% mortality rate.

32.2.7 SHIGELLOSIS (*SHIGELLA* SPECIES)

Shigellosis is caused by infection with *Shigella* species, a Gram-negative bacillus. As with the other members of the Enterobacteriacea family, the organisms colonize the GI tracts of many species of animals. Several species of shigella are further divided into 45 serogroups: *S. sonnei* (group D) accounts for over 65% of shigellosis in the U.S.; *S. flexneri* (group B) accounts for the rest (about 450,000 total unconfirmed cases in the U.S. each year). *S. dysenteriae* type 1 and *S. boydii* are rare, although they continue to be important causes of disease in the developing world. Over 150 million cases of shigellosis occur annually worldwide.[*] As with salmonella infections, fecal-oral transmission of contaminated food is the major route of transmission.

Children account for 70% of shigellosis cases. The syndrome is characterized by abdominal cramps, diarrhea (often containing abundant blood and mucus), fever, and stomach cramps. The onset is 1 to 2 days and duration is self-limiting in 5 to 7 days. Severe infections with high fever are associated with seizures in children less than 2 years old. Asymptomatic carriers are contagious by shedding organisms in the feces.

Diagnosis and pathogenicity is similar to salmonellosis. Although the disease is self-limiting, antibiotic treatment shortens the duration of illness and prevents the spread of the organism. Ampicillin, trimethoprim/sulfamethoxazole, nalidixic

---

[*] Epidemics of *S. dysenteriae* type 1 have occurred in Africa and Central America with case fatality rates of 5 to 15%. In addition, *S. dysenteriae* produces an exotoxin (Shiga toxin) that damages intestinal epithelium and glomerular endothelial cells.

acid, or fluoroquinolones are indicated. As with salmonellosis, about 3% of patients with S. *flexneri* infections develop Reiter's syndrome, lasting for months or years. Vaccination and preventive measures are similar to those recommended for salmonellosis.

32.2.8 *ESCHERICHIA COLI* O157:H7

This Gram-negative enteropathogenic bacteria is an emerging cause of foodborne illness. The *Escherichia* genus consists of five species, of which *E. coli* is the most common and clinically important. Approximately 73,000 cases of infection occur annually in the U.S. *E. coli* possesses a broad range of virulence factors, exotoxins, and adhesion molecules, allowing the organisms to attach to the GI and urinary tracts.

A large number of enteropathogenic groups of *E. coli* inhabit the small and large intestines of healthy cattle and are further classified according to their serologic serotypes. Most *E. coli* strains are part of the normal human bacterial flora. *E. coli* serotype O157:H7, however, is not. In fact, it is one of the most virulent strains responsible for producing fatal enterotoxins.[*]

E. coli is the most common microorganism responsible for sepsis and urinary tract infections. It is also a prominent cause of neonatal meningitis and gastroenteritis in developing nations. Strains of *E. coli* responsible for gastroenteritis are subdivided into six groups: enterotoxigenic, enteropathogenic, enteroinvasive, enterohemorrhagic, enteroaggregative, and diffuse aggregative. Each is responsible for a variety of diseases, including traveler's and infant diarrhea, dysentery, intra-abdominal infections, hemolytic uremic syndrome (HUS),[**] and hemorrhagic colitis.

The organism's ability to invade intestinal epithelial cells, its capacity to release exotoxins, and its ability to express adhesion molecules, confers the properties necessary for producing gastroenteritis. The disease is characterized by acute dysentery accompanied by abdominal cramps with little or no fever.

Infection is acquired through ingestion of poorly cooked ground beef, consumption of unpasteurized milk and juice, sprouts, lettuce, salami, and contact with cattle. Waterborne transmission occurs through swimming in contaminated lakes, pools, or drinking inadequately chlorinated water. The organism is easily transmitted from person to person and has been difficult to control in child day-care centers.

Stool cultures and serology confirm the presence of *E. coli* O157:H7 in suspected infections. With the exception of severe complications, most infections are self-limiting in 5 to 10 days. Antibiotic treatment is unwarranted and may actually precipitate kidney infections. Antidiarrheal agents, such as loperamide, should also be avoided.

Thorough cooking and proper handling of ground beef and hamburger are effective in preventing *E. coli* infections. Raw meat should be kept separate from ready-to-eat foods. Hands, counters, and utensils should be washed with hot soapy water after they contact raw meat. Drinking unpasteurized milk, juice, or cider should be avoided. Fruits and vegetables should be washed thoroughly to avoid exposure.

---

[*] The serotype designation (O:, H:) refers to the expression of surface and fimbrial antigens, respectively, that uniquely characterize this genus.
[**] Chronic kidney failure and neurologic impairment are frequent complications of HUS.

32.2.9 CHOLERA (*VIBRIO CHOLERAE*)

Cholera is an acute, diarrheal illness caused by intestinal infection with the Gram-negative, facultative anaerobic bacterium *Vibrio cholerae*. Many species of this curved bacillus are also implicated in human infections (*V. parahaemolyticus* and *V. vulnificus*), although *V. cholerae* is the best-known member of the genus. The species are further subdivided into over 200 serogroups, on the basis of their somatic O antigens. *V. cholerae* serogroup O1 or O139 is responsible for classic epidemic cholera, and it produces cholera toxin.

Although the infection is often mild or asymptomatic, approximately one in 20 infected persons has severe disease, which is primarily due to the secretion of the toxin. The cholera toxin is similar to the heat-labile enterotoxin of *E. coli*. During infection, the toxin binds to receptors on intestinal epithelial cells, stimulating hypersecretion of water and electrolytes. Within 2 to 3 days of ingestion, copious watery diarrhea, vomiting, rapid loss of body fluids, and leg cramps develop. The symptoms eventually progress to dehydration, metabolic acidosis, shock, and cardiovascular collapse. The condition is fatal (25 to 50%) if untreated (interestingly, the organism is not flushed from the intestinal tract during a diarrheal episode but adheres to the mucosa via attachment pili).

Like other enterobacteria, cholera is acquired by ingesting contaminated water or food. Large epidemic outbreaks are related to fecal contamination of water supplies or street-vended foods. The organism is occasionally transmitted through eating raw or undercooked shellfish that are naturally contaminated. While 0 to 5 cases per year are reported in the U.S., there are no identifiable risk groups. Risk is extremely low (1 per million), even in travelers. It is a major cause of epidemic diarrhea, however, throughout the developing world. It is responsible for a global pandemic in Asia, Africa, and Latin America for the last four decades. A modest increase in imported cases since 1991 is related to an ongoing epidemic that began in 1991 in South America. The disease is acquired or carried back in contaminated food by travelers to endemic countries. A few cases have occurred in the U.S. among persons who traveled to South America or ate contaminated food brought back by travelers.

Fluid and electrolyte replacement is effective in preventing death, but the logistics of delivery in remote areas during pandemics renders this option difficult to achieve. Doxycycline, trimethoprim-sulfamethoxazole, and furazolidone reduce the bacterial burden and toxin production. Eradication of *V. cholerae* is very unlikely, since the organism is found in natural estuarine and marine environments and is associated with chitinous shellfish.

Because of advanced water and sanitation systems, cholera is easily prevented and treated and is not a major threat in industrialized nations. Currently available killed parenteral vaccines offer incomplete protection of relatively short duration and have been discontinued; no multivalent vaccines are available for O139 infections. Newer killed, whole cell, oral vaccines for the O1 strain may offer some protection, but neither is available in the United States (Dukoral® from Biotec AB and Mutacol® manufactured by Berna).

32.2.10 SMALLPOX

Naturally occurring smallpox (*variola major*) is a member of the *orthopoxvirus* family, the largest and most complex family of viruses. It is easily transmissible via close person-to-person contact. The virus accounted for 7% to 12% of all deaths in eighteenth-century England. The last case of smallpox in the U.S. occurred in 1949, and in the world, in Somalia in 1977. Routine vaccination in the U.S. was stopped in 1971; the World Health Organization (WHO) determined in 1980 that smallpox had been successfully eradicated from the world.

Smallpox virus was inhaled and replicated in the respiratory tract. Dissemination occurred via lymphatics, resulting in viremia. The lymphatic vessels provide the pathways for the virus to spread to the spleen, bone marrow, liver, and skin (characteristic rash). A second viremia caused the development of additional lesions. Depending on which of the two variants of smallpox was contracted, mortality ranged from 15% to 40% (for variola major) to 1% (variola minor).

The incubation period for variola was about 7 to 17 days. Initial symptoms include high fever, fatigue, and head and back aches. The characteristic lesions (*pocks*) appear in 2 to 3 days on the face, arms, and legs. Lesions become pus-filled and begin to crust early in the second week. Eschar develops, separates, and sloughs off after 3 to 4 weeks.

Smallpox is very contagious through the respiratory/salivary route and infects humans only through accidental or occupational exposure. Individuals are most contagious during the first week of signs and symptoms corresponding to high viremic periods.

Although routine vaccination against smallpox ended in 1972, the level of continuous immunity among persons vaccinated before 1972 is uncertain. Recently, the threat that smallpox could be used as a weapon of bioterrorism has prompted the development of new vaccination strategies for both military personnel and civilians. Vaccinia, a form of cowpox, is used for the production of smallpox vaccine. The procedure consists of scratching live virus into the patient's skin and observing for the formation of vesicle and pustules. In October 2002, the FDA approved a new 100-dose kit for smallpox vaccine (Dryvax®, Wyeth), the only currently licensed smallpox vaccine. All supplies of Dryvax® for civilian use are under CDC control. Complications and potential risks related to vaccination occur primarily in immunocompromised individuals and, more recently, in persons with preexisting cardiovascular disorders. The most serious of complications are encephalitis, progressive infection (vaccinia necrosum), and myocardial infarction.

32.2.11 TULAREMIA (*FRANCISELLA TULARENSIS*), Q FEVER (*COXIELLA BURNETII*), AND VIRAL HEMORRHAGIC FEVERS (VHF)

Tularemia is caused by the Gram-negative coccobacillus, *Francisella tularensis*. Humans acquire the zoonotic infection through ticks (arthropod vectors), rabbits, and domestic pets. About 100 cases annually are reported in the U.S. Clinically, tularemia is a plague-like, glandular, typhoidal disease. GI and pneumonic syndromes are characterized by fever, chills, headache, myalgia, and malaise. Streptomycin and gentamicin are the antibiotics of choice. A live-attenuated vaccine is available but rarely used.

Q fever is caused by an obligate intracellular bacteria, *Coxiella burnetii*, closely related to *Francisella*. Most human infections are acquired through inhalation from contact with animal reservoirs (arthropods are not important vectors with Q fever). The infection is characterized by acute onset of an influenza-like syndrome (fever, headache, malaise), followed by pneumonia, hepatitis, endocarditis, and pulmonary disease. Tetracyclines are the drugs of choice for acute infections; rifampin plus doxycycline is used for chronic infections. Vaccines are protective if administered before contracting *C. burnetii*.

Viral hemorrhagic fevers (VHF) are a clinically related group of viral diseases with a diverse etiology. The family of Filoviridae includes the Marburg and Ebola viruses. Similarly, the family of Bunyaviridae includes the hantavirus and bunyavirus (primarily causes encephalitis in humans). All are RNA viruses endemic in Africa and, with the exception of the bunyavirus, cause severe or fatal hemorrhagic fevers. The condition is characterized by acute onset of fever, headache, generalized myalgia, conjunctivitis, and severe prostration, followed by various hemorrhagic symptoms. The organism facilitates the destruction of endothelial cells leading to vascular injury and increased capillary permeability, leukopenia, and thrombocytopenia. Antiviral therapy has not been shown to be clinically useful.

Arenaviruses, including the Lassa, Junin, and Machupo viruses, are endemic in Africa and South America. The organisms stimulate cell-mediated inflammatory responses following an incubation period of 10 to 14 days. The syndrome is manifested by fever, petechiae, cardiac, hepatic, and splenic damage. No vasculitis or neuronal damage is observed. The recently approved antiviral drug, Ribavirin®, has demonstrated some activity against Lassa fever, which has a 50% mortality rate if untreated.

32.3 CHEMICAL AGENTS AS THREATS TO PUBLIC SAFETY

32.3.1 NERVE GASES

The nerve gases were developed during World War II as possible chemical warfare agents, the first compound of which was tetraethyl pyrophosphate (TEPP). The biological action of the nerve gases, such as sarin (GB),[*] tabun (GA), and soman (GD), is similar to, but more toxic than the organophosphate (OP) insecticides (see Chapter 26, "Insecticides"). The clear, colorless, tasteless liquids inhibit the action of acetylcholine esterase (Ach-Σ) by forming an **irreversible** OP–Ach-Σ complex, rendering it incapable of hydrolyzing acetylcholine (Ach). Inhibition of the enzyme results in accumulation and overstimulation of Ach at autonomic and somatic receptors. Excessive stimulation of nicotinic receptors is followed by skeletal muscle

---

[*] The deliberate release of sarin in a Tokyo subway in 1995 by a terrorist organization was responsible for 12 deaths and 5000 casualties.

paralysis. These circumstances account for the toxic manifestations of OP insecticides as well as the nerve gases.

Soman, a methylphosphonofluoridic acid ester, is miscible with organic solvents and water. It is readily absorbed through skin. Soman is the most toxic of the three "G" agents and one of the most toxic compounds ever synthesized, with fatalities occurring with an oral dose of 10 µg/kg in humans. **Sarin**, a methylphosphonofluoridic acid ester, and **tabun**, a dimethylphosphonofluoridic acid ester, are also miscible with organic solvents and water, and are readily absorbed through skin (tabun possesses a bitter almond smell). Recently, however, **VX** (methylphosphonothioic acid ester) has emerged as a more toxic nerve agent. Its chemical and biological properties satisfy the requirements for VX as a chemical bioterrorist threat. The odorless, tasteless, oily liquid was originally developed in the U.K. in the 1950s. Unlike more volatile aromatic and aliphatic hydrocarbons, heating VX liquid renders it suitable for inhalation, dermal, or ocular contact with the airborne vapors. Contamination of food and water supplies is also possible. Of concern are its ability to accumulate in physiological compartments, its slow metabolic degradation, and its high density, enabling it to spread throughout low-lying areas.

Onset of symptoms is seconds for inhalation of vapors, and hours for dermal contact or oral ingestion. In addition, they all decompose in the presence of bleach (or base). As with all the nerve agents, VX produces a severe cholinergic syndrome, terminating in convulsions, respiratory failure, and death with high doses. Recovery from mild or moderate exposure to a nerve agent is possible. Treatment relies on removal from exposure, supportive measures, decontamination, and rapid administration of atropine (antimuscarinic) and pralidoxime (Ach-Σ reactivator). The FDA has recently approved pyridostigmine bromide, an anticholinesterase agent, as a prophylactic drug for U.S. military personnel to increase survival after exposure to soman poisoning during combat use.

Nerve agents are metabolized quickly in air and soil and, after several hours, in water, incurring a low incidence of environmental accumulation. The risk for accidental exposure to the general population is low, except for military personnel or individuals working in or around storage plants.

32.3.2 VESICANTS, CHEMICAL ASPHYXIANTS, AND PULMONARY IRRITANTS

Vesicants, such as nitrogen mustard compounds, are capable of causing tissue necrosis upon extravasation. These alkylating agents have a delayed onset of action (about 6 to 8 h), although cellular necrosis ensues immediately. Inhalation produces a typical pulmonary irritation. The toxicity of vesicating agents is more severe than lacrimating agents, the latter of which were subsequently developed for domestic law enforcement. Sulfur mustard compounds (H, HD, HT; "mustard gas") possess a garlic odor, although they are sometimes odorless. The compounds are generally colorless or yellowish liquids, do not accumulate in the environment, and are not a threat for accidental public exposure.

Lacrimating agents (benzyl bromide), simple asphyxiants (inert gases), chemical asphyxiants (carbon monoxide, cyanide), and pulmonary irritants (carbon disulfide, phosgene), are now recognized as potential chemical bioterrorist threats. Most of the clinical toxicity of these compounds is discussed in detail in Chapter 23, "Gases." Some of their applications as bioterrorist weapons are further entertained below.

Cyanide has risen on the high priority list for bioterrorist threats, although its toxicity is recognized historically. Also known by the military designations AN (for hydrogen cyanide) and CK (for cyanogen chloride), cyanide may also have been used during the Iran-Iraq war in the 1980s. It was probably incorporated along with other chemical agents against the inhabitants of the Kurdish city of Halabja in northern Iraq. The compounds are released in air, soil, or water as industrial waste products in the electroplating and metallurgical industries. Additional uses of cyanides include photographic development, fumigating ships, and use in the mining industry. Cyanides are also metabolic products of bacteria, fungi, algae, and plants.

As a terrorist threat, AN gas is most toxic. The colorless gas has a faint bitter almond odor. The EPA allows a maximum contaminant level of 0.2 mg/l of cyanide in drinking water. It requires the reporting of spills or accidental releases into the environment of 1 lb or more of cyanide compounds. The clinical toxicity and treatment of cyanide poisoning are discussed in Chapter 23.

32.3.3 RICIN (*RICINUS COMMUNIS*)

Ricin is derived from the processing of the castor bean and its seeds (*Euphorbiaceae*) in the extraction of castor oil.* The seeds, plant, fruit, and constituents are stable in extreme hot or cold temperatures. The plant is indigenous to temperate and tropical India, Africa, and South America. The seeds have been found in Egyptian tombs. The oil appears to have had only technical use until the eighteenth century, when its medicinal application was explored.

Ricin is composed of two lectins found in the seeds, ricin I and II. The compounds, especially ricin II, bind to and inactivate the 60S ribosomal subunit in somatic cells, thus blocking protein synthesis. The potent cholinergic properties of the oil have rendered it useful for decades as an "over-the-counter" laxative. It is one of the most potent of plant toxins.

Ingestion of intact castor bean seeds is unlikely to cause deleterious effects for several days, although ingestion of chewed castor beans rarely results in significant morbidity. Gradually, however, it produces nausea, vomiting, dyspnea, and diarrhea. Gastroenteritis follows and is characterized by severe bloody diarrhea, vomiting, and dehydration. Mental confusion, seizures, and hyperthermia complicate the scenario.

Inhalation of ricin powder likely produces a cough, dyspnea, nausea, and vomiting within a few hours. Pulmonary congestion and cyanosis could soon follow. **Injection** of a lethal amount of ricin (estimated to be about 500 µg) at first would cause local muscle paralysis and lymph node necrosis near the injection site. Massive stomach and intestinal hemorrhaging would ensue, followed by multiple organ failure. Death occurs within 36 to 48 h and is due to focal necrosis of liver, spleen, lymph nodes, intestine, and stomach.

---

* Ricinus is Latin for tick; the seed resembles some arthropods in shape and markings.

Ricin is otherwise not an environmental metabolic product, and unintentional ricin poisoning is highly unlikely. Its presence therefore suggests deliberate contamination; hence, the bioterrorist concern.[*] The manufactured material can be dissolved in water, vaporized, or injected, thus facilitating its exposure through oral, respiratory, or parenteral routes.

Antidotes are not available for ricin poisoning. Treatment necessitates supportive emergency measures, including maintenance of respiration and renal perfusion, and gastric decontamination.

REFERENCES

SUGGESTED READINGS

Borio, L. et al., Hemorrhagic fever viruses as biological weapons: medical and public health management, *JAMA*, 287, 2391, 2002.

Broad, W.J., A Deadly Weapon for Beginners (Ricin), *New York Times*, Jan. 12, 2003.

Broad, W.J. and Miller, J., Threats and Responses: The Bioterror Threat; Health Data Monitored for Bioterror Warning, National Desk, *New York Times*, Jan. 27, 2003.

Center for Drug Evaluation and Research, U.S. Food and Drug Administration. Center for Biologics Evaluation and Research, *Anthrax Vaccine*, 2001.

Drazen, J.M., Perspective: smallpox and bioterrorism, *N. Engl. J. Med.*, 346, 1262, 2002.

Public Health Emergency Preparedness and Response, Centers for Disease Control and Prevention, http://www.bt.cdc.gov.

Recommendations of the Advisory Committee on Immunization Practices: Use of Anthrax Vaccine in the United States." *Morbidity Mortality Wkly. Rep.*, 49, 1, 2000.

USAMRIID's Medical Management of Biological Casualties Handbook, U.S. Army Medical Research Institute of Infectious Diseases, Centers for Disease Control and Prevention, 2003.

REVIEW ARTICLES

Agency for Toxic Substances and Disease Registry (ATSDR), Toxicological Profile for Mustard Gas. Draft for Public Comment, U.S. Department of Health and Human Services, Public Health Service, Atlanta, GA, 2001.

Bozeman, W.P., Dilbero, D., and Schauben, J.L., Biologic and chemical weapons of mass destruction, *Emerg. Med. Clin. North Am.*, 20, 975, 2002.

Dixon, T.C. et al., Anthrax, *N. Engl. J. Med.*, 341, 815, 1999.

Franz, D.R. and Zajtchuk, R., Biological terrorism: understanding the threat, preparation, and medical response, *Dis. Mon.*, 48, 493, 2002.

Hamburg, M.A., Bioterrorism: responding to an emerging threat, *Trends Biotechnol.*, 20, 296, 2002.

Henretig, F.M., Cieslak, T.J., and Eitzen, E.M., Jr., Biological and chemical terrorism, *J. Pediatr.*, 141, 311, 2002.

---

[*] In 1978, Georgi Markov, a Bulgarian writer and journalist, died of severe gastroenteritis and multiorgan failure after he was attacked in London by a man with an umbrella suspected of containing ricin pellet at the tip. Other reports have implicated use of ricin during the Iran-Iraq war in the 1980s.

Karwa, M., Bronzert, P., and Kvetan, V., Bioterrorism and critical care, *Crit. Care Clin.*, 19, 279, 2003.

Kimmel, S.R., Mahoney, M.C., and Zimmerman, R.K., Vaccines and bioterrorism: smallpox and anthrax, *J. Fam. Pract.*, 52, S56, 2003.

Lashley, F.R., Factors contributing to the occurrence of emerging infectious diseases, *Biol. Res. Nurs.*, 4, 258, 2003.

McQuiston, J.H., Childs, J.E., and Thompson, H.A., Q fever, *J. Am. Vet. Med. Assoc.*, 221, 796, 2002.

Nyamathi, A.M. et al., Ebola virus: immune mechanisms of protection and vaccine development, *Biol. Res. Nurs.*, 4, 276, 2003.

Olsnes, S. and Kozlov, J.V., Ricin, *Toxicon*, 39, 1723, 2001.

Orloski, K.A. and Lathrop, S.L., Plague: a veterinary perspective, *J. Am. Vet. Med. Assoc.*, 222, 444, 2003.

Rosenbloom, M. et al., Biological and chemical agents: a brief synopsis, *Am. J. Ther.*, 9, 5, 2002.

Sandvig, K. and van Deurs, B., Entry of ricin and Shiga toxin into cells: molecular mechanisms and medical perspectives, *EMBO J.*, 19, 5943, 2000.

Slater, L.N. and Greenfield, R.A., Biological toxins as potential agents of bioterrorism, *J. Okla. State Med. Assoc.*, 96, 73, 2003.

Slater, M.S. and Trunkey, D.D., Terrorism in America. An evolving threat, *Arch. Surg.*, 132, 1059, 1997.

Spencer, R.C., Bacillus anthracis, *J. Clin. Pathol.*, 56, 182, 2003.

Terriff, C.M., Schwartz, M.D., and Lomaestro, B.M., Bioterrorism: pivotal clinical issues. Consensus review of the Society of Infectious Diseases Pharmacists, *Pharmacotherapy*, 23, 274, 2003.

Wenzel, R.P., Recognizing the real threat of biological terror, *Trans. Am. Clin. Climatol. Assoc.*, 113, 42, 2002.

Index